SECOND EDITION

Wellness Practitioner

Concepts, Research, and Strategies

Carolyn Chambers Clark, EdD, ARNP, is founder of The Wellness Institute and *The Wellness Newsletter*. She currently has a private wellness practice and serves as a wellness consultant. She is Editor of *Alternative Health Practitioner: The Journal of Complementary and Natural Care* (Springer Publishing Company), and is on the editorial board of *Health Care for Women International.*

SECOND EDITION

Wellness Practitioner

Concepts, Research, and Strategies

Carolyn Chambers Clark, EdD, RN

Wellness Theory
Facilitating Movement Toward Wellness
Positive Relationship Building
Stress Management
Nutritional Wellness
Exercise and Movement
Self-Care, Touch, and Wellness
Environmental Wellness
Community Wellness Programs
Research and Wellness Theory

SPRINGER PUBLISHING COMPANY

First edition published as *Wellness Nursing,* 1986.

Copyright © 1996 by Carolyn Chambers Clark

Springer Publishing Company, Inc.
536 Broadway
New York, N.Y. 10012-3955

Cover design by Tom Yabut
Production Editor: Pamela Ritzer

96 97 98 99 00 / 5 4 3 2 1

Library of Congress Cataloging-in-Publication Data

Clark, Carolyn Chambers.

    Wellness practitioner : concepts, research, and
strategies / Carolyn Chambers Clark, — 2nd ed.
      p.   cm.
    Rev. ed. of Wellness nursing / Carolyn Chambers Clark. c1986.
    Includes bibliographical references and index.
    ISBN 0-8261-5151-5
    1. Health promotion. 2. Health education. 3. Nursing.
I. Clark, Carolyn Chambers   Wellness nursing. II. Title. [DNLM. 1.
Nursing Theory. 2. Health Promotion. 3. Patient Education.
4. Alternative Therapies.
    WY 86 C592w 1986
    RT90.3. C48   1996   613—dc20
    DNLM/DLC   CIP
    for Library of Congress   95–47784

Printed in the United States of America

Any medical, health, or therapeutic agent or procedure described in this book should be applied by the practitioner under appropriate supervision in accordance with professional standards of care and the unique circumstances of each situation.

CONTENTS

For Tony

PREFACE

Any new theory is first attacked as absurd; then it is admitted to be true, but insignificant; finally—it seems to be important, so important that its adversaries claim that they themselves discovered it!

—Henry James

Wellness practitioners are interested in enhancing their own wellness or someone else's. Although this book was developed to teach wellness practitioners—who may include traditional health care professionals such as nurses and physicians, or alternative health practitioners—it can just as well be used to a great extent by the lay public.

This book shares some of the ideas I have about what wellness is, how it provides a framework for change, and how we can change ourselves and facilitate wellness in others. Many of the interventions are new to wellness practitioners; others have been alluded to in the literature or are not widely practiced. I believe all add a different and needed dimension to wellness practice. I have apprenticed myself to expert practitioners in many areas to learn approaches which I believe every practitioner must master to participate in an integrated wellness practice. Each of these approaches appears in the book with suggestions for use with self, peer, and clients. Most, if not all, interventions can be completed by the client or the client and a peer who has mastered the procedure. A major emphasis of wellness practice is assisting the client to be independent and able to provide self-care measures to enhance wellness.

The idea of health promotion is not a new one, but the idea that the client is the expert in his or her own wellness *is*. Giving up the expert role (at least in the traditional sense) to work on one's own wellness, to role model wellness for clients, and to allow clients to make their own informed decisions (even when we disagree with their choices) is difficult but challenging. Practitioners *and* clients are responsible for keeping up-to-date on the constantly changing information sources relevant to wellness; practitioners are not the dispensers of information, they are the teachers of clients about how to access information systems, and the recipients of knowledge from clients.

Another theme (or paradox) pervading this book is the essential uniqueness, yet similarity of practitioners and clients. We're all on the journey to wellness together—no one totally lacking it and no one totally attaining it, but all managing a brief glimpse of total wellness potential. Students, teachers, practitioners, and clients are all learners and teachers of one another.

Another theme is the importance of self-awareness and planned interventions in each wellness dimension. Nutritional wellness, fitness/movement maximization, stress management, positive relationships, coherent beliefs, and environmental sensitivity interact to provide purposeful movement toward wellness.

Strong societal forces support the wellness movement which has proven itself to be more than a fad. Wellness practitioners as leaders in this movement will seize the first available opportunity to start wellness practices in schools, hospitals, industry, and communities.

"Integrative Learning Experiences" at the end of each chapter have been developed to provide a challenge both to the novice and expert practitioner; many can be used as they are with clients, or they can be practitioner adapted for use. It is suggested that the practitioner try out each experience prior to using it with clients. Case studies provide a focus for discussion and a synthesis of information.

As you read through the book and complete the learning exercises, remember to be easy on yourself. You are a unique being; give yourself understanding, nurturance, and time to blossom.

Carolyn Chambers Clark

CAROLYN CHAMBERS CLARK
St. Petersburg, Florida

LIST OF ILLUSTRATIONS

LIST OF TABLES

1

INTRODUCTION TO WELLNESS THEORY

This chapter discusses the following topics:

- The definition of wellness
- The importance of arriving at a stated purpose for practice through wellness theory
- Societal factors supporting the use of wellness theory and practice
- Definition of terms and their relevance to wellness theory
- Assumptions underlying the wellness model
- Boundaries of wellness theory

One purpose of this book is to provide evidence for using wellness as the guiding purpose for practice. To do this, the parameters of wellness must be defined.

WELLNESS PRACTICE DEFINED

Dunn (1961) coined the term, "high-level wellness." Key concepts include maximizing one's potential, having direction and purpose in life, meeting the challenges of the environment, looking beyond the needs of self to the needs of society, and doing it all with joy or a zest for life. Wellness practitioners help clients and themselves move toward a higher level of wellness. *Wellness Practice* is focused on a joint assessment of client needs; application of theory; facilitation of whole person healing and self-healing/self-care measures; and joint evaluation of client movement toward wellness. Practitioner–client interactions are based on the (apparent) paradox, "You alone do it, but you don't do it alone. There is no wellness practitioner but you, the individual person" (Pilch, 1981, p. 18). Thus, the health care practitioner is not the person who stands back, assesses, plans, and evaluates, but a *facilitator* who teaches clients how to self-assess, decide on wellness goals, plan on actions to meet those goals, and self-evaluate success.

Wellness practice deals with how the flow of energy between subsystems of mind/body/spirit is interrupted or blocked and how the flow of energy is reopened or rechanneled. The practitioner facilitates the removal of obstacles to energy flow among subsystems, resulting in enhanced well-being and self-actualization of potentials.

Motivation is intrinsic to the model; the client is the one who chooses a goal of meaning to him or her; compliance becomes irrelevant because the client is responsible for decisions. The process of moving toward wellness is more important than the product, wellness. Ensuring that the client does what is "good" for him or her becomes facilitating movement toward a goal chosen by the client. Such a change may require a change in belief systems. The model suggests that practitioners (as whole persons) also examine their belief systems for consistency, especially in terms of the model. Additionally, the model requires that practitioners also be engaged in moving toward wellness by choosing, facilitating, and evaluating their own movement toward wellness goals.

Figure 1.1 exemplifies practitioner client interactions from a wellness perspective. In this model, both practitioner and client are complete systems that interact within themselves [inputs, throughputs (activities within the system), and outputs], and interact with each other (intersystems) across interfaces to achieve jointly planned and achieved goals and feelings of well-being.

Figure 1.2 (p. 5) shows the relationships between biological, historical, social, and cultural factors, environment, and the whole person. The whole person evolves toward wellness by learning to:

- manage life experiences
- seek out challenges
- relate to others in a flexible, differentiated, assertive manner
- use self-care strategies
- examine and readjust beliefs and practices into an integrated, goal-directed whole
- develop coping strategies that produce success

During the evolutionary process of moving toward wellness, whole persons interact with stressors in a more rational, efficient way by perceiving and managing situations differently. Biological, historical, social and cultural factors can also be affected (and affect whole persons) in the process: for example, childhood perceptions that affect adult behaviors can be reevaluated and readjusted in adulthood; the immune system (genetic given) can be strengthened (or weakened) by using (or not using) self-care strategies.

THE IMPORTANCE OF ARRIVING AT A STATED PURPOSE FOR PRACTICE THROUGH WELLNESS THEORY

If wellness practitioners are to seize control of their practice, a theory base is necessary. Theory can provide professional autonomy and a power base.

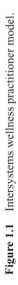

INPUTS
- food
- water
- stressors
- unique historical, social, cultural, and biological factors

positive nutrition
stress management
environmental sensitivity
coherent beliefs

PRACTITIONER THROUGHPUTS

positive relationship skills

fitness activities

OUTPUTS

Movement toward wellness, including:
- setting and moving toward own nutritional, fitness, belief system, stress management, environmental, relationship, and self-care goals
- role modeling wellness
- facilitating wellness behaviors in client

(energy, information, and materials exchanged)

INTERFACE

INPUTS
- food
- water
- stressors
- unique historical, social, cultural, and biological factors

inconsistent belief systems
stress overload
destructive relationships

CLIENT THROUGHPUTS

environmental distress

lack of fitness
illness/disease
under/over-nutrition

OUTPUTS

Movement toward wellness, including:
- setting fitness goals/actions to meet goals
- increasing coherency in belief systems
- increasing ability to function in social and work roles
- setting nutritional goals/actions to meet goals
- increasing ability to use self-care and self-healing strategies
- setting stress management goals/actions to meet goals

JOINTLY PLANNED AND ACHIEVED GOALS
FEELINGS OF WELL-BEING

Figure 1.1 Intersystems wellness practitioner model.

Wellness theory may be the theoretical base that can unite practitioners. Wellness practitioners claim their practice is based on health promotions, yet many of the terms used and practices observed are based on medical terms and practices and are disease-focused. Wellness theory can support practice that is consistently focused on health promotion. It can also increase cohesiveness among practitioners providing a broad base for practice. It can be argued that the profession that possesses theoretical knowledge about wellness is most likely to provide wellness-enhancing services for clients. As knowledge about wellness accrues practitioners will value their knowledge and find access to resources such as money, space, and people more readily. Additionally, arguments over the purpose of practice among practitioners would become less predominant and cohesiveness would increase. Practitioners who use a wellness theory base are on firmer ground when their ideas are challenged (Chinn & Jacobs, 1994).

When practitioners become wellness role models and take action to move toward wellness in their own lives, not only will they be a visible encouragement to clients and consumers, but they will have a greater potential for being effective leaders.

SOCIETAL FACTORS SUPPORTING THE USE OF WELLNESS THEORY AND PRACTICE

Convergence of practice toward wellness theory will also result in a more relevant response to societal demands. There is growing disillusion with medical care as the treatment of choice for many. Consumers are becoming increasingly aware of the effect of lifestyle on well-being and level of wellness. Self-care is deeply rooted in cultural tradition. Surveys indicate that more than 75% of all symptoms today are treated without professional assistance. The self-care movement is shifting the locus of decision making away from professional dominance and toward consumers (Gross et al., 1991).

The disillusionment with medical care has also led to the use of alternative or complementary practices which are wellness-oriented, less intrusive, and have fewer side effects (Clark, 1995; Class, 1993; Downer, 1994; Eisenberg et al., 1993). The federal government has followed suit by establishing the Office of Alternative Medicine within the National Institutes of Health, after a push from Senator Tom Harkin and Representative Berkley Bedell (Rubik, 1995).

Increasing scientific study is being directed to mind-body interactions, particularly to the interrelationships between the brain and the immune system (Halley, 1991). This work provides support for the interactive nature of systems and pulls interest away from the mechanistic/medical model which asserts that body organs can be removed without any effect on total body functioning.

Insurance companies have responded to accumulating evidence that lifestyle is the key to well-being and wellness by offering reduced premiums to non-smokers and to those engaging in fitness programs. The Stay Well program offered by Blue Shield of California pays members to stay healthy by reward-

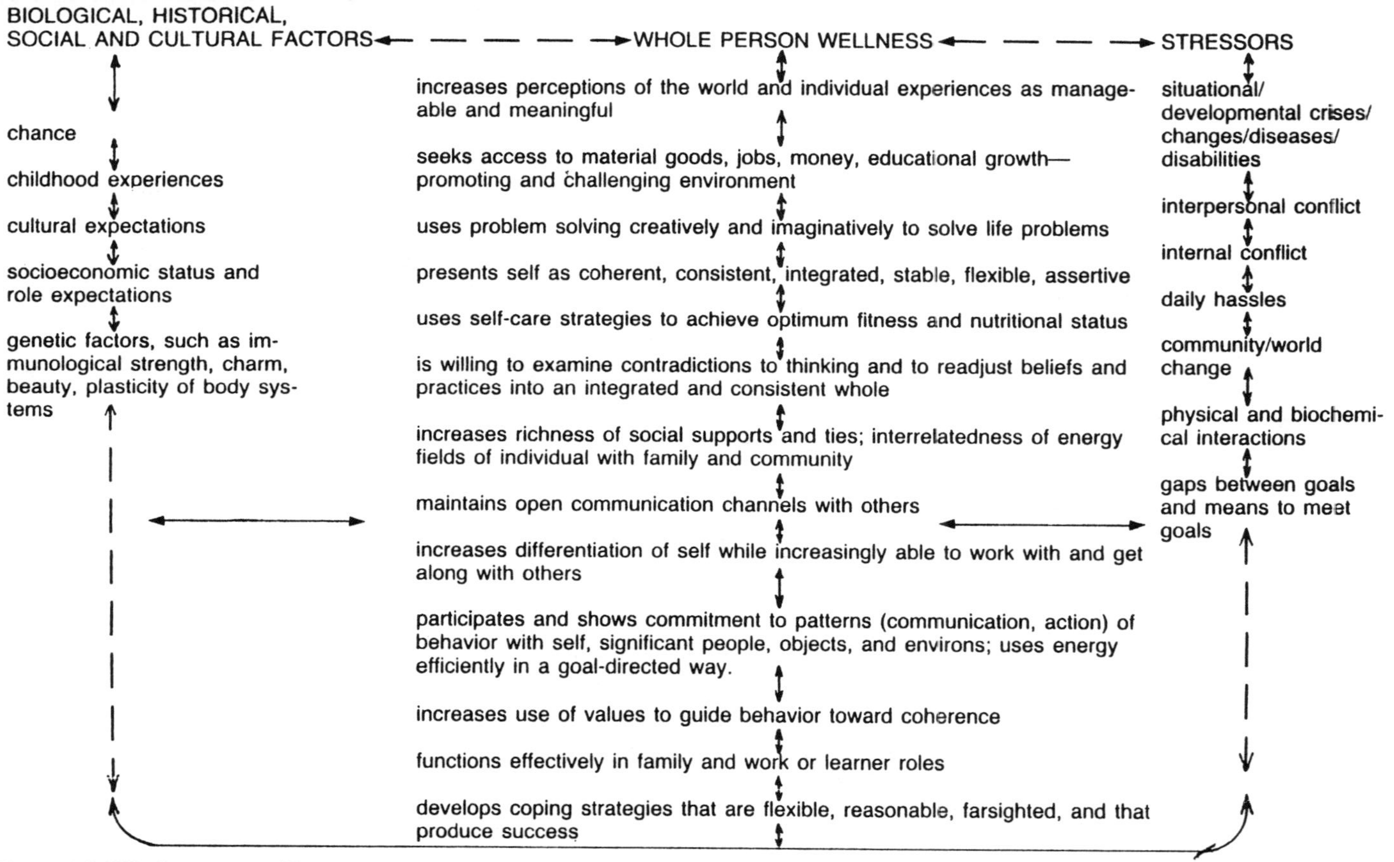

BIOLOGICAL, HISTORICAL, SOCIAL AND CULTURAL FACTORS ←→ **WHOLE PERSON WELLNESS** ←→ **STRESSORS**

Biological, historical, social and cultural factors:
- chance
- childhood experiences
- cultural expectations
- socioeconomic status and role expectations
- genetic factors, such as immunological strength, charm, beauty, plasticity of body systems

Whole person wellness:
- increases perceptions of the world and individual experiences as manageable and meaningful
- seeks access to material goods, jobs, money, educational growth—promoting and challenging environment
- uses problem solving creatively and imaginatively to solve life problems
- presents self as coherent, consistent, integrated, stable, flexible, assertive
- uses self-care strategies to achieve optimum fitness and nutritional status
- is willing to examine contradictions to thinking and to readjust beliefs and practices into an integrated and consistent whole
- increases richness of social supports and ties; interrelatedness of energy fields of individual with family and community
- maintains open communication channels with others
- increases differentiation of self while increasingly able to work with and get along with others
- participates and shows commitment to patterns (communication, action) of behavior with self, significant people, objects, and environs; uses energy efficiently in a goal-directed way.
- increases use of values to guide behavior toward coherence
- functions effectively in family and work or learner roles
- develops coping strategies that are flexible, reasonable, farsighted, and that produce success

Stressors:
- situational/developmental crises/changes/diseases/disabilities
- interpersonal conflict
- internal conflict
- daily hassles
- community/world change
- physical and biochemical interactions
- gaps between goals and means to meet goals

Figure 1.2 Whole person wellness.

Source: This figure suggested by the work of Ahmed and Coelho (*Toward a New Definition of Health*. New York. Plenum, 1979); Antonovsky (*Health. Stress and Coping*, San Francisco, Jossey Bass, 1979); and Dunn (*High Level Wellness*, Arlington, VA, Beatty, 1961.)

ing their policyholders with up to $500 if they do not use insurance coverage. The ideal is to have insurance reimbursement for wellness activities; however, providers are reluctant to pay until there is conclusive evidence that a specific weight loss or exercise program is appropriate for reimbursement. To date, some health insurance policies reimburse for health promotion services if ordered by a physician (Hosokawa, 1984). As more nurses qualify for third party reimbursement, they will be in a better position to be reimbursed for wellness nursing activities.

"Employee medical costs in American companies are rising so fast—20% a year, compounded—that within eight years they will offset after-tax profits in the average large corporation" (Daniel, 1985, pp. 74–79). Because of this problem, many companies have begun to establish wellness programs for employees because these programs save money. Herzlinger, a professor of business administration at Harvard's Business School, counsels that business must "Go far beyond their largely token programs in disease prevention and health promotion into massive, action-oriented education for employees, their families and communities" (Daniel, 1985, pp. 74-79).

Herzlinger cautions that "Band-Aid" responses like Diagnostic Related Groups (DRGs) will simply inflate charges.

> You know, DRGs were tested in New Jersey, and the federal government wants to get out of the experiment there—chiefly bcause DRGs don't work . . . Heart disease costs us $65 billion a year. Add in cancer and arteriosclerosis and by conservative estimate the country spends $160 billion a year on disease highly correlated with life style. (Daniel, 1985, pp. 74–79)

The American Hospital Association (AHA) jumped on the wellness bandwagon in 1978. The AHA created the Center for Health Promotion. By 1982, a representative of the AHA reported receiving 60 to 90 requests/month from hospitals for assistance in developing health promotion/wellness programs for businesses.

There is increasing evidence that educational, organizational, and environmental interventions can be effective in keeping people well and in preventing many chronic diseases. Wellness is also important in containing medical costs, in guiding consumers to use the health care system appropriately, to take a more active role in their own wellness, and to know what they are paying for when they receive medical and nursing services. If practitioners can respond to the challenge, wellness may indeed be the focus of practice in the twenty-first century.

DEFINITION OF TERMS AND THEIR RELEVANCE
TO WELLNESS THEORY

Concepts can range from the empirical to the highly abstract (Chinn & Jacobs, 1994, p. 53). For example, height and weight are directly observable, and thus are relatively empirical concepts. Wellness cannot be directly observed and it is a relatively abstract concept; it must be inferred from other more observable concepts. Wellness is so abstract that it can be thought of as a *construct* (because it is constructed from multiple sources).

A primary purpose of this chapter is to develop a systematic view of the concepts and interrelationships among them so that eventually this view can be used to describe, explain, predict, and/or control wellness practice.

The model for practice used in this book is a systems model: it is an organized set of dynamically interrelated parts. *Systems* exchange information, matter, and energy at the interface between systems. Chaos may ensue when a system is knocked off balance. However, a higher, more adaptive level (of wellness) can occur after this imbalance, resulting in a new steady state. Thus, chaos is not to be avoided, because out of it may come more adaptive and complex capacities (Barton, 1994).

In the model, *whole persons* are conceptualized as energy systems of mind/body/spirit oscillating in a spiraling course through time and space from conception to infinity. Whole persons are in constant change as they move between and within dimensions toward and away from illness, disease, aggressive acts, and withdrawal. The spiral movement continues through time and space as whole persons evolve toward high level wellness and self-actualization. Whole persons are believed to have innate self-healing and self-repair abilities which may lie dormant or become blocked in the process of interrelating with the environment. Practitioners and clients are examples of whole person systems; both can become *integrated* whole persons as they move toward wellness.

As a whole person, the practitioner is also in constant flux between the dimensions of wellness. The practitioner's role in assisting the client toward wellness is to:

- be an effective role model for wellness
- facilitate consistent client involvement in the assessment, implementation, and evaluation of wellness goals
- teach clients to perceive life experiences as manageable and meaningful by increasing self-responsibility and commitment to self-care
- teach and facilitate client self-care strategies to enhance fitness, nutritional status, stress management, positive relationship building, coherent belief systems, and their environment
- facilitate client creative problem solving to enhance wellness
- facilitate client assertive behavior
- teach clients effective communication skills
- assist clients to differentiate themselves from the practitioner and significant others
- facilitate richness of client social supports
- facilitate effective learner, family, and work role behaviors in clients

Whole persons are in constant flux between fitness and lack of fitness; over/undernutrition; positive and negative/destructive relationships and positive, satisfying ones; stress management and stress overload/deprivation; clear life purpose, consistent belief systems, lack of commitment to self-care; environmental distress/unawareness and environmental sensitivity/comfort. Each of these dimensions will be discussed in detail in subsequent chapters.

Wellness is a process of moving toward greater awareness of and satisfaction from engaging in activities that move the whole person toward fitness, positive nutrition, positive relationships, stress management, clear life purpose, consistent belief systems, commitment to self-care, and environmental sensitivity/comfort. The wellness process can be pursued by clients to prevent illness, facilitate rehabilitation, or enhance the quality of life and more fully actualize potential when ill, dying, or overcoming disability.

Differentiation of self is an important concept in the model; actualization of this concept enables a clear boundary development between the emotional and intellectual subsystems of a whole person, leading to enhanced problem-solving ability, flexibility in behavior, intimacy in relationships, and a higher level of wellness. *Pseudo-self*, or that which has not been processed through a value clarification process, is the part of a whole person at the whim of the emotional system of others and leads to manipulation of the whole person. *Solid self* increases as a consistency between beliefs, feelings, and actions is actualized through the value clarification process (Gilbert, 1992). The value clarification process and its relationship to wellness are presented in detail in Chapter 2.

Environment is external to whole persons; it is a changing field that is continuous and contiguous with whole persons. Environment can be modified by whole persons as well as modify whole persons.

Self-care can be defined as those activities and programs whole persons perform for themselves. Barry et al. (1979, p. 5) contend that *self-care* has been unclearly defined and can include such divergent activities and programs as:

- learning experiences teaching clients how to diagnose and treat common ailments
- groups which help consumers modify their lifestyles toward positive nutrition and to smoking and alcohol cessation
- teaching the chronically ill how to manage their conditions without the continual care of a physician or nurse
- lay-initiated clinics, especially women's clinics
- non-Western or otherwise nontraditional techniques, such as yoga, biofeedback, meditation, acupressure, and Tai-Chi.

The wellness model presented in this book provides a middle ground definition of self-care; to the far right are those self-care programs which are initiated and developed within a profession; at the other extreme are self-care activities developed in lieu of practitioners. In the model presented, the practitioner is involved in self-care activities, but the decisions about goals, actions, and evaluations are the client's.

ASSUMPTIONS UNDERLYING THE WELLNESS MODEL

The wellness model has been developed based on the following assumptions about whole persons, who:

- are capable of self-assessing their own wellness needs
- are capable of taking action to meet their wellness goals
- are capable of evaluating their progress toward wellness
- are in the process of moving toward wellness
- are capable of displaying characteristics of wellness even when ill, disabled, or dying
- have innate self-healing processes which can be activated to enhance wellness
- can learn to move to a higher level of wellness when facilitated by nurses well-grounded in wellness theory and practice
- can learn from modeling, clearly structured goals, means to meet those goals, and peer support.

BOUNDARIES OF WELLNESS THEORY

The boundary lines of a theory or model suggest that they are concerned with a particular area of inquiry, in this case, the intra- and interaction of the whole person and environment. *Boundaries* may be influenced to some extent by the retrictions of nurse attitudes and moral and cognitive complexity attainment.

According to Joyce and Weil (1972), a person at a high level of *cognitive complexity* is able to negotiate rules and take responsibility for his or her own learning and structure. Kohlberg (1975) speaks to the issue of moral development. Practitioners must be at a high level of moral development in order to negotiate contracts with clients and respect the dignity of individuals. Although many practitioners may not have attained this level of functioning, moral reasoning and cognitive complexity can be influenced in the direction of higher levels by exposing people to them. As practitioners are exposed to the next higher stage of reasoning, contradictions to the current level of reasoning can be identified in the value clarification process, discussed in Chapter 2.

Wellness theory is not restricted by level of health. Wellness theory is appropriate to persons who are ill, disabled, dying, or relatively well.

Wellness theory is not restricted by age or setting. School programs focusing on wellness and the knowledge of one's body are now being developed for very young children. Practitioners who work with families in community settings can also affect the wellness of newborns and even fetuses by facilitating parent wellness.

This chapter has provided a conceptual basis for wellness practice. Chapters 2 and 3 are transitional chapters; they are designed primarily to assist practitioners to enhance their level of wellness and positive role model status. "Integrative Learning Experiences" at the end of this chapter and other chapters provide other avenues for enhancing wellness; some are most useful for practitioners, while others can be used, or adapted for use, with clients.

Integrative Learning Experiences can assist you in putting into practice the concepts described in each chapter. Completing the experiences can help you move toward wellness; the process will also assist in understanding the process clients will need to pass through to move toward wellness. Once you have completed the experiences you can adapt them for use with clients. Beginning level experiences are most appropriate for the beginning wellness practitioner, students and practitioners who are relatively unfamiliar with wellness practice. Advanced level experiences are most appropriate for more advanced wellness practitioners, e.g., graduate students who are proficient in basic wellness skills and advanced wellness practitioners.

INTEGRATIVE LEARNING EXPERIENCES

1. Set aside a notebook for journal writing. Always date your entries and write nonjudgmentally. After finishing an entry, read what was recorded and write any additional thoughts, avoiding judging what has been written. Use the following statements to explore wellness and you.

A. Wellness is related to your idea of life. Explore your life goal, your reason for living.

B. Wellness is related to your idea of life's authentically satisfying and fulfilling human pleasures. Which of life's pleasures do you deny yourself? Cherish? Which ones give you the most pleasure? How do you get fun out of living? What else could you do to get more fun out of living? Do you want to get more fun out of living?

C. Wellness hinges on your freedom to determine the course of your life; who runs your life? Are you able to make a free decision? Would you like to be freer? What is getting in your way of being freer? How can you overcome that obstacle?

D. Wellness is related to your motivation. Explore how you get yourself started in wellness behaviors, how you keep it going, what you need from others to keep it going, and how you can get what you need. Does your religion encourage you to practice wellness? What does your religion say about the body, about relationships, etc.? How could you relate your religious beliefs to wellness so they could provide support for practicing wellness? Do you want to?

E. Wellness requires change. Explore how comfortable you are with change in your life. Where in or on your body do you locate your wellness and worseness? Does this change? Could it? Under what conditions? What threatens your level of wellness, what lowers its level and what enhances it? What can you do to enhance it? Write down wellness teachings from your sacred literature; are these teachings reflected in your day-to-day life? What changes would enhance these reflections? Do you want to change them?

F. Wellness often depends on getting support for wellness behaviors. Discuss who has helped you move toward wellness and the specifics of what that person or persons did to help.

G. Wellness may depend on reworking painful feelings and experiences so well-being can exist. How have you reworked painful feelings? What else could you do to rework them? Are you ready to?

H. Wellness is related to integrating attachment to others with separateness and differentiation of self. Do you "belong" to too many others or things? Are you detached, engaged, seeking, plugged-in, rooted, tied at the umbilical cord to someone or something? Are you happy with your degree of attachment? What would you want to change? How could you go about changing? What is your index of separateness or differentiation? Do you have time and space for yourself? Do you want more? How can you get it? Do you allow your inner world time and space for imagination, fun, fantasy? Would you like to allow it more? How can you? What do you need and how can you get there? Are you ready to begin?

I. Wellness is related to a high degree of self-esteem. How have you defined yourself till now? Are you comfortable with this definition? Do you want to change it? What prevents you? How can you overcome this?

J. Wellness depends on positive relationships with others. As you write, it may become clear to you that you have specific unfinished business with one or more other people in your life. Write a dialogue with one or more of them about the unfinished business. When you are finished, reread the dialogue and see what insights you have. Finally, decide whether you want to open a dialogue with the person in real life. If so, set a time and place for doing so.

K. Wellness is related to your level of fitness; write about your fitness level.

L. Wellness is related to what you take into your body—food, chemicals, liquids, cigarette smoke, etc. Write about your level of nutrition.

M. Wellness is related to your environment; write about what in your environment affects you positively and negatively.

N. Wellness is related to your ability to stand up for your rights and assert yourself. Write about your level of assertiveness.

O. Wellness is related to your ability to manage stress; write about your stress management needs and skills.

P. Wellness is related to "quality of life." What specific things do you think increase your quality of life? What can you do to enhance your quality of living? What things can others do to enhance your quality of living? Are you ready to enhance your quality of living?

Write in your journal at least once a week. As you work, identify wellness goals for yourself. Prioritize them, choosing a goal that is attainable and that you are sure you are ready to pursue. Be sure your goal is specific and written in behavioral terms (e.g., practice assertive skill of broken record with Ms. Jones in meetings at least twice a week).

Find a peer at work (if possible) or someone you can talk to on the phone whenever it is necessary to obtain support and facilitation; writing notes to one another has also been shown effective. This person will be your peer facilitator.

- Write in your journal weekly about your movement toward wellness and your relationships with your peer facilitator.
- Choose one specific wellness goal and write it in behavioral terms in your journal. Examine your readiness and motivation for choosing that goal. If you are not ready to work on the goal or are motivated to work on it because you think you "should" rather than because you want to, choose another goal.
- Write in your journal about ways you might try to sabotage yourself from attaining your goal; write down observable actions you will take to make sure you avoid sabotaging yourself.
- Write down any questions you have or assistance you want from your peer facilitator and share this information with him or her. Be sure to make a specific plan to meet, talk on the telephone or write to one another weekly so you can attain your goal.
- Each week write in your journal concerning progress made, how your peer has been helpful or unhelpful and share the information with your peer facilitator each week.

(This exercise was developed by adapting material from the following sources: Pilch, John J., *Wellness, Your Invitation to a Full Life*. Minneapolis, MN: Winston Press, 1981; and Progoff, Ira., *At a Journal Workshop, The Basic Text and Guide for Using the Intensive Journal*. New York: Dialogue House Library, 1975; and empirical experiences teaching others to develop personal wellness goals.)

2. Identify a situation when you felt challenged by another person. Close your eyes and imagine yourself handling the interaction by remaining relaxed and confident, and giving a rationale for your actions based on a wellness conceptual model.

3. Write in your journal about your feelings and thoughts about seizing control of wellness practice.

4. Write in your journal about your current or potential status as a wellness role model. What would you have to do to be one? In what ways are you already?

5. Brainstorm with your peer facilitator about how wellness practitioners can get "a piece of the funding action," or with a client about how consumers can have a greater voice in funding decisions.

6. Write a critique of the wellness model presented in this chapter, including ideas about how concepts need further refinement, etc. Make some efforts at refining the model.

7. Compare and contrast your ideas about selfcare with those presented in this chapter. What would you have to do to accept the concept as presented here?

REFERENCES

Barry, P. et al. (1979). *Self-Care Programs. Their Role and Potential.* Chapel Hill, NC: The University of North Carolina.

Barton, S. (1994). Chaos, self-organization, and psychology. *American Psychologist* (January): 5–4.

Chinn, P., & Jacobs, M. (1994). *Theory and Nursing, A systematic approach* (4th ed.). St. Louis: C.V. Mosby.

Clark, C.C. (1995). What is alternative health practitioner about? *Alternative Health Practitioner: The Journal of Complementary and Natural Care* 1(1): 3–4.

Class, P. (1993). Transforming nursing leadership. *The Nursing Spectrum* (December 6): 6–7.

Daniel, J. (1985). Health costs: why the blue chips see red. *American Health* (January/ February) 4(1):74–89.

Downer, S.C. (1994). Survey of alternative therapies used by cancer patients. *British Medical Journal* 309 (July): 86.

Dunn, H. (1961). *High Level Wellness.* Arlington, VA: Beatty Press.

Eisenberg, D., Kessler, R.C., Foster, C., Norlock, F.E., Calkins, D., & Relbanco, T. (1993). Unconventional medicine in the United States. *The New England Journal of Medicine 328*: 246–252.

Gilbert, R.M. (1992). *Extraordinary Relationships: A New Way of Thinking About Human Interactions.* Minneapolis, MN: Chronimed Publishing.

Gross, P.A., Halperin, J.L., Lipkin, M., Marks, J.H., Rivlin, R.S., & Wise, T.N. (1991). *Managing Your Health Strategies for Lifelong Good Health.* Yonkers, NY: Consumers Union.

Halley, F.M. (1991). Self-regulation of the immune system through biobehavioral strategies. *Biofeedback and Self-Regulation 16* (1): 55–73.

Hosokawa, M. (1984). Insurance incentives for health promotion. *Health Education,* (October/November):9–12.

Joyce, B., & Weil, M. (1972). *Models of Teaching.* Englewood Cliffs, NJ: Prentice-Hall.

Kohlberg, L. (1975). The cognitive-developmental approach to moral education. *Phi Delta Kappan 56*(10):670–677.

Pilch, J. (1981). *Wellness: Your Invitation to a Full Life.* Minneapolis, MN: Winston Press.

Rubik, B. (1995). The NIH office of alternative medicine: What has it accomplished in its two years? *Alternative Health Practitioner: The Journal of Complementary and Natural Care* 1(1): 7–11.

2

BEGINNING TO MOVE TOWARD WELLNESS

This chapter explores the following topics and their relationship to wellness:

- Differentiation of self
- Value clarification
- Centering
- Facilitating movement toward wellness

As role models for wellness, practitioners learn to differentiate intellectual from emotional systems and take on a wellness value system. Theory and procedures for accomplishing this task, suggestions for use with clients, and additional procedures for facilitating client wellness are presented in this chapter.

DIFFERENTIATION OF SELF

Bowen suggests there are emotional and intellectual systems in the brain; these two centers are probably connected by neural tracts, but there is variation among people in the connections. At a low level of differentiation the *intellectual* center (which allows people to think about their lives and plan and control their behavior) is not well differentiated from the *emotional* center. At a high level of differentiation, the intellectual center is well developed and screens stimuli from the emotional center. People who are less differentiated have a high level of fusion between their emotional and intellectual systems, with the latter controlling decisions and behavior (Gilbert, 1992).

> Bowen uses the term differentiation to refer to the degree to which the intellectual system is differentiated from the emotional system as well as to explain the extent to which people are differentiated from each other in their emotional relationship system. (Gilbert, 1992, p. 186)

Although Bowen considers people to be on a continuum from low level differentiation to high level differentiation, it may be more useful to consider people as moving back and forth between various levels, depending on the amount of anxiety they are experiencing; high levels of anxiety short-circuit the intellectual system and lead to overly emotional responses. For example, when experiencing anxiety, practitioners may over-react to a situation; their emotional systems take precedence over their intellectual systems and perceptions, and self-talk similar to the following might occur: "Oh, oh, time to panic!" or "I can't handle this, I'd better get out of here" or "How dare she say that!"

If practitioners are at a higher level of differentiation, the intellectual system screens noxious stimuli, and thoughts and perceptions may be more like the following: "Keep calm," "I can handle this," "What am I getting so excited about? This isn't the end of the world; I can handle this."

It is clear that responding at a lower level of differentiation is more likely to be associated with increased stress, fatigue and burnout; thus, measures to enhance relaxation and decrease stress can enhance level of differentiation, e.g., centering and measures discussed in Chapters 3, 4, and 5.

Some signs that are associated with low level differentiation during stressful situations with clients include increased blood pressure, pulse, and respiration, and decreased ability to focus on the work at hand. (Physiological correlates of high anxiety and lack of the relaxation response have been known for many years. See Peplau, 1952; Selye, 1956, 1974; and Simmons, 1950; among many others.)

CASE STUDY: *Wellness Practitioner Mary S. Demonstrates a Low Level of Differentiation*

Mary S., an experienced practitioner was working with Mr. White. Suddenly, a student practitioner appeared in the room, marched up to Mary S., and stated very loudly: "What are you doing? You're doing that wrong! Let me show you how to do it right!" Mary S. turned beet red, experienced rage sufficient to trigger murder, and asked the other woman to step outside. What happened next remains censored. Had Mary S. remained differentiated, she would have been able to perceive that the new practitioner was seeking to meet her own needs, albeit in a somewhat hostile manner. Instead, Mary S. responded to the comment in an emotionally overreactive way and experienced increased stress.

CASE STUDY: *Wellness Practitioner Mary S. Moves to a Higher Level of Differentiation*

Mary S. brought the above example to her supervisor the following day and was able to identify how angry she had become and how the anger was blocking her from collaborating with the new practitioner. The supervisor was able to help Mary see how her anger had led to an undifferentiated response, and suggested she go out and hit a tennis ball (her favorite sport) until her anger had been dissipated. She also suggested Mary write in her wellness journal and explore her anger more deeply. The next week Mary S. came to the supervisor all smiles and reported that the other practitioner had "pulled a similar maneuver, but I remained calm." The supervisor congratulated Mary on her movement toward wellness.

When families demonstrate a *low level of differentiation*, there is a tendency for two or more family members to act (emotionally) as one. They may have difficulty differentiating their feelings and show anger (or other feelings) if another family member does, or try to live through one another by controlling life choices or events. Bowen refers to this phenomenon as "fusion" (1978). A family with a high level of fusion does not permit self-actualization in individuals. Practitioners using a wellness framework for practice seek to increase differentiation of self in themselves and in their clients.

Becoming differentiated is a lifelong process requiring commitment and ongoing evaluation of movement. Bowen notes that the more differentiated one is, the more *solid self* one has:

> The solid self is made up of clearly defined beliefs, opinions, convictions, and life principles. These are incorporated into self from one's own life experiences by a process of intellectual reasoning and careful considering of the alternatives involved in each choice. In making a choice, one becomes responsible for self and the consequences. Each belief and life principle is consistent with all the others, and self will take action on the principles even in situations of high anxiety and duress. (1978, p. 365)

In family systems theory, the ability to make a responsible decision or choice is called the "I position." The pseudo-self has not been acquired through conscious consideration; people who have more pseudo- than solid self guide their reactions by emotional shifts in their relationships, and may see others only as resources for meeting their needs.

Bowen developed a profile of differentiation from low (basing decisions on feeling responses, being comfortable and loved, and reducing anxiety) to high. At the low level of differentiation, chronic dysfunction, high dependency on others, living by moving from one crisis to another, and institutionalization are found.

At the *moderate level of differentiation,* people are more able to function (as in work settings), but life pursuits are focused on relationship systems. Pleasing the teacher or the boss or gaining relationship status from one who knows is more important than learning subject matter or the quality or value of the work itself. Pseudo-self may be large; principles and beliefs may be a helter-skleter assortment of ideas, collected under the pressure of pleasing others. They may have mastered a body of knowledge, but they are unable to use it in intense relationships. Some characteristic behaviors noted in people at a moderate level of differentiation include the tendency to be a rebel or a disciple, to search for the perfect relationship and to fuse or distance oneself emotionally (due to increased anxiety about intimacy) when a relationship is found.

The *moderate to good level of differentiation* is characterized by the ability to make decisions not dominated by the emotions; although outbursts may occur, during periods of calm the ability to reason is used to develop principles and beliefs that are then used to overcome automatic, emotional responses in situations of high anxiety; lives are orderly because there is energy available to plan; relationships are freer because solid self does not fuse with the self of the other person and create anxiety; marriage is a functional partnership; intimacy is possible because fear of loss of self is not a threat; all family members take responsibility for their behavior and decisions rather than blaming one another for their failures or crediting one another for successes; there is no need to attack one another's beliefs or principles; people are able to develop life goals based on their own interests, not someone else's.

The *highest level of differentiation* may be more hypothetical than real. At this level, people are the most free to engage in intense emotional responses because they are not compelled to react in a specific way; choice is available. There is the greatest freedom from automatic reactions and the least tension when relating with others. Wellness practitioners can encourage differentiation in themselves by learning and practicing centering, assertiveness, and stress reduction procedures; they can encourage differentiation to the client by teaching them these measures and encouraging them to use them.

Differentiation of self affects the ability to parent. Samaroff (1980) describes the differentiation of self in parenting from *symbiotic* (low differentiation) to *perspectivistic* (high differentiation):

1. *Symbiotic:* There is no separation of the other's responses from one's own, e.g., "You are angry because I am."
2. *Categorical:* Traits and characteristics of the child are viewed as separate from those of the parents, e.g., "The child is stubborn," "My boss is stupid," "The teacher is unfair."
3. *Compensating:* Traits are viewed as age-related, e.g., "The child is stubborn because he or she is a toddler," "Jane is rebellious because she is a teenager."
4. *Perspectivistic:* Behavior stems from individual experiences in specific environments, e.g., "Jeremy, perhaps you behaved that way because you were with friends who egged you on."

People who show lower levels of differentiation tend to get drawn into rigid three-person *triangles*.

A triangle works as follows: two people are involved in a relationship of emotional significance; anxiety or stress builds up between them; and another person, issue or object is pulled in to decrease discomfort. (Miller, 1982, p. 26)

Triangles occur in all families (and in other social and work situations in which there is high anxiety). In the less-differentiated family or person, triangles are more rigid and more automatic. Here are some typical triangles:

1. Husband and wife plan a vacation without their child; child becomes ill. More-differentiated couples can cope with conflicting demands and roles and will problem-solve to meet all role relationships satisfactorily. Less-differentiated couples will sacrifice one role, usually the husband–wife one, to focus on the child.

2. Partners have an argument. In less-differentiated families, one partner may form a triangle by pulling in the child (and complaining or arguing with him or her), their job, or school ("And if you hadn't gone back to school, we

wouldn't have this problem"), or some other object or person, including in-laws, alcohol, drugs, or food. In more-differentiated families, partners will stick to the issue of the argument and find a way to resolve it that suits both people.

3. A client is anxious about his or her ability to get answers from a physician and triangles in the wellness practitioner to talk to the doctor. Variants on this triangle are 1) a practitioner who questions his ability and triangles in the supervisor, and 2) a novice practitioner who questions his ability to work with a client and triangles in the experienced practitioner to do his talking for him.

4. There is a change in a work or school system, such as the hiring or firing of a new boss or the introduction of a new procedure or a new curriculum without sufficient collaboration with those involved. As stress in the work or school system increases, others (usually those with less power) are triangled in; students may be criticized, practitioners may triangle in supervisors when uncomfortable about the client's reactions; supervisors may battle with one another, leaving the wellness practitioner in the middle; or stress may appear in the form of illness in an important system member.

CASE STUDY: *Low Level of Differentiation in the White Family*
Ms. White lives with her two children, Jeremy, aged 1, and Jessica, aged 2 months. Birth control methods were explained to Ms. White after her last pregnancy, but she feels like a "somebody" when she invests love in caring for her children, and so became pregnant again. She is constantly with the children and anticipates their every need, frequently assuming their feelings; for example, she covered Jessica's head with a towel one day, "because she was angry with me." Whenever Jeremy tries to assert his independence, his mother starts talking about Jessica.

CASE STUDY: *A Student with a Moderate Level of Differentiation*
Nancy K. is working toward her baccalaureate degree. She has been married for 10 years, but feels isolated from her husband: "I always expected Joe would be my knight in shining armor, but now I'm not so sure he is." Nancy and Joe have two teenage daughters who are "going through that rebellious stage." Nancy was devastated at school the other day when she got a paper back with a C on it, and she exclaimed: "How could I get a C when I worked so hard and learned so much doing it! Can't I ever please that teacher?"

CASE STUDY: *A Family at a Good Level of Differentiation*
The Mays have encountered many stressors lately, and they have been arguing more often than usual, but when the storm is over, they are able to think and talk about the issues and to come to an understanding. The parents, Barb and Jo May, have a close relationship and they go to dinner and dancing once a week and take the children on a weekend trip every week. All three children are responsible for specific chores and are expected to develop their own life interests. Every Wednesday evening, the Mays have a family meeting to share problems and achievements, and to disagree with each other without attacking. The family members describe themselves as "happy" and they have few colds and other illnesses.

In addition to understanding what issues trigger anxiety in specific situations, it is important to maintain an "I" position or a good level of differentiation of self. There are a number of measures that practitioners can take to increase their level of differentiation, including value clarification and centering.

VALUE CLARIFICATION

Value clarification can assist practitioners and clients to develop larger portions of solid self, and thus become more differentiated. The steps of value clarification and their attendant processes are the following (Raths et al., 1966, pp. 63–65; Kirschenbaum & Simon, 1974, pp. 264–266; Kirschenbaum, 1975, pp. 102–104).

Prizing

1. Prizing and cherishing. At this step in the process, nurses learn to set priorities, become aware of what they are for or against, begin to trust their inner experiences and feelings, and examine why they feel as they do.
2. Clearly communicating one's values and actively listening to others'.

Choosing

1. Choosing freely by examining values others have imposed on them.
2. Choosing thoughtfully between alternatives by examining the process by which they choose, and considering the possible consequences of each choice.

Acting

1. Trying out the value choice includes developing a plan of action and trying it out; contracts to act may be drawn up between the nurse and self or others.
2. Evaluating what happened when action was taken and making plans to reinforce actions that support their values. (Integrated Learning Experiences, Beginning Level, p. 44, Nos. 6–11, provide value clarification experiences for each value clarification process; they can be adapted for use with clients.)

CASE STUDY: *Clarifying Values about Assertiveness Issues*

All students in a seminar were asked to bring an assertiveness issue that they wanted to work on to class. (Choosing freely) The instructor helped each student discuss when he or she might want or not want to be assertive in a situation brought to class. (Prizing and Cherishing; Examining alternatives and consequences of action) Students selected another student to pair up so as to practice role playing the assertiveness situation. Some students decided to contract with one another to try out the situation in real life and to receive positive reinforcement from one another for doing so. (Trying out; contracting; reinforcing change). All students were encouraged to try their new assertive behaviors out in real life situations and to report back to the class by evaluating their performance. (Evaluating)

CASE STUDY: *Assisting a Client to Clarify His Values*

Theresa F., a wellness practitioner, was working with Mr. Thomas who was overweight and smoked a pack of cigarettes a day. Although Theresa's first impulse was to tell him to quit smoking and lose weight, she restrained herself and decided to try value clarification instead. One of their conversations follows:

PRACTITIONER:	What kinds of things about yourself are you most concerned about?
CLIENT:	I'm afraid I'll have another heart attack. (choosing freely)
PRACTITIONER:	Anything else? (encouraging choosing from alternatives)
CLIENT:	My wife's nagging; she's always trying to get me to stay on a diet, but the same time, she bakes cakes and pies!
PRACTITIONER:	Perhaps we should get your wife in here too to work on this. (Goes out and brings wife into the room.) Your husband was just telling me about your concerns about his staying on a diet.
WIFE:	The doctor told him to lose weight and I try, but he's always sneaking goodies.
PRACTITIONER:	Are you interested in losing weight, Mr. Thomas?
CLIENT:	Well, if it would make my wife happy. . .
PRACTITIONER:	I'm wondering what would make you happy.
CLIENT:	Not having a heart attack again.
PRACTITIONER:	What do you know about preventing a heart attack?
CLIENT:	The doctor says losing weight, exercising regularly, and stopping smoking, but it seems like a lot to me.
PRACTITIONER:	What if you could choose one of those to begin with; which would it be?
CLIENT:	Exercising. I've always been active in construction and baseball until this heart attack laid me low.
PRACTITIONER:	Suppose we find an exercise plan for you and your wife agrees to exercise with you? How does that sound?
CLIENT:	Sounds good to me, but can you get her to stop nagging me?
PRACTITIONER:	I can teach you both how to support each other without nagging. We can start by using assertiveness skills such as "I" messages and other communication skills that have been found useful by some of my other clients. How does the plan sound to you, Mrs. Thomas?
WIFE:	O.K. I guess.

(Discussion continues as practitioner proceeds through rest of value clarification processes and makes plans with the couple to try out new behaviors and evaluate them.)

CENTERING

Centering refers to

quietly becoming aware of your own breathing . . . As you access these different levels of your being, you will become aware of an enveloping stillness . . . in which personal insights may emerge. (Krieger, 1993, p. 19)

Centering is a powerful, easily achieved skill for enhancing differentiation of self and thereby freeing practitioners from becoming too personally identified with the client's life issues. When practitioners are not centered, they are apt to feel fatigued, stressed, depressed, or angry when working with a client who displays these qualities. Centering allows the practitioner to be separate from yet open to input from clients. By differentiating oneself from clients through the act of centering, many blocks to listening drop by the wayside, including:

- *Comparing* (only partially listening to clients because of trying to assess who is smarter, more competent, more emotionally healthy, or suffering more)
- *Mind Reading* (not paying attention to what is being communicated; trying to figure out what the client is *really* thinking and feeling, rather than listening closely to what is being said)
- *Rehearsing* (not listening because of rehearsing what to say next; some people rehearse whole chains of responses, e.g., "I'll say, then he'll say, then I'll say")
- *Filtering* (listening to only part of what is said, e.g., what will relieve the guilt, threat, or unpleasantness)
- *Judging* (not paying attention because the client's comments have already been labeled as stupid, nuts, or unqualified)
- *Dreaming* (not listening because the client says something that triggers a chain of private associations)
- *Identifying* (taking what the client says and referring it back to one's own experience, e.g., his pain reminds you of yours)
- *Advising* (not listening for a full expression of the issue, or acknowledging the other's pain prior to suggesting what one should do)
- *Sparring* (looking for ways to disagree, discount, or put down what the other person says)
- *Being Right* (unable to listen to criticism because mistakes cannot be acknowledged)
- *Derailing* (changing the subject when bored or uncomfortable; joking or quipping is a common derailing technique)
- *Placating* (agreeing with everything to be pleasant and nice)

(McKay, Davis, & Fanning, 1995, pp. 16–19)

As a center of stability is achieved through centering, these blocks to communication are not necessary and real listening can occur.

Centering can be achieved while standing or sitting, but beginning efforts produce the best results in a sitting position.

1. Sit in a comfortable chair with feet flat on the floor and hands resting quietly in your lap; close your eyes.
2. Check out your body for tension spots and relax these areas as you exhale.
3. Inhale easily, filling your body with relaxation.
4. Exhale, moving your breathing to your center, about the level of your navel.

5. Continue breathing in this manner until you feel calm, integrated, unified, and focused.
6. (Optional) Picture the body surrounded by a protective shield that allows positive energy in, but keeps negative energy out. The shield may be conceived as a color, light source, or spiritual sense.

Centering takes little time once the idea is mastered. Wellness practitioners have reported to the author the following ways of using centering:

- "I take a moment, go to the rest room, and get centered between clients."
- "I center myself as I'm walking down the hall on the way to my next client."
- "I center myself when I'm with the client; I ask the client to center herself or himself and we do it together. I find we both have a lot more energy to concentrate on the tasks ahead when we do."

Clients can also be taught to use centering. For example, they may find it helpful to use prior to any anxiety-provoking situation in the hospital, at home, in social situations, or at work. The steps in entering remain the same. Directions given for the practitioner can be copied or adapted for use with clients.

FACILITATING MOVEMENT TOWARD WELLNESS

Once practitioners have attempted to raise their level of differentiation through centering and value clarification, they are ready to proceed with clients. Facilitating movement toward wellness with others includes the use of a number of approaches: evaluating the effect of change toward wellness, resistance to and readiness for change, and use of contracting, self-assessments, belief scales, imagery, structured relaxation, affirmation, and neurolinguistic programming.

Evaluating the Effect of the Proposed Change

Movement toward wellness requires change. One reason people resist change is because the new is unfamiliar. If movement toward wellness is viewed as a threat to current status, existing ways of life, job, or money, familiar habits, or autonomy or free will, resistance to change can be expected. When facilitating movement toward wellness, it is useful to ask the following questions:

- What other factors in the person's life will be affected as a result of changing?
- What forces are operating to inhibit change at this time?
- What information or experiences must precede the change?
- What new procedures or experiences will need to be developed as a result of the change?
- Who is likely to suffer from the change?
- How will power, influence, custom, or lifestyle be affected by the change?

- How aware is the client of the need for change or of its purpose?
- Is the client sufficiently involved in planning for the change?
- What past experiences between the nurse and the client might be influencing resistance to change now?
- How open has the client been to the introduction of change in the past?

The best developed model for assessing readiness for change is the *Health Belief Model*. It is used to predict the likelihood that individuals will seek help or change behavior in order to avoid illness. The model asserts that even when individuals recognize personal susceptibility they will not take action unless they believe illness would bring serious physical or social repercussions. The Health Belief Model is based on the idea of avoiding negatively-valued outcomes or personal threats, such as illness disability, nonproductivity, discomfort, and death. It is questionable to what extent a model based on avoidance is adequate to explain self-actualization and maximalization of potential.

Pender (1987, p. 66) has developed a *Health Promotion Model* based on a synthesis of the wellness and health promotion literature. In Pender's Model, individual factors [importance of health/wellness, perceived control, desire for competence, self-awareness, self-esteem, definition of health (actualization vs. stabilization), perceived health status, and perceived benefits of health-promoting behaviors] interact with modifying factors (demographic variables such as age, race, sex, ethnicity, education, income), interpersonal variables (expectations of significant others, including health care professionals), situational variables (prior experience with health promotion and options available), perceived barriers (unavailability, cost, inconvenience, extent of life change required), and cues to action (advice from others, mass media, awareness of potential for change and growth) to influence the likelihood of behavior change.

A factor to assess when examining client responsibility is the level of dissatisfaction with current lifestyle and the readiness for change. A client who is constantly slightly depressed and lacking in energy and who has tried all medical treatments may be dissatisfied enough to be ready to try jogging or another form of exercise as a treatment. Another client who has tried all the fad diets available in an effort to lose weight may be ready to try a long-term weight management program if it seems enticing and if support is provided. Another client who is in chronic pain that is not touched by strong medication may be willing to learn self-hypnosis as a last resort.

There may be a number of times clients are most open to taking responsibility for wellness. One is childhood. This is an age when beliefs about illness and wellness may not yet be well formed.

Another time of openness is the mid–life crisis, ages 35-45. At this time, people begin to see they are alone, mortal, and are searching for internal, not institutional, validation. It is a time when people can move out of roles defined by others and into self-fulfillment (Sheehy, 1974).

There may be other times when people are open to taking responsibility for their wellness. Times of crisis are times when change is possible and clients may be more willing to accept responsibility or to try a change in lifestyle.

Decreasing Resistance to Change

Once sources of resistance to change have been identified, steps can be taken to reduce it. If anxiety or threat are the source of resistance to change, clients can be taught to practice centering.

Resistance to change will be decreased if rewards for changing are given and problem solving is used. The first step in learning more effective behavior is to identify the behavior to be changed. Behavior is an action, not a feeling, attitude, or mood. Behaviors must be pinpointed and expressed in such a way that they can be counted. Table 2.1 shows examples of behaviors that can and cannot be counted.

Table 2.1 Examples of Behaviors That Can and Cannot Be Counted

Countable behaviors	Noncountable behaviors (general behaviors or internal states)
Jogging	Being neat
Brushing and flossing teeth	Being motivated
Drinking fluids	Being angry
Losing weight	Being depressed
Gaining weight	Feeling guilty
Smoking a cigarette	Improving communication
Practicing relaxation exercises	Being noncompliant
Attending a yoga class	Grieving
Eating complex carbohydrates	Being hostile

Once the behavior is expressed in countable terms, *baseline data* can be gathered. These data consist of information gathered prior to treatment; the pinpointed behavior is counted or measured to see how often it occurs now. These data can be charted and hung in the client's home or elsewhere, and can be recorded on the treatment chart, in the client's journal, or wherever agreed upon. Data from this "before" or baseline phase can be used later to check progress toward the goal. There are a number of ways to count behavior: frequency, rate over time, or how long the behavior continues. The method used to count depends on the behavior. For example, the frequency method might be best for participating in relaxation exercises, the rate over time to measure weight gain or loss, and the duration method to measure jogging. A notebook, graph, chart, or journal can be used to gather baseline data.

The next step in increasing desirable behavior is to find out what is rewarding and depriving to the particular client. Table 2.2 shows reinforcers for a student who was chronically late to class. Clients, too, can be asked to make such a list. There are some nearly universal rewards sch as attention, smiles, praise, and candy or other sweets. If the client is unable to state a reward, a universal reward can be used or the chart can be read to find hints. Of course, giving sweets to someone with diabetes or who wants to lose weight would be self-defeating. A reward cannot be used if control cannot be established over when the reinforcer is dispensed. For example, if a family lets a child watch TV whether or not the child participates in family meetings, watching TV cannot be used as a reward for the child's participating in family meetings. If the client is hospitalized, more rewards can be controlled. If the client is at home, fewer rewards are under nursing control. It is wise to enlist the aid of families, other personnel, and whoever it is who dispenses rewards; the best way to do this is to reward them for helping by giving them attention, not scolding them when they do not comply, and by using whatever other things seem to be rewarding to them. When operating from a wellness framework, keep in mind that self-modification or client choice in applying behavior modification principles and voluntary changes in selected aspects of their own behavior is the focus, not changing the behavior of others through the manipulation of rewards and punishments (Pender, 1987, p. 80).

Table 2.2 Reinforcers for One Student

Positive, rewarding reinforcers	Negative, depriving reinforcers
Eating ice cream	Watching cartoons
Seeing a movie	Working overtime
Sleeping late on weekends	Being reminded that I'm late
Talking with other students	Doing dishes
Going dancing	Doing reports
Reading mysteries	Eating cottage cheese

In order to increase the occurrence of a goal-directed behavior, the reward must immediately follow movement toward that behavior. Giving the client words of praise 2 days after he or she walked around the block is less likely to increase walking behavior than praising right after the walk.

In some cases it may be unrealistic or impossible to provide the reinforcer immediately following the occurrence of the goal-directed behavior. In that case, a written contract, wall chart, token system, or some other method can be used to indicate a reward is due. For example, a wall chart could be used to show participation in planned exercise. A mark could be used to indicate 30 minutes of TV time or crossword puzzle work that could be collected that evening or on the weekend for each time 30 minutes of exercise is accomplished. Or, clients can be given tokens to indicate completion of a behavior; a specified number of tokens can be used to purchase a reward.

Some desired behaviors may occur at random or very rarely. In those cases, shaping techniques to reinforce approximations to the target behavior can be used. For example, telling the client the exact words to say and then praising the behavior, or asking the client to avoid smiling when talking are ways of *shaping behavior*. When shaping client behavior, nurses act as sculptors, helping clients to approximate the behavior that will be successful for them.

CASE STUDY: *Helping a Client Start an Exercise Program*

Mr. Sconce had just been discharged from the hospital and had been advised to begin an exercise program by his physician. The client revealed his anxiety about beginning such a program to the wellness practitioner, Ms. Joshua. The practitioner began by listing the steps in an exercise program (learn how to take pulse, learn warm-up and cool down exercises, choose a suitable type of exercise, set up rewards and a way to chart movement toward exercise goal). Next, the practitioner demonstrated the steps, ignoring any statements of fear of failure and praising any positive attempts. (The use of the negative reinforcer of not commenting verbally or nonverbally on fears will extinguish that behavior in time if used consistently.) Next, Ms. Joshua asked Mr. Sconce to copy what she did, and praised him for each step successfully completed. Ms. Joshua also enlisted Mrs. Sconce in the effort and both client and spouse soon were actively engaged in a walking program together. Ms. Joshua taught the Sconces how to make a contract with one another for changing behavior. Table 2.3 shows the contract the Sconces used.

Whether wellness practitioners work with clients, peers, family members, or self-contracts to achieve wellness goals, the *contracting process* remains the same:

1. *Mutual exploration of wellness interests.* Questions to ask include: Is this goal realistic for me now? Why is this goal being chosen now? Has this goal been chosen before and what were the results, things learned, barriers encountered? Does this goal have a high personal priority or was it chosen to please others? How appropriate is this goal now? How specifically written is the goal? Has only one goal been chosen?

   NOTE: The more specific, realistic, appropriate, and attainable the goal, the more likely it is to be attained; be sure only one goal is worked on at a time.

Table 2.3 A Behavioral Contract for Mr. and Mrs. Sconce

Wellness Goal: To walk briskly for 30 minutes every day

I, Adolph Sconce, promise to walk briskly with Edith Sconce 30 minutes every day for a period of 2 weeks, whereupon Edith and I will treat ourselves to a movie. I understand that if I do not fulfill this contract, the designated reward (movie) will be withheld.

Signed: _____
                          (Client)

           _____
                        (Facilitator)

           _____
                   (Wellness Practitioner)

           _____
                          (Date)

---

2. *Identification of actions needed to accomplish the goal.*What countable behaviors are involved in meeting the goal? (The more clearly and specifically actions are stated, the easier it is to evaluate progress toward the goal.)
3. *Establishment of reward(s) for movement toward goal.* What is reinforcing and realistic as a reward?
4. *Division of responsibilities.* What responsibilities are involved? Who is responsible for which ones? What specific assistance will the facilitator give the other person?—e.g., encouragement, phone calls, assertive asking about how the wellness goal is going, weekly meetings to discuss the goal.
5. *Time limit.* What mutually agreed upon time limit is set to accomplish the goal and/or evaluate movement toward the goal?
6. *Evaluation of movement toward goal.* How will movement toward the goal be evaluated? By whom? When? What consequences will accrue as a result? What additional assistance does the goal writer need from the facilitator in order to move toward goal attainment? What barriers are interfering with movement toward the goal and how can they be surmounted?
7. *Modification, renegotiation, or termination of the contract.* If a goal is met, a new one is reset. If a goal proves inappropriate, a new goal is found.

Facilitators for wellness goals can be wellness practitioners but they can also be peers, family members, other health professionals, or anyone who agrees to learn and follow the procedure for contracting. Self-contracting can also be used, but research and empirical knowledge have shown that people with low self-esteem or little perceived control over what happens to them may not take responsibility for carrying through on a contract (Pender, 1987, p. 190).

Table 2.4 shows possible wellness goals. This self-assessment can be used to assist in the choice of a wellness goal.

Table 2.4 Wellness Self-Assessment

Directions: Read the statements for each dimension of wellness; circle the number which most appropriately resembles the importance of each statement to you and your well-being and current interest in changing your life style as follows:

1. I am already doing this. (Congratulate yourself!)

2. This is very important to me and I want to change this behavior now.

3. This is important to me, but I'm not ready to change my behavior right now.

4. This is not important in my life right now.

Nutritional Wellness				
I maximize local fresh fruits and uncooked vegetables in my eating plan.	1	2	3	4
I minimize the use of candy, sweets, sugar, and simple carbohydrates.	1	2	3	4
I eat whole foods rather than processed ones.	1	2	3	4

Table 2.4 (*continued*)

	1	2	3	4
I avoid foods that have color, artificial flavor, or preservatives added.	1	2	3	4
I avoid coffee, tea, cola drinks, or other substances that are high in caffeine or other stimulants.	1	2	3	4
I eat high fiber foods daily.	1	2	3	4
I have a good appetite, but I eat sensible amounts of food.	1	2	3	4
I avoid crash diets.	1	2	3	4
I eat only when I am hungry and relaxed.	1	2	3	4
I drink sufficient water so my urine is light yellow.	1	2	3	4
I avoid foods high in saturated fat, such as beef, pork, lamb, soft cheeses, gravies, bakery items, fried foods, etc.	1	2	3	4
I use bottled water or an activated carbon filtration system to insure safe drinking water.	1	2	3	4

Fitness and Wellness

I weigh within 10% of my desired weight.	1	2	3	4
I walk, jog, or exercise vigorously for more than 20 minutes at least 3 × / week.	1	2	3	4
I seem to digest my food well (no gas, bloating, etc.)	1	2	3	4
I do flexibility or stretching exercises daily and always prior to and following vigorous exercise.	1	2	3	4
I am satisfied with my sexual activities.	1	2	3	4
When I am ill, I'm resilient and recover easily.	1	2	3	4
When I look at myself nude, I feel good about what I see.	1	2	3	4
I use imagery to picture myself well and healthy every day.	1	2	3	4
I use affirmations and other self-healing measures when ill, injured, or to enhance my fitness.	1	2	3	4
I avoid smoking and smoke-filled places.	1	2	3	4

Stress and Wellness

I sleep well.	1	2	3	4
I have a peaceful expectation about my death.	1	2	3	4
I live relatively free from disabling stress or painful, repetitive thoughts.	1	2	3	4
I laugh at myself occasionally, and I have a good sense of humor.	1	2	3	4
I use constructive ways of releasing my frustration and anger.	1	2	3	4
I feel good about myself and my accomplishments.	1	2	3	4
I assert myself to get what I need instead of feeling resentful toward others for taking advantage of or intimidating me.	1	2	3	4
I can relax my body and mind at will.	1	2	3	4
I feel accepting and calm about people or things I have lost through separation.	1	2	3	4
I get and give sufficient touch (hugs, etc.) daily	1	2	3	4
I live with a sense of joy and a zest for life.	1	2	3	4

Wellness Relationship and Better

I have at least one other person with whom I can discuss my innermost thoughts and feelings.	1	2	3	4
I keep myself open to new experiences.	1	2	3	4

I listen to others' words and the feelings behind the words.	1	2	3	4
What I believe, feel, and do are consistent.	1	2	3	4
I allow others to be themselves and to take responsibility for their thoughts, actions, and feelings.	1	2	3	4
I allow myself to be me.	1	2	3	4
I live with a sense of purpose.	1	2	3	4

Wellness and the Environment

I have designed a wellness support network of friends, family, and peers.	1	2	3	4
I have designed my personal living, playing, and working environments to suit me.	1	2	3	4
I work in a place that provides adequte personal space, comfort, safety, direct sunlight, fresh air; and limited air, water, or material pollutants; or I use nutritional, exercise, or stress reduction measures to minimize negative effects.	1	2	3	4
I avoid cosmetics and hair dyes that contain harmful chemicals.	1	2	3	4
I avoid pesticides and the use of harmful household chemicals.	1	2	3	4
I avoid x-rays unless serious disease or injury is at stake, and I have dental x-rays for diagnostic purposes only every 3 to 5 years.	1	2	3	4
I wear a good sunscreen ointment when exposed to the sun.	1	2	3	4
I use the earth's resources wisely.	1	2	3	4
I meet the challenges of my environment.	1	2	3	4

Commitment to Wellness

I examine my values and actions to see that I am moving toward wellness.	1	2	3	4
I take responsibility for my thoughts, feelings, and actions.	1	2	3	4
I keep informed on the latest health/wellness knowledge rather than relying on experts to decide what is best for me.	1	2	3	4
I wear seat belts when driving and insist that others who drive with me also do so.	1	2	3	4
I ask pertinent questions and seek second opinions whenever someone advises me.	1	2	3	4
I know which chronic illnesses are prominent in my family and I take steps to avoid incurring these illnesses.	1	2	3	4
I work toward achieving a balance in all wellness dimensions in order to enhance my sense of well-being and satisfaction.	1	2	3	4
I look beyond my needs to the needs of society.	1	2	3	4

Using Self-Assessments to Promote Wellness

Self-assessments (such as Table 2.4) may be more appropriate to wellness facilitation than risk appraisals for several reasons. Self-assessments generally point the way to goals; they also may point out, and reinforce, positive behaviors. Since they are self-assessments, clients self-assess their wellness. The practitioner may discuss findings with the client or use them to assist clients to develop wellness goals, but the choice is the client's.

Health Hazard/Health Risk Appraisals (HHA/HRA) are focused on risks that may have negative effects on life outcomes; an individual's health-related behaviors and personal characteristics are compared by a professional to mortality statistics and epidemiologic data to estimate risk or dying versus the amount of that risk that could be eliminated if lifestyle is changed. Often, a score is provided indicating risk and chance of death if the behavior is continued.

Based on a review of available studies and discussions with HHA/HRA developers, Wagner et al. (1982) concluded that the scientific basis for them is problematic due to impreciseness in measurements and inaccuracies in client-supplied information. Also, beliefs in the ability of HHA/HRAs to motivate behavioral change cannot be substantiated from evidence; additionally, adverse effects have been noted. For example, depressive responses to life expectancy predictions have occurred. Another problem with HHA/HRAs is that they may be touted as behavioral change motivators in themselves; the relationship between facilitator and client has been demonstrated to be the crucial variable, not the sophistication of the assessment tool. Finally, although self-assessments can be used to engender guilt, when used from a wellness perspective the object is not to upset or evoke guilt in the client, but rather to assist the client to decide whether change is a high priority for that client. Since risks are not stated in number or word form, the chances are that clients are probably less likely to respond negatively to self-assessments.

Client Assessment Questions that Can Assist in Movement Toward Wellness

A wellness framework implies that the responsibility for the client resides with the client, unless there is a life threatening situation in which the client cannot decide. It also implies that a wellness goal chosen by the client may not have high priority for the practitioner. For example, an obese client may have high priority on stress management, while the practitioner thinks weight loss should be the first priority. A wellness framework assumes the client sets the goal, not the practitioner.

Stepping out of the caretaking role may be difficult. However, consider the following. If the client takes self-responsibility for body/mind/spirit in one small issue, the process has been learned and it can be transferred to other issues, including those of high priority for the practitioner. Also, if the practitioner is able to demonstrate how success in attaining (life) goals can be accomplished, trust can be established and the client is more apt to agree to pursue a wellness goal of agreed upon high priority.

Practitioners may not be working in situations in which clients have a great deal of energy to invest in setting and striving toward wellness goals. For example, practitioners working in acute care settings may wonder how wellness can be encouraged in their settings.

A beginning step is to adapt assessments to fit a wellness framework, e.g.:

1. What goals would you like to work on?
2. What are your strong points and special abilities?
3. What kind of help do you want from me?
4. What do *you* think you need?
5. Why do you think you are having this problem *now* in your life?
6. What does this weight (symptom, worry, etc/.) mean in your life?
7. What would you have to give up or take on to get rid of this problem (weight, symptom, worry, etc.)?

The Wellness Belief Scale

Another measure wellness practitioners can use to facilitate wellness includes assisting clients to examine their wellness beliefs. Table 2.5 shows a *wellness belief scale*. The scale was modeled after Rotter's original work (1966) on *internal locus of control* or the degree to which people believe they have control over what happens to them. The purpose of the belief scale is to measure client responsibility for wellness, by measuring degree of internality. Those who score 21 are at a high point of internality. Beliefs about wellness can influence the degree to which people take responsibility for their wellness. Numerous studies support the idea that people with strong beliefs about their ability to control destiny are more likely to be alert to information in the environment, place greater value on skills or achievement rewards, be more concerned about this ability (especially if the ability is lacking), and be resistive to subtle attempts to influence them. Rotter referred to these two basic stances as internal- and external-orientation. For example, Brown et al. recently reported that people who believe they have little personal control over events that happen to them do not engage in health promotion activities (1983). Boyd (1993) developed a scale to measure children's participation in their own health care.

Table 2.5 The Clark Health/Wellness Belief Scale

These questions can be used to find out how different people feel about health and wellness. Each item consists of a pair of statements, a and b. Select the statement for each pair which you most strongly agree with or think is true, not the one you think you should choose. There are no right or wrong answers; this scale is a measure of what you believe. For some items, you may find you believe both statements or neither one. In such cases, be sure to select the one you most strongly believe by checking one "agree" for each number. Try not to be influenced by your previous choice.

AGREE

1. A.	I carry the key to my own well-being in the way I choose to live.	_____
B.	Health and illness are both luck and beyond my control.	_____
2. A.	Wellness is a lifelong effort.	_____
B.	If I wait, medical science will develop cures for all illnesses.	_____

Table 2.5 *(continued)*

3. A. It matters little whether my health care practitioner pursues wellness as long as he or she looks after mine.   _____

    B. I think it's important to steer clear of health care practitioners who are not pursuing their own wellness by not smoking, by keeping their weight down, etc.   _____

4. A. No matter how hard I try, I think I'll probably still get ill (won't be able to quit smoking or lose weight), so I might as well do what I want to do.   _____

    B. I have faith in my ability to increase my wellness.   _____

5. A. I think that if I'm going to be ill, I'm going to be ill.   _____

    B. Trusting to fate about my wellness doesn't work. I find I have to take a definite course of action.   _____

6. A. Staying well is a matter of hard work, and luck has little or nothing to do with it.   _____

    B. Staying well is a matter of being born under the right condition and being in the right place at the right time.   _____

7. A. Environmental factors have little effect on whether I get ill or not.   _____

    B. Heredity plays a major role in whether I get ill or not.   _____

8. A. I can influence governmental decisions about wellness.   _____

    B. Politicians, business people, and scientific experts make the decisions about my wellness.   _____

9. A. When I devise a wellness plan, I am pretty certain I can make it work.   _____

    B. I don't make long-term wellness plans because I don't think they work.   _____

10. A. Sometimes I don't think I can control my state of health.   _____

    B. It is hard for me to believe that my state of health is always due to luck or chance.   _____

11. A. I might as well decide my wellness goals by flipping a coin.   _____

    B. Getting what I want in terms of wellness has little or nothing to do with luck.   _____

12. A. With enough effort I think I can decrease the anti-wellness parts of my environment.   _____

    B. I think it's difficult and perhaps impossible to decrease the anti-wellness factors in my environment.   _____

13. A. A good health insurance plan ought to include incentives for staying well.   _____

    B. A good health insurance plan should be inexpensive, covering catastrophes like chronic illnesses and heart attacks.   _____

14. A. It doesn't really matter what I eat since wellness is unrelated to my food.   _____

    B. I should choose what I eat carefully, because it contributes to my wellness.   _____

15. A. I should work at being physically and mentally fit because both contributed to my wellness and health.   _____

    B. It doesn't matter whether I'm fit or not since wellness is due to luck and my doctor's prescription.   _____

Table 2.5 *(continued)*

			AGREE
16.	A.	Stress is due to factors beyond my control.	_____
	B.	I can learn to reduce my stress level and thereby be healthier.	_____
17.	A.	If I heal when I'm hurt or ill, it's because something outside me helped me to heal, like an antiseptic or medicine.	_____
	B.	I can learn to use my own healing potential and thereby enhance my wellness.	_____
18.	A.	I think it's important to stand up for my rights when I feel others are trampling on them.	_____
	B.	It doesn't pay to stand up to others since they don't listen anyway.	_____
19.	A.	I think it's important to question health care practitioners, lawyers, and anyone from whom I purchase a service because I share the responsibility for what happens to me.	_____
	B.	I assume doctors, lawyers, nurses, and other authorities know what I need better than I do.	_____
20.	A.	Meeting new friends is a matter of luck and being in the right place at the right time.	_____
	B.	Meeting new friends is up to me to go places, introduce myself, and suggest we spend time together.	_____
21.	A.	Pain is something that has to be endured and it will pass.	_____
	B.	When I am in pain, I can take action to reduce my pain.	_____

People who are internally oriented are more likely to take responsibility for wellness; others are apt to let a health care practitioner or fate determine level of wellness. Most people fall along a continuum from externality (0 = take little responsibility for own wellness) to internality (21 = take a great deal of responsibility for own wellness).

Once the client completes the belief scale, a discussion about what the answers mean to the client can ensue. Writing down what is peripherally known can often clarify thoughts and feelings and can be the basis for change. When responses are discussed in a group, lively debates and (sometimes) changes in beliefs can occur.

Some research suggests that locus of control *(internality-externality)* can be changed. In one study, student counselors changed their locus of control from external to internal after becoming more aware of their muscles' activity by receiving electromyographic feedback (Scalese, 1978). This study suggests that learning to tune in to internal body processes increases the belief of control over one's own fate.

Coller (1977) reported that clients became more internal in their locus of control as a result of a specific kind of group counseling called the *EPIC model*. The EPIC groups followed six exercise units consisting of perception and feedback skill training; self-disclosure; self-explanation skill building; assessment and understanding of self; personal contracting for change and growth; development of programs for achieving personal growth; and achieving and assessing personal goals and growth. This research suggests that structured exercises that help clients focus on themselves, develop goals, and work toward them can increase internality.

A study by Rotter (1966) looked at the effect of training in success-oriented learning situations with preadolescents. He examined the idea that if people receive enough training in success-oriented learning situations to counteract their previous learning, they will begin to attribute successes and failures to their own behavior; in other words, they would become more internal. The results of the study were that externally-oriented individuals who were exposed to success at learning tasks did become more internally-oriented. It may be that clients who are exposed to success at learning may affect their internality and their movement toward wellness in a positive way.

Relaxation Techniques

There are a number of techniques that can assist in relaxation and enhance change toward wellness. Relaxation of the muscles reduces pulse rate and blood pressure and decreases perspiration and respiration rates. The body responds to anxiety provoking thoughts and events with muscle tension. Physiological tension increases the subjective experience of anxiety. Muscle relaxation is incompatible with anxiety; learning to respond with one blocks the habit of responding with the other. Relaxation teachniques have been found useful in the treatment of muscular tension, anxiety, insomnia, depression, fatigue, irritable bowel, muscle spasms, neck and back pain, high blood pressure, milk phobias, and stuttering (Davis, Eshelman, & McKay, 1995). Most people do not realize which of their muscles are chronically tense nor think about how the constriction may be affecting their circulation, movement, or tendency to develop chronic illness or discomfort. Working while relaxed with a relaxed client also allows the practitioner and client to be more open to one another, to listen, and to learn more easily. Kern and Stejskal (1983) found that relaxation in the classroom reduced students' anxiety and improved their learning and recall.

Relaxation is a skill requiring practice and daily sessions to achieve mastery. Table 2.6 presents several types of relaxation exercises.

Table 2.6 Relaxation Exercises

Progressive Relaxation

1. Lie down in a comfortable spot or sit in a comfortable chair.
2. Close your eyes. Follow steps 3–10, tensing for 5–7 seconds and relaxing for 20–30 seconds. Allow yourself to deeply experience bodily changes.
3. Tense all the muscles of your hands, forearms, and upper arms.
4. Let all the tension out of the muscles of your hands, forearms, and upper arms.
5. Tense all the muscles of your head, face, throat, and shoulders, including the forehead, cheeks, nose, eyes, jaw, lips, tongue, and neck.
6. Release all the tension in your head, face, throat, and shoulders.
7. Tense all the muscles in your chest, stomach, and lower back.
8. Release all the tension in your chest, stomach, and lower back.
9. Tense all the muscles in your thighs, buttocks, calves, and feet.
10. Release all the tension in your thighs, buttocks, calves, and feet.

Taking a Trip in Your Mind's Eye

1. Find a comfortable, quiet spot and assume a relaxed position.
2. Close your eyes.
3. Let your breathing begin to move lower in your body, moving toward your abdominal area. Each time you exhale, your breathing moves lower in your body toward your abdominal area.
4. Take yourself on a trip in your mind's eye to a place that is comfortable and relaxing, somewhere you have been or somewhere you would like to be. See all the sights associated with your quiet, relaxing place. Hear all the sounds associated with your quiet, relaxing place. Smell all the smells associated with your quiet, relaxing place. Taste any tastes associated with your quiet, relaxing place. Fully experience all the sensations associated with your quiet, relaxing place.
5. Totally immerse yourself in your quiet, relaxing place until you are ready to return, then gradually return from your trip, keeping the relaxation and calmness with you for as long as you wish. Then gradually open your eyes and resume your day.

Quick, Total Relaxing Exercise

1. Find a door with a strong door knob. Close the door tightly and grasp the door knob.
2. Place your feet shoulder distance apart, 2 to 3 feet from the doorknob, depending on the length of your body; the distance should be adequate to allow you to totally stretch out but not strain your body.
3. Let your body totally relax, and let your head drop toward your chest.
4. Hold this position until you feel your body relaxing; stand up, take a few deep breaths, and repeat steps 2–4.

Note: Relaxation tapes may be needed to learn the process since it is difficult to read while trying to learn to relax. They can be purchased at many bookstores or personally developed.

Imagery

Everyone has had experiences with self-generated images: dreams, day-dreams, and fantasies may contain strong images generated by the right side of the brain. Experiences in the present may evoke images of past experiences that were similar. Most children have a well-developed sense of imaging. As they age, their skills may lie dormant as the logical, rational side of their brains is used in schoolwork and linear thought processes.

Imagery is a powerful tool for self-use or for engaging the client in movement toward wellness. The power of the approach is derived from its right-brained source. The right brain, which controls the left side of the body, is primarily responsible for orientation in space, body image, artistic endeavor, and recognition of faces. The right hemisphere deals with visual, holistic, intuitive, nonlinear thought. The left side of the brain is involved with analytic, logical thinking, particularly verbal and mathematical functions (Ornstein, 1972, p. 52). Imagery or visualization allows direct access to the subconscious and the autonomic nervous system functions, bypassing the left brain and its tendency to try to solve problems through logical processing. Unfortunately, logical processing can go awry and lead to ruminating or repetitive worrying that increases stress. Imagery can cut through rumination to the essential core of issues and thus lead to effective problem solving, decreased anxiety in interpersonal situations, and increased healing potential.

Through imagery it is also possible to learn to control functions previously thought to be under involuntary control, such as body temperature and heart rate. The power of imagery goes far beyond controlling physiological responses.

> Everyone has had some awareness of how the images and thoughts he holds in his mind can affect the world around him. Probably everyone has noticed that if he awakens cheerfully, with a positive image of himself and the coming day, that image will manifest itself in the external world. People he meets will also tend to be cheerful and happy, or will become so in the presence of his positive attitude. Events that draw his attention are likely to be positive, or he will tend to see something positive in them. (Samuels, 1975, p. 70)

Since imagery is a right-brain process, it is difficult to describe in a linear, left-brained written description. To grasp the power of imagery, it is necessary to try out different kinds of imagery exercises. Use Tables 2.7–2.10 to understand the process; if necessary adapt the exercise and read "yourself" instead of the word "client." Imagery can be used in a number of ways, including : (1) to solve problems, Table 2.7; (2) prepare for upcoming situations, Table 2.8; (3) enhance healing, Table 2.9; (4) decrease the influence of negative feelings and relationships, Table 2.10.

Table 2.7 Using Imagery to Solve Problems

1. Find a quiet spot and sit in a relaxed position; close your eyes.

2. Clearly define the problem. Use 3–5 words to state the problem succinctly. If you are having difficulty defining the problem, picture yourself telling the problem to a friend.

3. Ask, "Am I ready to solve this problem?" and wait for an answer. If the answer is "yes," proceed to step three; if "no," choose another problem.

4. Place the clearly defined problem in a frame using your choice of color to create a border around the problem.

5. See the solution in a frame using your choice of (a different) color to create a border around the solution.

Table 2.8 Using Imagery to Prepare for an Upcoming Situation

1. Decide on an upcoming situation for practice. Choose a situation you are anxious about, one whose outcome you are worried about or need practice in handling.

2. Assume a comfortable position with body relaxed and eyes closed.

3. Use the contraction/relaxation exercise to attain relaxation.

4. Imagine yourself as the director of a movie that you are going to run in your mind's eye. As director, you can stop or start the movie at any point that discomfort occurs.

5. Begin the situation, imagining everything about the situation: what is said, what you feel, what the other person(s) in the situation say and do. When you notice yourself becoming uncomfortable, stop the movie in your mind and go back to focusing on relaxing your body. When relaxed again, begin the movie at a spot a little before you felt anxious. Continue the movie until you feel uncomfortable or displeased with what occurs and return to relaxing. Work back and forth between the movie in your mind and relaxing until you can complete the whole situation while remaining relaxed.

Note: Your mind does not differentiate between an *image* of a situation and the actual experience of being in the situation, so a great deal of learning can occur using imagery and it will be much easier to remain calm and relaxed in the real-life situation once you have used the movie of the mind technique.

CASE STUDY: *Assisting a Client with the Movie of the Mind Technique*

Sarah K., a recent college graduate, expressed her anxiety about confronting her boss about obtaining a pay raise. Don W., a wellness practitioner, talked to Sarah about using imagery to prepare for the confrontation. Sarah agreed to try the technique. Don W. played a relaxation tape for Sarah K.; he asked the client to signal by raising the index finger of her right hand when she was relaxed. Don sat opposite Sarah and watched for the finger signal for relaxation; when Sarah raised her finger, Don asked her to imagine herself as the director of a movie with her as the star and her boss as the supporting actor. Sarah was asked to go on with the scene until she felt uncomfortable and then signal by raising the index finger of her left hand. Don worked with Sarah in this manner until she opened her eyes and exclaimed: "I got through the whole situation without feeling fearful!" Don then asked her to continue the practice at home and told her she would notice that it became easier and easier to get through the scene and as that happened it would be even easier to talk to her boss about a raise.

Table 2.9 Using Imagery to Enhance Healing

The following universal images can be used for:

Asthma or upper chest congestion: image of cool throat and warm chest

Hemorrhoids or anal pain: image of heavy, cool anus and warm pelvis

Itching or pain: image of coolness or picture an ice cube in the area

Low back pain: image of a heavy spine

Gynecological disorders: image of warm pelvis

Viruses: image of immune system (for example, white blood cells imagined as knights on horseback attacking the illness-producing cells and carrying them off to be excreted from the body)

Anger, resentment, etc.: image of peace, love, harmony

Headache: image of a hole in the head near the area of the headache; on exhalation of breath, imagine the pain going through the hole as a color

Chronic sinus problems: imagine tubes opening and draining, e.g., a sink unclogging in the area

Tense areas: imagine the muscles in the area getting wider and longer, unknotting or relaxing

Hot areas: imagine coolness, e.g., submersing the area in cool water

Moist areas: imagine the area becoming dry, e.g., a desert growing in the area

Dry areas: imagine the area becoming moist, e.g., a spring or fountain growing in the area

Fatigue: picture energy and vitality entering the area

CASE STUDY: *Helping a Client Develop a Healing Image*

Rebecca S., a wellness practitioner had just learned about the use of imagery to assist healing and wanted to try it out with a client with low back pain due to tension and stress. She told her client about the method, who soon agreed, stating, "These pain pills just don't work anymore and I'm at the end of my rope." Rebecca asked the client to close her eyes and listen to the relaxation tape she had brought. When the tape finished, Rebecca asked her client to keep her eyes closed and picture what her lower back looked like in her mind's eye. The client reported that her lower back looked like, "Tight, twisted red hot ropes." Rebecca asked the client to imagine her lower back becoming relaxed and healthy. The client opened her eyes after a few minutes and said, "I just imagined dumping ice cubes on those red hot ropes and untying the knots in the rope; now my back looks healthy and feels good." Rebecca suggested the client use imagery whenever she began to feel the pain return.

Table 2.10 Using Imagery to Decrease Painful or Negative Feelings

1. Help the client relax using either a taped relaxation exercise or instructions in Table 2.6.
2. Ask the client to picture the painful or negative feelings.
3. Ask the client to think of a container and picture it vividly.
4. Ask the client to put all the painful or negative feelings in the container, put a tight lid on it, and lock it tightly.
5. Ask the client to put the locked container in a place where it can no longer influence the client.
6. Ask the client to open her/his eyes when the task has been completed.
7. Ask the client to discuss what happened during the treatment.

Note: Clients may have difficulty with any of the following: finding the right container, keeping the lid on it, and putting it somewhere where it can no longer influence them. Often, clients will automatically recognize they are not yet ready to give up their painful or negative feelings when difficulty is encountered in the containerization process.

The wellness practitioner may wish to ask the client to verbalize the process by which healing was enhanced or may allow the client to complete the process without verbalizing unless he or she wishes to. The verbalization does not aid in the process for the client, but can give the practitioner clues about the client's ability to visualize and need for additional help.

A major asset of imagery as an intervention is that the client need not expose situations that may be anxiety-provoking or embarrassing, or discuss the process; this is a major advantage when using the approach in a group or when working with a client with whom a deep level of trust has not yet been established. Frequently showing the client that the practitioner can be of assistance without establishing an intimate relationship can build trust. Additionally, imagery interventions allow the practitioner to work with clients who are unable or unwilling to establish an open, working relationship. Clinical outcomes show that imagery works best in situations when the practitioner gives the broadest directions, allowing clients to develop their own images.

Affirmations

An *affirmation* is a positive thought that you consciously choose to immerse in your consciousness to produce a desired result (Ray, 1976, p. 14). The following guidelines are suggested for use of affirmations:

- Provide a relaxing, sharing atmosphere. Consider using a relaxation exercise as a prelude to the affirmation process.
- Obtain information from the client about health issues he/she is concerned about.
- Dialogue with the client to see whether the affirmation is best stated in the attitude, feeling, or action mode. If affirmations are stated too quickly in the action mode, clients may be unable to benefit from them; ask the client, "Are you ready to start thinking about changing or are you ready to use affirmations to take action to change?" Sometimes clients may be unsure themselves and *think* they want to change, but may find during the affirmation process that they are not yet ready to change and are really at the contemplation stage; affirmations are useful for either stage, but should be stated in the appropriate way, e.g., "It's getting easier and easier to smoke 10 cigarettes a day" (behavior mode) vs. "It's getting
- Assist the client to state the affirmation in his/her own words. Actively listen to the client until it is clear how an affirmation might be stated, but then keep checking with the client until it suits him or her. ("It sounds as if an affirmation for you might be, 'It's getting easier and easier to let go of my angry feelings toward Cora.' How does that sound to you?") Affirmations are best stated in the becoming mode, e.g., "It's getting easier and easier to . . ." or "I'm becoming more comfortable with the idea of . . .".
- Once an affirmation has been agreed upon, ask the client to write or say the affirmation 10 to 20 times each day while listening to one's inner, gut response to hearing it said or writing it. (Practice this process with the client

at least once together. Ask the client to say the affirmation then ask, "What is your reaction to hearing yourself say that?" Ask the client to say the affirmation again, and ask, "How does it sound this time?" Continue working with the client this way; clients usually begin by responding with inner responses such as, "I'll never be able to do it"; with repetition, their inner responses begin to move toward, "maybe I can do it.")

- Clients can be advised to carry their chosen affirmation with them on a 3×5 card and place it in a briefcase, purse, or car dashboard where it will be read throughout the day. Underscore how hearing oneself on tape, viewing oneself saying the affirmation, or writing and reading it back provides two kinds of feedback and thus is more powerful than simply saying the affirmation to oneself. Stress the importance of trying all methods of doing affirmations and choosing the best one for that individual client.
- Clients can record their affirmations and play them back or look in the mirror and say the affirmation until they see themselves saying it, maintaining good eye contact and having a relaxed expression.
- Clients can also practice with the nurse or with a supportive peer in the following way: Sitting across from one another, say the affirmation to your partner until you are comfortable doing so. Ask for feedback from your partner after each statement or your affirmation, e.g., "Did I squirm, fidget, or was I unclear or contradictory in what I said and how I looked?" Next, have the partner say the affirmation to the client using the second person, e.g., "Sarah, you're finding it easier and easier to . . ."
- Provide, or have the client provide, an ongoing method reinforcement for continuing the affirmation.
- Use affirmations to support other medical, nursing, or related therapies the client has chosen to participate in.
- Present affirmation as a new method that has proved useful for many clients with many different kinds of problems. Ask for the client's full participation in working with you to develop useful affirmations.
- Provide support if the client becomes frustrated, lacks skills, or expects too much, e.g., "This is difficult, but you *will* get it." "Keep trying, you're making progress." "Don't expect to change patterns you've taken years to develop overnight."

CASE STUDY: *Using affirmations*

Judy T., a wellness practitioner, asked John H., a client who was having difficulty following through with his exercise regime, if he wanted to try affirmations. He agreed and Judy T. proceeded to help John phrase an appropriate affirmation. At first it seemed he was ready to develop an affirmation to exercise; as they talked, it became clear he had not taken personal responsibility for exercise. They phrased the following affirmation, "I, John, am finding it easier and easier to accept the idea of exercising to get better." The first few times John repeated the affirmation, he seemed negative about accepting the idea; when he said it the fourth time, he smiled and said, "You know, maybe exercising would help!" John continued saying his affirmation and he carried the written form of it with him on a 3×5 card whereever he went; Judy observed him reading it several times during her shift. The following week, John said he had mastered the affirmation and was ready to develop an affirmation about exercising.

Neurolinguistic Programming

Neurolinguistic programming (NLP) is a useful way of establishing rapport with clients and assisting them to overcome parts of themselves that are resistive to the idea of wellness. NLP is a way of reframing information so it is more acceptable or helpful to the individual (Wight, 1995). *Reframing* is changing the frame from which events are perceived in order to change the meaning or the context. Reframing is a powerful communication tool that can assist the nurse to enhance wellness. An assumption of NLP is that no behavior is in and of itself useful. All behavior will be useful somewhere. Identifying *where* is context reframing.

Richard Bandler and John Grinder (1982), the originators of NLP, provide examples of reframing that have been adapted for use:

- A practitioner helps a father reframe a "stubborn" daughter to think of her as having a priceless gift that will protect her when others try to take advantage of her. (changing the context used to evaluate behavior)
- A practitioner reframes the dreaded event of the client passing out in a shopping mall to a paradoxical prescription of, "Now I know this is an important thing for you to do; it's something that can help you. I want you to go out every day to a different mall and pass out." (changing the meaning of the behavior to a controlled event)
- A client who conceives of himself as "devious" is assisted by the practitioner to rename the behavior as, "Your ability to be creatively constructive." (changing meaning of behavior)
- A student who dwells on how "greedy" for money she is is helped by the practitioner to be greedy about learning about wellness. (changing context for behavior)
- A client who complains there were too many wellness workshops scheduled at once was told by the practitioner, "I understand, but one of the nice things about it is it gives you extra practice in the decision-making process." (changing meaning of behavior)
- A client who complained wellness is too much work was told by the practitioner, "It must make you feel really good about yourself to realize you have so much perseverance." (changing meaning)
- A client who was angrily yelling and complaining was told, "I want to tell you that I know you are angry; you look angry and you sound angry. One of the important things a person can do is know that he feels the feelings he has and can express them directly." (changing meaning)
- A client angry with her son calls him "stupid"; the practitioner comments, "Some people use stupidity as a way to learn a tremendous amount. Some people use stupidity to get people to do things for them. That's pretty smart." (changing meaning)

In addition to reframing, the practitioner can learn to speak the client's language by observing and responding to client *representational systems*. People link experience to sensory input and tend to recall information based on their preferred representational system. Hover (1983) points out there are no practitioner client communication failures or resistant clients, only inflexibility in the practitioner. If the practitioner is willing to try something new there are limitless possibilities for meaningful practitioner–client interaction. Some ways to speak the client's language are:

1. *Listen to clients' word choices regarding sensory representation and use them too:*
   If clients say, "From my point of view . . .," or, "I can see . . .," use visual words like, "see," "observe," "view," or "focus" with the client.
   If clients use words such as "hear," "harmonize," or "sounds like . . .," use auditory language to match theirs.
   If clients use words such as "I'm in touch with . . .," "I feel . . .," or "I'm pressured," use kinesthetic words like "sense," "feel," "touch," "texture," or "pressure."

2. *Observe client eye and breathing movements, validate your observations, and then use them to establish rapport and understanding.*

- Clients who look up and to the left are often having a remembered (past) image. Check this out by saying, "I'm wondering if you're picturing something in your past."
- Clients who look up and to the right are often having a constructed (future) image. Check this out by asking, "I wonder if you're seeing something that could happen in your future."
- Clients who look down and to the left are often hearing a remembered voice. Check this out by saying, "I'm wondering if you're hearing someone's voice from the past."
- Clients who look to mid-right are often hearing a constructed auditory experience, such as making up a song. Check this out by saying, "I'm wondering if you're hearing how something might sound."
- Clients who look down and to the right are often reliving a kinesthetic, olfactory or gustatory experience. Check this out by saying, "I'm wondering if you're recalling a feeling experience."

Asking clients to describe a recent good experience or tell you what they do well and then ask them how they know they do it well will elicit additional information about their representational system.

When the practitioner observes and matches client verbal predicates (see, hear, feel, smell, taste) and nonverbal cues (breathing rate, voice tone, posture or gestures), rapport can be established rather quickly. Clients can also be taught to speak each other's language and gain enhanced rapport with family members, friends, coworkers, peers, etc.

Example

RUTH:	I resent you leaving all your dishes in the sink after you cook those disgusting vegetarian meals.
PRACTITIONER:	When you see that stuff, what does it remind you of?
RUTH:	I see the whole house a mess. It's overwhelming.
PRACTITIONER:	Robert, what do you feel overwhelmed about in this relationship?
ROBERT:	I worry about Ruth's smoking. I know I can't do anything to make her quit, but I think I should be able to.
PRACTITIONER:	So when Ruth sees the dishes in the sink she feels just as helpless and overwhelmed as you do, Robert, about Ruth's smoking.
RUTH:	I never knew you felt that way.
ROBERT:	Me either.

In NLP, *anchors* are sensory experiences that help the client organize experience. For example, if the client is very depressed and does not seem to have the energy to complete the agreed upon exercise program, the practitioner can help develop an anchor. The following steps can be used:

1. Assist the client to attain a relaxed state by using one of the structured relaxation exercises.
2. Ask the client to "Picture a time in your life when you had a lot of energy and enthusiasm. Signal me by raising your right index finger when you have it vividly in your mind's eye."
3. When the client signals, tap lightly on the top of his or her shoulder. This will anchor the experience and make it easily accessible in the future when those feelings need to be called forth. The client or nurse or a trusted other person can be taught to tap lightly on that spot to elicit the energy and enthusiasm needed.

The purpose of NLP is to assist clients to feel better about themselves, organize internal information in a more congruent fashion, and break out of the boundaries of their self-restricting behavior. As such, NLP is a creative addition to wellness practice.

The reader is referred to the following sources for additional information on NLP by Bandler and Grinder and published by Real People Press, Moab, Utah: *Frogs Into Princes, Trance-Formations, Reframing.*

INTEGRATIVE LEARNING EXPERIENCES

Beginning Level

1. Write in your journal about your experiences with the following:

A. comparing	C. rehearsing	E. judging
B. mind reading	D. filtering	F. dreaming

G. identifying   I. sparring   K. derailing

H. advising   J. being right   L. placating

2. Practice the following exercise with a peer:

   A. Ask your peer to talk with you for 3 minutes about an event that hap-
       pened recently that has personal significance.
   B. At the end of 3 minutes, make some notes about what you heard, no-
       ticed, and how you felt.
   C. Now, center yourself; when ready, ask your peer to talk with you for 3
       more minutes about the chosen event.
   D. Write down (and then discuss with your peer) any differences noted in
       you, her or him, or what was heard.

3. Practice centering until you have mastered it. Try it out in several practitioner–client situations and write in your journal about the results, including
   1A–1L.

4. Identify your level of differentiation in various practitioner–client situations
   and devise a plan for moving to a higher level of differentiation.

5. Identify triangles you engage in and develop a plan for taking the "I" position
   more frequently.

6. Write in your journal about what is important to you as a practitioner; set
   priorities and communicate the essence of what you've written with at least
   one other person.

7. Write in your journal about values your parents, teachers, peers, or significant others have taught you; examine each and choose freely those you totally
   agree with. Devise a plan for reducing the importance of values not freely
   chosen.

8. Consider all possible consequences of your value choices.

9. Devise a plan for trying out your value choice. Consider writing a self-con-
   tract to implement your value choices.

10. Evaluate what happened when you tried out your value choice. Note any in-
    consistencies between affirmed values and actions; make plans to reinforce
    actions that will support prized values.

11. Identify a situation that you think requires change. Write down all the pos-
    sible resistances to change in that situation. Devise a plan for reducing resis-
    tance to change.

12. Identify a client you are working with and draw up a behavioral contract. Try
    out the approach and write about your experience in your journal.

13. Identify a problem you wish to solve; use the steps in Table 2.7 to solve it.

14. Try out the problem-solving steps in Table 2.7 with a peer; one of you act as a
    practitioner, the other as a client. Discuss what happened and any learning
    that occurred. Identify how you might apply the procedure with clients.

15. Try out the problem-solving steps in Table 2.7 with a client who needs to solve
    a problem or make a decision. Write about the results in your journal.

16. Identify an upcoming situation that you feel apprehensive about. Use the steps in Table 2.8 to assist you to perform competently in the situation. Write about your experience in your journal.
17. Work with a peer who has an upcoming anxiety-provoking situation. Take the practitioner's role in replicating the situation in Table 2.8. Write in your journal about the experience.
18. Work with a real-life client who has an upcoming anxiety-provoking situation using the information in Table 2.8. Write in your journal about your findings.
19. Use the information in Table 2.9 to enhance healing in yourself.
20. Help a peer devise a healing image for an identified problem. Write in your journal about your findings.
21. Help a client devise a healing image for an identified problem. Write in your journal about your findings.
22. Use the information in Table 2.10 and information on NLP to decrease the influence of negative feelings in your life. Write in your journal about the experience.
23. Take the practitioner's role with a peer and use the information in Table 2.10 to assist him or her to decrease the influence of negative feelings. Write in your journal about the experience.
24. Use the information in Table 2.10 to assist a client to decrease the influence of negative feelings. Write in your journal about your findings.
25. Identify a situation in your life that could be helped by using affirmations. Devise an affirmation and write about the results in your journal.
26. Work with a peer to help him or her develop a useful affirmation and practice it until it has become integrated with the person (as evidenced by comments such as "I can . . ." or "It is getting easier. . ." or "I believe it").
27. Work with a client using affirmations. Describe the experience in your journal including any learning that occurred, obstacles and how you overcame them or could overcome them, and successes.

Advanced Level

1. Complete 1–27 above if not already completed.
2. Teach a client how to center.
3 Teach a client how to identify triangles that may produce difficulty.
4. Teach a client the value clarification process.
5. Teach another practitioner or student practitioner the following procedures:
   A. behavioral contracting
   B. imagery for problem solving
   C. imagery for performing competently
   D. imagery for healing
   E. imagery for decreasing the influence of negative feelings
   F. affirmation

6. Devise research questions and carry out the research for the following:
   A. relationship of centering to active listening
   B. relationship of level of differentiation to client healing
   C. relationship of value clarification to willingness to change
   D. relationship of behavioral contracting to change
   E. relationship of imagery problem solving to decision making
   F. relationship of Movie of the Mind procedure to future competence
   G. relationship of healing images to healing
   H. relationship of affirmation to lifestyle changes

REFERENCES

Bandler, R., and Grinder, J. (1982). *Reframing*. Moab, UT: Real People Press, pp. 1–37.

Bowen, M. (1978). *Family Theory in Clinical Practice*. New York: Jason Aronson.

Boyd, B.C. (1993). Children's self-responsibility health scale. *Dissertation Abstracts International,* 55-02B.

Brown, N. et al. (1983). The relationship among health beliefs, health values, and health promotion activity. *Western Journal of Nursing Research,* 5(2): 155–163.

Collar, C.F. (1977). The effective personal integration model and its impact on locus of control. Unpublished doctoral dissertation, Denton, TX: North Texas State University.

Davis, M., Eshelman, E., and McKay, M. (1995). *The Relaxation and Stress Reduction Workbook.* (4th ed.). Oakland, CA: New Harbinger.

Gilbert, R.M. (1992). *Extraordinary Relationships—A New Way of Thinking About Human Interactions.* Minneapolis: Chronimed Publishing.

Hover, D. (1983). Enhancing family communication using neuro-linguistic programming. In *Family Health: A Theoretical Approach to Nursing Care,* Ed. by I. Clements and F. Roberts. New York: Wiley, pp. 83–91.

Kern, D., and Stejskal, J. (1983). Relaxation in the classroom: reduce your students' anxiety while improving their learning and recall. *Journal of Holistic Nursing,* 1(1): 17–20.

Kirschenbaum, H., and Simon, S. (1974). Values and the future movement in education. In *Learning for Tomorrow: The Role of the Future in Education,* Ed. by A. Toffler. New York: Vintage Books, pp. 257–271.

Kirschenbaum, H. (1976). Clarifying values clarification: Some theoretical issues and a review of research. *Group and Organization Studies,* 1(1):99-115.

Krieger, D. (1993). *Accepting Your Power To Heal—The Personal Practice of Therapeutic Touch.* Santa Fe: Bear & Company.

McKay, M., Davis, M., and Fanning, P. (1995). *Messages, the Communication Book.* 2nd ed. Oakland: New Harbinger.

Ornstein, R. (1972). *The Psychology of Consciousness.* San Francisco: W.H. Freeman and Co., p. 52.

Pender, N. (1987). *Health Promotion in Nursing Practice.* 2nd ed. Norwalk, CT: Appleton-Century-Crofts.

Peplau, H.E. (1952). *Interpersonal Relations in Nursing.* New York: G.P. Putnam, pp. 119–157.

Raths, L., Harmin, M., and Simon, S.B. (1966). *Values and Teaching.* Columbus, OH: Charles E. Merrill Books.

Ray, S. (1976). *I Deserve Love.* Millbrae, CA: Les Femmes.

Rotter, J. (1966). Generalized expectations for internal vs. external control of reinforcement. *Psychological Monographs,* 80(1):1–28

Samaroff, A.J. (1980). Issues in early reproductive and care-taking risk: Review and current status. In *Psychosocial Risks in Infant Environment Transactions,* Ed. by P.B. Savin et al. New York: Brunner/Mazel, pp. 343–359.

Samuels, M., and Samuels, N. (1975). *Seeing with the Mind's Eye.* New York: Random House.

Scalese, V. (1978). *Effects of electromyographic feedback training on the perception of locus of control and accuracy of person perception.* Unpublished doctoral dissertation, Kalamazoo, MI: Western Michigan University.

Selye, H. (1956). *The Stress of Life.* New York: McGraw-Hill.

Selye, H. (1974). *Stress Without Distress.* Philadelphia and New York: J.P. Lippincott.

Sheehy, G. (1974). *Passages: Predictable Crises of Adult Life.* New York: E.P. Dutton, p. 251.

Simmons, L. W. (1950). The relation between decline of anxiety reducing and anxiety resolving factors in a deteriorating culture and its relevance to bodily disease. *Proceedings of the Association of Research Neurological and Mental Disease,* 29:127.

Wagner, E. et al. (1982). An assessment of health hazard/health risk appraisal. *American Journal of Public Health,* 72(4):347–352.

Wight, P.S. (1995). Strategies in times of conflict. *Advance for Nurse Practitioners,*

3

POSITIVE RELATIONSHIP BUILDING

This chapter explores two important aspects of relationship building:

- Empathy
- Assertiveness

Humans are social beings who require interaction with one another to grow. Two important skills for wellness practitioners and clients are empathy and assertiveness: one allows understanding of others, and the other allows individuals to stand up for their own thoughts, feelings, and desires. At the beginning level, the practitioner struggles to be empathic and assertive; at the advanced level, the practitioner is ready to begin modeling and teaching clients these skills. The Integrative Learning Experiences at the end of this chapter, Case Studies, and Clinical Examples mirror this differentiation of beginning and advanced skills. The practitioner models and teaches clients to use these critical skills for positive relationship building.

EMPATHY

Empathy is the ability to accurately perceive the feelings and meanings of others. When working with others, empathy forms the basis for a helping relationship. Empathy is the opposite of telling others, "I know what your health problems are" or "I know why you're having a hard time attaining wellness." When being empathic, the practitioner does not lose separateness from others and take on their feelings or views (sympathy), but does try to understand what their feelings and views are. Empathy can be rated from low to high (Carkhuff, 1969; McKay, Davis, & Fanning, 1995).

Assessing Empathy

Table 3.1 gives examples of different levels of empathy and the kinds of comments the nurse may make to convey these different levels of empathy.

Table 3.1 Levels of Empathy

Low Empathy:	The other's feelings are ignored or their full meaning is not grasped.
Example 1:	

PRACTITIONER:	You should exercise more.
CLIENT:	Why? I'm as healthy as you are.
PRACTITIONER:	You'll be sorry when you're older!
CLIENT:	I can't see running around getting a heart attack.
PRACTITIONER:	Well, if you're not going to exercise, let's talk about something else.

Example 2:

CLIENT:	I'd like more information on nutrition.
PRACTITIONER:	You'd like more information so you can lose weight? (*assumption*)
CLIENT:	Yes, but I wonder why I get tired and my skin feels crawly after I eat certain foods. It kept me up all night—I was at my wits' end and . . .
PRACTITIONER:	(interrupting) As I told you before, this book will help you with that small matter (*plays down client's perception of the importance of his feelings*)

Beginning Empathy:	The practitioner conveys an accurate awareness of the conspicuous current feelings and their meaning to the client.
Example:	

CLIENT:	I've noticed I feel very tired and groggy lately, and I get depressed a lot.
PRACTITIONER:	What's your reaction to this? (*gets more information*)
CLIENT:	Well, I wonder if I should go get a prescription from my doctor for an antidepressant.
PRACTITIONER:	You're wondering if medicine will help? (*reflects client's ideas*)
CLIENT:	Yes, but I tried them once before and they didn't help. Maybe there's something wrong with my attitude or the way I eat. I've been dieting to lose weight so I cut out bread and cereal and live pretty much on cottage cheese. Yesterday, I really got scared. I got very dizzy and saw black spots before my eyes.
PRACTITIONER:	You were really scared yesterday when you got dizzy. (*reflects feeling verbally conveyed by client*)
CLIENT:	Yes, I suppose I better plan a better reducing diet. Maybe I can find one that allows me to feel good while I lose weight.
PRACTITIONER:	You want to find a reducing diet that allows you to feel good. I think I can help you with that.

Table 3.1 (*continued*)

High Empathy:	The nurse communicates accurately and confidently the current conspicuous and deeper feeling of the client.
Example:	
CLIENT:	You're so high and mighty, always telling us what to eat and what to do! (*angrily*)
PRACTITIONER:	You really feel angry when I tell you what to do. (*reflects feeling tone of client through own tone of voice*)
CLIENT:	Yes! Since I was little someone has always been telling me what to do! I can take responsibility for myself—that's why I'm in this class.
PRACTITIONER:	You're feeling angry because you want to take more responsibility for yourself.
CLIENT:	Yes, you got it.

When the wellness practitioner *assumes* the client's meaning, low empathy occurs. Judging others' current feelings based on past experiences or the expectation of how others always act, feel, or think is invalid in an empathic relationship. Empathy allows the wellness practitioner to understand another's feelings while still maintaining differentiation of self. For example, the practitioner can be empathic with a crying client without resorting to sympathetic tears and helplessness. Empathy provides a balance between emotional acceptance and intellectual objectivity.

Empathy provides an emotional mirror for the reflection of others' feelings. Empathic people learn to use the words and language of those they care about and reflect feelings and ideas back (McKay, Davis, & Fanning, 1995) to check whether this is how the client feels. Advice is not given unless it has been asked for, and then only if there has been an attempt to solve the problem together. Behavior is not labeled as "childish" or "crazy." Instead, the tone of voice or mood conveyed by the client is used. Reflection does not take on the tone, "Here is what you are saying"; it is made in a tentative manner, such as, "It sounds as if you're really angry," unless there is no doubt about the matter.

Sometimes it is difficult to understand the other's point of view. Using a relaxation and imagery exercise may help in these cases. Find a quiet spot and focus on relaxing. Picturing yourself as the client may provide help in learning how clients view situations; to do this effectively, it is necessary to be totally immersed in the thoughts, feelings, and actions of clients—to walk in their shoes, so to speak.

Empathy requires the ability to listen actively and to reflect the essence of the client's communication. Although listening seems simple and passive, it is difficult to stop trying to solve other people's problems for them, telling them what you would do under similar circumstances, or pooh-poohing the problem by discounting its importance ("What are you worrying about, look at Mr. Jones over there."). In most conversations, the person who is not speaking is often not listening very carefully to what is being said, but instead is getting ready to interrupt, preach, moralize, boast, discount what the other has just said, convince, reassure, or give advice. Many conversations sound like double monologues, with both wanting to be listened to, but neither listening to the other person.

When the practitioner is an active listener, there is a conscious desire to listen attentively without preconceived notions, trying to understand not only the words but also the emotions and body movement of what the other person is communicating. Active listening is necessary to produce reflective communication. Reflective communication helps the client clarify what is really being experienced. To be effective, reflective communication combines a statement of the words and emotional content just conveyed by the other person. Although it sounds simple, it is not easy to do without sounding like a parrot.

Reflective communication acknowledges that clients may often ask for advice but seldom take it, or if they do, there is no permanent change or growth unless they have come to alter their way of thinking by increasing their ability to see their options. Reflective communication provides a sounding board against which clients learn to be more independent while experiencing a sense of caring, closeness, and help in clarifying their thoughts and feelings, expanding their consciousness and wholeness as people, and working out their own solutions.

Helping Clients Develop Empathy

There are a number of measures to help clients develop empathy, including:

1. Paraphasing. Ask clients to "say back to me what you heard me say." The paraphrased information can then be discussed in terms of what was not heard or recalled. Clients can tape record the initial words and the paraphrase and compare them for accuracy. Once clients understand that they are not listening actively, they may be ready to work on their empathy skills.

2. Providing reading material on empathy and its use. After clients have read the material, the practitioner and client can discuss what was read and identify examples of empathy (or its lack) in further conversations.

3. Analyzing practitioner empathy. (This is a more difficult skill and requires a willingness to take criticism.) The client can be asked to tell the practitioner whenever client meaning is overlooked or not acknowledged. A signal system can be used to encourage client participation. For example, the practitioner can provide a card the client can hold up whenever the nurse misses the client's meaning, overlooks a feeling, changes the subject, etc. Once the practitioner demonstrates willingness to examine self-empathy, the client will probably be more willing to do so also.

ASSERTIVENESS

Assertiveness is the ability to stand up for thoughts, feelings, or desires. It means being able to define and stand up for reasonable rights, while being respectful of others' rights, setting goals for wellness, acting on these goals by following through consistently, and taking responsibility for the consequences of actions.

"I" -Messages vs. "You"-Messages

Being assertive requires taking a risk by clearly stating what is expected from others and what they can expect from the nurse. "I" messages are used, e.g., "I would like to . . .," "I suggest we settle it by . . .," "I feel angry when I'm called lazy."

Contrarily, aggressiveness has an element of control or manipulation. "You"-messages, such as "Why didn't you . . .?," "You should have. . .," "I think you are crazy" prevail when aggressiveness occurs. A common pattern that develops when assertiveness is missing is the avoidance of a confrontation or wellness issue, build-up of resentment, blow-up or angry outburst, feelings of guilt and recrimination, and a return to avoidance. Thus, aggressiveness/avoidance are intimately connected, and assertive behavior is in a different realm in which issues are addressed, thoughts and feelings are expressed when they occur, and action is taken to enhance wellness.

Sometimes "You"- aggressive messages masquerade as assertive ones, e.g., "I think *you're* wrong!," "I feel *you* ought to change," "I want *you* to do as I say." In these messages, the speaker tries to control the listener by judging behavior, or attempting to force change or action; *these messages are aggressive and avoid the responsibility each person has for his or her behavior* (Clark, 1994).

Some "We" -messages can also be assertive, especially if they imply collaboration, such as "We can meet and work this out." (Undifferentiated messages, such as, "Let's do our exercises," when only the client is exercising are *not* assertive *or* collaborative.)

"You"-blaming messages are apt to put others on the defensive; for this reason alone they ought to be deleted. In addition, they absolve the speaker of his or her responsibility in the issue at hand. Examples of this type of aggressive statement are: "Why didn't you take care of that?," "Why can't you do it right?," "I think this is your fault," "Why are you going around upsetting everyone?"

Some assertive messages do use the word *you*, but there is neither blame nor coercion attached to assertive "you" -messages. ("Would you like to tell me your point of view?," "I want to thank you," "I thought I heard you say. . . .)"

Assertiveness is a useful practitioners' skill for several reasons: practitioners can role model for clients and assist them to be more assertive; assertive communication also lets both parties know where they stand and frees energy to deal with the situation as it really is instead of being used to decipher what the other person *really* means.

Assertiveness and Stress

Assertiveness is also useful as a stress reduction measure. People who are unable to express their thoughts and feelings directly or who feel unappreciated or exploited often report having psychosomatic complaints such as headaches or stomach problems. Assertive people often report increased feelings of self-confidence, reduced anxiety, decreased bodily complaints, and improved communication and response from others. There are a number of strategies to use to become more assertive.

Controlling Anxiety, Fear, and Anger with Relaxation Procedures

One way to reduce anxiety and fear about being assertive is to regularly practice relaxation exercises (see Chapter 2). Assertiveness requires presenting oneself in a confident, self-assured manner. When body musculature is tense and constricted, a self-confident presentation is difficult. A relaxed body increases the probability that others will be approached in a direct, open manner.

Techniques for Enhancing Assertiveness

Wellness practitioners may not be aware of how they come across to others. There are a number of strategies that can be used to provide feedback about presentation of self. Mirror practice gives feedback about facial expression, posture, and whether words fit with gestures and body position. It can also be helpful in rehearsing assertive statements prior to trying them with the real-life person. This kind of rehearsal can build confidence so that assertiveness in the real-life situation is more likely.

Audio- and videotape recorders also provide excellent practice in assertion. Audiotape provides clues about whether there are sufficient pauses, whether tone of voice is assertive, whether statements are made too quickly, if words are said with sufficient firmness and authority, and whether the issue is stated clearly and adhered to. Tape recorders are also useful for recording (and providing instant replay about) ability to limit interruptions, express feelings appropriately, take a stand on an issue, disagree, admit a mistake, reward or thank another person, give positive criticism, say no, express distress about the way a relationship is moving, and ask for collaboration. Some statements to record on a tape recorder and evaluate for effectiveness are:

- I cannot talk to you now. I'll talk to you at 1 o'clock.
- I feel really angry about this!
- I have made up my mind on this.
- I see your point, but I disagree.
- I *did* make an error.
- Let's sit down and work this out together.

- No, I will *not* reconsider this; this item is not negotiable.
- I'm upset about our relationship and I'd like to talk with you about it.
- I appreciate your help.
- We agreed your report would be on my desk yesterday. What happened?

Another use of audiotape is to record relaxing or reward messages that can be played back at a later time. Relaxation exercises can be found in Chapter 2; some rewarding messages to consider recording are:

- You are working toward wellness in a useful, helpful way. Congratulations on your effort. Keep up the good work.
- Congratulations on not smoking. Give yourself a hug or find someone to hug. Be proud of yourself. Allow yourself to feel good about your accomplishment.
- Congratulations on meeting your fitness goal. Treat yourself to a reward and be sure to allow yourself to feel good about your accomplishment!

Videotape feedback adds the extra information of eye contact, body posture and positioning, gestures, facial expressions, verbal responses that are too quick or hesitant, conciseness of statements, and confidence of presentation. Probably the best use of videotape is to record upcoming or past situations. Scripts can be written for two people and then recorded and evaluated according to each of the information components. Table 3.2 provides a completed guide for assessing an assertive presentation of self that has been videotaped. (The "Goals for Next Role Play" can be used if working with a partner.)

Another way to use videotape is for *role playing*. In this approach, one person tells the other about an upcoming or past situation. (It is best to choose two-person situations, avoiding those with a long history of emotional overlay; strive for choices that are likely to end in a successful role play, not in frustration because deep-seated issues are involved.) The first person gives the other a description of what is to be said, which role each person will take, how the other should act to approximate the real-life situation, and how the interchange will end and begin. A 3-to-5-minute script is sufficient when extraneous discussions are omitted and the issue is adhered to. The other role player needs to be coached to be helpful and should be told that making it easy for the other person is *not* helpful. Being as aggressive or avoiding as the real life person will provide much better practice and will prepare the other person in a better way. Some directions that might be given are: "Be sure to try to make me feel guilty about saying no," or "Every time I try to stick to the issue, you change the subject," or "Use a really angry tone of voice, but pretend you're not angry."

Using a script and trying it out will help the practitioner identify areas that require further practice or more information. For example, if asking for a raise or a decision of some type, it is necessary to "do one's homework," coming up with alternate solutions for problems and providing adequate information for the other person to support a point of view. Merely asserting without having

Table 3.2 Assertiveness Assessments

Nonverbal Presentation of Self	Examples/Comments
Frequent and direct eye contact	"I kept looking at the ceiling when talking. I crossed my arms and looked angry when talking about being pleased."
Speaking loudly enough and firmly enough	
Open, direct body communication	
Gestures match words said	

Verbal Presentation of Self

"I let her lead me away from my goal and we started talking about her sore leg instead of my raise. I used the following blaming messages:

I think you should give me a raise.
I feel you overlooked me."

Remain on the point of discussion without changing topics

Use "I" messages, e.g., "I can't help you now," "I feel angry when . . .," I'd like to talk with you about . . .," I don't like to be shouted at . . .," "I realize you're concerned, but please don't make decisions for me," "I did make a mistake." "Thank you." "I'd like to do a joint evaluation with you." "I think we can work this out."

Refrain from using "You-blaming" messages, e.g., "You didn't. . .," "You should have. . .," "It's your fault that. . .," "You aren't doing that right."

Goal(s) for Next Role Play
1. Maintain eye contact
2. Uncross my arms
3. Tell my partner I feel angry instead of giving an inconsistent message
4. Get feedback from partner

---

appropriate data to support a stand is less likely to end in a positive resolution. All of the procedures discussed as applicable for the practitioner are also appropriate when assisting clients to be more assertive.

What Prevents Wellness Practitioners From Being Assertive

Practitioners may fear being assertive because they fear not being liked, being rejected, being retaliated against, etc. It is important to be aware of which of these fears (or others) may be preventing assertiveness and take action to dispel them (see Chapter 5 for additional stress reduction measures to use to dispel irrational beliefs).

The same fears seem to operate in both sexes; both can be fearful of rejection and tend to bend over backwards to please. When asked what prevents them from being assertive, they often say, "I don't want to hurt their feelings." Male practitioners are less concerned with hurting others' feelings and are more apt to confess, "I don't want them to get the better of me, so I end up being aggressive." They also report that they feel pressured by females to "be strong and never show our feelings."

These reactions can be traced back to early family experiences in which girls are raised to be nice, not fight, not show anger, and (often) are judged on how they look or socialize, not on their competence in the task. As a result, many girls grow up to be women who underestimate their achievements, attribute their success to luck, and doubt their ability even when highly competent. Men assume they are competent and readily set out to prove it (Rivers, Barnett, & Baruch, 1979, pp. 106–107).

Early school experiences also influence the assertiveness of men and women. Dweck (1975) found that teachers expect boys to be rowdy and inattentive about schoolwork, but girls are expected to be well-behaved, dutiful, and exerting their best effort. When boys fail, they are told to try harder (a motivation problem), but girls are just told they have done something incorrectly (may be interpreted as a lack of ability).

Assertiveness appears to be situational. Some practitioners may feel more comfortable being assertive at work, while others feel more comfortable being assertive at home. Perhaps one of the few generalizations that can be made is that everyone has some assertiveness issue to deal with; no one is totally unassertive nor totally assertive. There is a continuum.

CASE STUDY: *Assertiveness With Peers*

> Bob Smith was working to obtain his degree. When assertiveness was discussed in a seminar, he shared the following comment: "Why is it that everyone expects you to be strong and handle every situation?" As the discussion group helped Bob explore the issue further, it became clear that Bob's peers gave him verbal and nonverbal messages to be strong and not show any of the unsureness he felt about dealing with some nursing situations. It was suggested that Bob set up a time to talk with his female counterparts about how he felt and to share how difficult it was to always be the one who was expected to be strong and competent. The next week in class, Bob shared how he had met with his female peers and seemed surprised that they were surprised about how he felt; they decided to ask each time a stressful situation occurred how each one felt about taking responsibility in that situation. Bob reported feeling greatly relieved that "Things are now out in the open."

Assertive Strategies for Dealing with Criticism

There are three strategies for assertively responding to criticism: acknowledgment, clouding, and probing (McKay, Davis, & Fanning, 1995, pp. 124–128). Constructive criticism can lead to improvement; feedback from others can help you learn not to repeat the error. Extract the growth-promoting aspects of criticisms from others and use them to grow. Dispel irrational beliefs that criticism means failure or wrongness. Sometimes criticism is accurate, but not constructive.

Acknowledging. Whenever criticism is received, an assertive response includes acknowledging the critic's comment. Some examples are: (1) "You're right, I am half an hour late for work," (2) "You're right, I did misspell a lot of words," (3) "Yes, I am late in handing in this report."

Excuses and apologies are not part of an assertive response. Consider them automatic leftovers from childhood when excuses and apologies were demanded; parents and teachers expected an explanation and so one was compiled. As adults, individuals have the right to choose whether to give an explanation or not. Often, it is not advantageous to give an explanation because it provides further ammunition for the other person and does not present a picture of competence. Consider the two situations below; the first presents the wellness practitioner as blame-fixing, childlike, and incompetent; the second presents the practitioner as assertive and adult. The major difference between the two situations is that the practitioner gives an excuse in the first instance and does not acknowledge error; in the second instance, the practitioner acknowledges error and does not give an excuse.

Situation 1: Non-Acknowledging

SUPERVISOR:	You're late again! How long do you think I'm going to tolerate this?!
PRACTITIONER:	Oh, I'm so sorry, please forgive me, the car broke down again and my husband wouldn't give me a lift!
SUPERVISOR:	You've always got an excuse, but this time I'm not buying it. I'm writing you up and docking you for 15 minutes.

Situation 2: Acknowledging

SUPERVISOR:	You're late again! How long do you think I'm going to tolerate this?!
PRACTITIONER:	You're right, I am 15 minutes late.
SUPERVISOR:	I'm docking you for the 15 minutes.

Clouding. Clouding is a useful technique when nonconstructive, manipulative criticism that is disagreed with is received (McKay, Davis, & Fanning, 1995, p. 125). It allows practitioners to stand their ground while continuing to communicate with the other person. Clouding requires careful listening to what is being said to find something that can honestly be agreed with, either in part, in probability, or in principle. The idea is to agree with the part of the person's statement that makes some sense, but not agree to change.

Situation 1: Agreeing in Part

SUPERVISOR:	You always have an excuse for not working overtime. What's the matter with you anyway?
SUPERVISEE:	Yes, I do have many family responsibilities.
SUPERVISOR:	You don't seem to care for the patients here at all.
SUPERVISEE:	You're right; I guess it seems that way.

Situation 2: Agreeing in Probability

PHYSICIAN: Putting on a little weight, aren't you, sweetie?
NURSE: It may be that I've gained a few pounds.
PHYSICIAN: Time to put you on a reducing diet.
NURSE: You may be right that it is time.

Situation 3: Agreeing in Principle

TEACHER: If you don't study more than you do, you're going to fail.
STUDENT: You're right; if I don't study, I will fail.

Probing. Criticism is often used by others to avoid important feelings or wishes. Assertive probing assists in determining whether criticism is constructive or manipulative, and clarifies unclear comments. The first step in assertive probing is to listen carefully and isolate the part of the criticism that seems most bothersome to the critic. The next step is to ask the critic, "What is it that bothers you about . . . ?"

Situation 1: Assertive Probing

SUPERVISOR: You're not doing a very good job here. Your work is not up to par.
PRACTITIONER: What is it about my work that bothers you?
SUPERVISOR: Well, everyone else is working overtime, but you waltz out of here two out of three nights.
PRACTITIONER: What is it about my leaving on time when other people work overtime?
SUPERVISOR: I don't like working overtime either, but the work has to be done. It's not right that you just work by the clock.
PRACTITIONER: What is it that bothers you when I work by the clock?
SUPERVISOR: When you leave, someone else has to finish your work. I want you to make sure your work is completed before you leave.
PRACTITIONER: I see. Thanks for explaining the situation to me.

Additional Assertive Strategies

Broken Record. This approach is useful when others do not seem to hear or accept what is being said, or when an explanation would provide the other person with an opportunity to continue a pointless discussion. It is especially useful for saying no to others' requests.

The first step in broken record is to clarify exactly what the limits of what will be done are. The second step is to formulate a short, specific statement about what is wanted; avoid giving excuses or explanations since they give the other person ammunition to undermine the original statement. The third step is to use consistent body language that supports the statement, including main-

taining eye contact, standing or sitting erect, and keeping hands and arms qui
etly at the side of the body. The fourth step is to calmly and firmly repeat the
chosen statement as many times as necessary until the other person realizes
there is no negotiation possible. The first few times a statement is said, the
other person may give an excuse or attempt to derive a different answer. The
fifth step is an optional one and includes briefly acknowledging the other's
ideas, feelings, or wishes before returning to the broken record statement, e.g.,
"I hear you saying you're upset, but I don't want to work any more overtime."

Situation 1: Broken Record

PERSON 1:	I just got an opportunity to fly to Aspen to ski. Won't you help me out and switch vacation schedules with me?
PERSON 2:	How great for you. *No, I don't want to switch schedules.*
PERSON 1:	You mean you're not going to help me? What kind of a friend are you?
PERSON 2:	I understand that you're disappointed, but *I don't want to switch schedules.*
PERSON 1:	But I have to go to Aspen and you're the only one who can help me.
PERSON 2:	*No, I don't want to switch schedules.*
PERSON 1:	Boy, you're really hard hearted. What happened to you, you used to be so nice, now suddenly, Wanda the Witch.
PERSON 2:	*No, I don't want to switch schedules.*
PERSON 1:	Boy, you're not going to give on this, are you?
PERSON 2:	No.

Contents-to-Process Shift. When the focus or point of the conversation drifts
away from the original topic, the content-to-process shift can be used to shift
from the subject being discussed (the content) to what is occurring between
the two speakers (the process), e.g., "We're off the point now, let's get back to
what we agreed to discuss."

Content-to-process shift can involve self-disclosure of current thoughts or
feelings, e.g., "I'm feeling uncomfortable discussing this now, and I notice
we're both tense." This approach is especially useful when voices are raised
and anger is present: "We seem to be getting into a battle about this." The trick
is to comment neutrally about what is observed so an attack will not be experienced by the other person.

Momentary Delay. In many social situations there is a compelling aspect
to situations. There is often the implied command from the other person that a
question must be answered right away. Rather than being swayed by the emotion of the moment, the wellness practitioner can take a deep breath and
momentary (or longer) delay. This procedure allows for further understanding
and analysis of the pros and cons of each available response.

Situation 1: Momentary Delay

SUPERVISOR: I'd like you to read the riot act to the aides; they aren't doing their work. You have to do something right now!

PRACTITIONER: (takes a deep breath) I'll need more information before I can act.

Situation 2: Momentary Delay

SUPERVISEE: I think I deserve a raise; here is a summary of the things I have brought to this job and the outcomes I have achieved.

SUPERVISOR: There may be something in what you have to say; let me think about this for a few minutes.

Time Out. When the conversation reaches an impasse, but the discussion is an important one, the conversation can be delayed to a later time; time out is only assertive if a specific time in the near future is set to continue the discussion.

Situation 1: Time Out

TEENAGER: I think you're blaming me unfairly.

PARENT: We've been talking about this quite a while now and I don't think we're getting anywhere. Let's sleep on it and I'll see you at 9:00 a.m. tomorrow.

Joining and Circling the Attacker. This approach is derived from the martial art of Aiki, in which the attacked person accepts the attack and turns with it, letting the attacker pass in the direction he or she has chosen. According to Dobson and Miller (1978):

> One of the best ways to survive . . . is to . . . flow with them. Harmonize . . . Be the water not the rock . . . The water has direction and flexibility. Eon by eon the rock is worn down, until half-way through eternity it has become a pebble. If the rock would turn with the force of the water, still retaining its place in the stream bed, the rock would lose nothing; the water would continue past. (pp. 87–88)

As in the martial art, there is a pause the attacker takes just before a change in direction. That brief moment is when the attacker loses balance; it is at that precise moment that the defender takes charge and helps the attacker to a new, firmer, less aggressive balance.

> Most attackers are spoiling for a fight. They are overextended, and they need the victim to fight back and preserve their tenuous balance. So if you yell at a yeller, you help him stay upright. (Dobson & Miller, 1978, p. 102)

The focus of energy is on the resolution of conflict and the restoration of harmony, and problem-solving. In each attacking or conflict situation, there are six alternative ways to respond:

1. *Do nothing.* This is an appropriate response when time is needed, when more information is needed to find out what is behind the attack, when the attacked person does not want to dignify the attack by reacting (it is not necessary to answer charges unless the practitioner chooses to do so), or when the attack makes no sense. Doing nothing must be a conscious choice, not a response to fear, in order to be an assertive response.

2. *Use diversion, deflection, or humor.* This is an appropriate response to deflect or redirect an attack. "Most attacks . . . come at you along a fairly straight line. By employing . . . surprise you can break that line and cause the attack to misfire" (Dobson & Miller, 1978, p. 73). Changing the subject ("I see you're wearing a new suit") or absurd explanations can be used to create a diversion or deflection.

Situation 1: Using Deflection/Humor

A: You forgot to get that report in! What do you think you're doing?!
B: You're right; I'm sorry I didn't follow through on our agreement.
A: That's no excuse!
B: I would have finished it, but I was attacked by Martians from outer space.
A: That's absurd!
B: I know. So is continuing to rage at someone after he's apologized.

3. *Join with the attackers,* agree with their right to feel as they do. (This is Aiki, confluence, flowing-with; being the water, not the rock.)

Alternate Situation 1: Joining the Attacker

SUPERVISOR:	What have you done? You're the worst practitioner I've ever seen!!
SUPERVISEE:	I don't blame you.
SUPERVISOR:	What do you mean, I don't blame you?
SUPERVISEE:	It's not up to me to blame anybody for feeling the way they do. You're not happy, and I can't quibble with that.
SUPERVISOR:	(puzzled) But you think your work is up to par?
SUPERVISEE:	It can't be if you're not happy with it. My job is to work with you.
SUPERVISOR:	(confused) I don't understand.
SUPERVISEE:	If you don't think I should be fired outright, let's see if we can't work together on this thing and make it mutually acceptable. What are some of your complaints?

(The supervisee's use of surprise combined with joining the attack led to the supervisor losing his balance. The practitioner has joined the supervisor and is helping him; the practitioner does not take the attack personally, but objectifies the conflict; this leads to confusion. The practitioner then takes the lead and helps the supervisor to deal with the conflict as an adult instead of a child.)

4. *Withdrawal* is an appropriate choice when all else fails and an escape route is open or when the time and place for discussion is wrong. To use withdrawal well, it must be completed clearly and with a single intention. Being unclear about the right to leave the scene can result in confusion. It is important to withdraw with certainty, knowing that it is each person's right to stay out of destructive involvements.

5. *Parley* is most effective when involved in a no-win situation in which the other person has defined the encounter as a contest; in this case, the nurse can remain centered and turn the conflict around, offering a reasonable way out for both parties. Some parleying comments are:

"Shall we see if we can work out a compromise?"
"Let's see if we can't iron out the problem."
"Maybe we can figure out a way to solve both our problems by working together."

6. *Fighting back* is the response of choice when there is no other option, it is a question of life or death, or it is a question of serious priority. Fighting back could include expressing anger directly or standing up to an insult.

Situation 1: Fighting Back

SUPERVISOR:	(who has just cornered the practitioner in front of several other employees) Listen, kid, my time is too valuable to spend chasing all over the place to find that record just because you're so inefficient you can't get the simplest things through your pinhead! And another thing, where is that new book I ordered?
PRACTITIONER:	I won't stand here and be insulted. I resent being blamed for someone else's room assigning. We can argue or try to solve the problem together.
SUPERVISOR:	I don't have to take this from you! I can have you fired!
PRACTITIONER:	If you want to stop this, find the record and I'll find out about the book. (Exiting)

This response focuses the supervisor on the problem and its solution, yet allows the practitioner to stand up for her rights, which she has already decided are a high priority for her with this supervisor who has constantly humiliated her in public. If the practitioner loses her job (an unlikely but possible resolution), she has already decided she has no intention of continuing to work under these conditions. Most likely the job will not be lost and conditions could improve as the supervisor realizes he cannot bully the practitioner.

When the decision to stand up for one's rights has been made, it is important to make several assessments prior to acting, including:

- Does this person have nothing to lose by being aggressive? (If the answer is yes, the practitioner may choose to reconsider this response and choose another, since the other person maybe irrational in the interchange.)

- What is the minimum amount of energy needed in this situation to make my point? (use the minimum energy needed to restore harmony)
- What is the best time and place for the confrontation?
- What is the best way to stop an attacker's advance?
- What is the best way to focus the conflict on the problem and not on generalities or personalities?
- What do I want my face to say and how can I ensure it says that?
- What do I want my body to say and how can I ensure it says that?
- What spatial relationship to the other person is most likely to end in harmony?

Multiple Attack. An attack from several other people seems intimidating. Examining the geometry of forces, it can be seen that due to the nature of the force exerted by the attackers, they require one another's presence in order to continue the attack. Their forces create a balance due to focusing energy directly on the attackee. If the practitioner keeps an attacker between herself or himself, a shield will develop between the practitioner and the rest of the attackers, and the attack will be defused.

Situation 1: Multiple Attack

Sandra is a practitioner who believes in wellness. She tries to collaborate with her clients and help them to take responsibility for decisions about what happens to them. As a result, she spends more time talking with her clients than some of the other employees do. Her supervisor has noted her "wasting time" talking with clients a number of times and several employees have demonstrated impatience waiting for her. Sandra is in a bind. She believes in what she is doing but knows she is being evaluated negatively. She knows this cannot go on indefinitely, so she moves in on a straight line to bring the attacks into direct confrontation. She calls a meeting of employees and her supervisor to discuss the kinds of plans she's implemented. Sandra centers herself, which helps her to remember the supervisor is not there "to get her." She's anxious about their work and worried about time pressures and being evaluated positively by her supervisors.

Ms. Bart, the supervisor, is the most outspoken and demands that Sandra spend less time talking with clients and more time completing her paperwork. Sandra pays attention to breathing and keeps centered so she doesn't scream out, "Look here, I went to school to learn these special skills I have and I know what's the best way to practice!" Sandra realizes that Ms. Bart, in the best tradition of attackers, has attacked with such force that she has almost lost her balance. Sandra decides to slide around Ms. Bart toward the other attackers. She asks for comments from the other employees, thanks them for their concern about clients, and asks if all the employees agree with Ms. Bart about her spending less time talking to clients. The employees disagree with one another and raise unrelated questions. Sandra refrains from becoming defensive and continues to go back to Ms. Bart's demands, keeping the supervisor between herself and the employees. Sandra eventually offers to speak at the next staff meeting, sharing with the employees her wellness interventions and outcomes for various "difficult" clients.

Situation 2: Multiple Attack

Sue Anderson, wellness practitioner, is working with a client, Emily Weiss, who is constantly complaining her teenage kids seem to be down on her lately. They argue about performing household tasks and complain about her cooking and "nagging." As a result, Emily feels cut off and resentful. Sue suggests a family meeting to bring the attacks into direct confrontation. Emily resists at first, until Sue does some role playing with her to help her decide exactly what she wants to say to her family, Emily practices centering herself prior to the family meeting and resists becoming defensive when the complaints start. Emily pays attention to her breathing, thanks them for being so candid, slides around the children's attacks, and keeps her husband between herself and the kids. Emily offers to stop nagging them in exchange for their agreeing to each cook one meal a week. The next week she reports to Sue that things are better around the house.

Hidden Agendas. Hidden agendas are unstated issues that are played out through interaction with others. Hidden agendas are excellent defensive maneuvers for low self-esteem. They protect against rejection by creating the desired impression at the expense of intimacy and authenticity. Wellness practitioners and clients use them to put up a smoke screen of carefully selected stories and calculated remarks. Clues that hidden agendas are operating include making the same point again and again and trying to prove something. The problem with hidden agendas is that they are obstacles to authentic, positive relationships. Therefore, it is important to assess the tendency for operating from a hidden agenda and take steps to devise self-instructions to counteract the pretense.

McKay, Davis, and Fanning (1995, pp. 78–83) list eight major hidden agendas:

1. *I'm Good.* Many of the statements from a person using this agenda demonstrate how caring and sensitive the person is; a fine character is created, but not an authentic self. No one is entrusted with the parts of oneself that are less than wonderful. People who always present themselves as good, honest, loyal, generous, successful, powerful, strong, wealthy, self-sacrificing, etc., tend to bore other people, and an intimate relationship becomes difficult.

2. *I'm Good (But You're Not).* In this agenda, the person attempts to raise his or her self-esteem by showing how stupid, incompetent, selfish, unreasonable, lazy, frightened, or insensitive others are. One practitioner often complained, "Do you think I can ever get anyone around here to help me? I'm the only one doing the work!" This hidden agenda gives a temporary boost to self-esteem, but others feel threatened and put down and defensive maneuvers on their part soon follow.

3. *You're Good (But I'm Not).* People who constantly flatter others have this agenda. More complex forms involve worship of smart, beautiful, or strong people. This agenda can also be used to ward off anger, rejection, and high expectations; who expects much of someone who is incompetent and self-berating?

4. *I'm Helpless, I Suffer.* This agenda portrays the person as a victim who has suffered misfortune, injustice, and abuse. The implied message is that the person is helpless and not responsible for what happens. Variations include presenting a problem and then proving nothing will help resolve it, and trading "horror stories" with another to form a bond of sympathy.

5. *I'm Blameless.* This is the agenda of people who have innumerable excuses for their failures. The basic position is: "I didn't do it." ("The doctor did it . . . The patient did it . . . The family interferes . . . My boss is the problem . . .").

6. *I'm Fragile.* The basic stance is, "Don't hurt me, I can't take it." The person tells or shows others he needs protection from the truth. ("I don't want to talk about it, it upsets me," "You're giving me another of my headaches," and "This reminds me of my parents fighting, let's not get into it" are typical comments from this stance.) On most hospital units there is one person who does not do his or her work but is not confronted by others because "She's fragile and couldn't take it."

7. *I'm Tough.* A variation is the super practitioner whose communication is often a harried listing of things done or to do; the underlying message is "I work harder, longer, and faster than anyone." The purpose of the agenda is to ward off hurt and protect a fragile self-esteem.

8. *I Know It All.* This is the agenda of the perpetual instructor, constantly moralizing as a protection from re-encountering early experiences of shame of being inadequate and not knowing.

McKay, Davis, and Fanning (1995, p. 83) suggest using self-instructions for overcoming hidden agendas (see Table 3.3); the statements can be said as mantras over and over again, can be taped to a bathroom mirror, the inside of a briefcase or carried on 3 × 5 cards.

Table 3.3 Self-Instructions for Overcoming Hidden Agendas

Agenda	Self-instructional statement
I'm Good	"I'm a mixture of strengths and weaknesses; I can learn to be balanced."
I'm Good (But You're Not)	I don't have to put you down to make me feel good; I can feel good on my own."
You're Good(But I'm Not)	"I can get attention for my strengths without making excuses."
I'm Helpless, I Suffer	"I experience joy as well as pain; I can allow myself to experience both."
I'm Blameless	I'm responsible for what happens to me."
I'm Fragile	"I can learn to deal with upset."
I'm Tough	"I can be safe without being tough."
I Know It All	"I can learn a lot from others if I listen, watch, and ask questions."

INTEGRATIVE LEARNING EXPERIENCE

Beginning Level

1. Make a verbatim recording of a 3-to-5-minute conversation with three clients. Assess your level of empathy. Write higher level empathic responses for each client and demonstrate them with those clients or with three others.

2. Keep a record of your I-Messages and You-Messages for a week. Change the You-Messages into I-Messages and devise a plan for implementation of increasing the percentage of I-messages you use.

3. Choose an assertiveness interchange of high priority for you. Be sure the situation does not have a long history of emotionally-charged behavior and involves only you and one other person, and builds in success. Write an assertiveness script for the situation. Practice the situation using a mirror and assess and (based on your assessment) change your verbal and nonverbal behavior during mirror practice to approximate an assertive presentation.

4. Use the assertiveness situation you have perfected through mirror practice and practice the situation with a nursing peer, obtaining feedback from the other person about your tone of voice, facial expression, body position, words chosen, consistency between words and nonverbal presentation. Be sure to coach your peer to play the other person's role so you obtain helpful practice.

5. Use an audio recorder and practice saying no until your evaluation identifies assertiveness and you make no excuses and do not apologize for saying no. (NOTE: overplay this past the point you would speak in the real-life situation to give you practice in bluntly saying no; this will allow you to say no in the real-life situation with more ease once you have passed the point of your usual response and encountered no negative effects.)

6. Choose another assertiveness situation and complete the following:

   A. Write a script for a two-person situation of high priority for you.
   B. Find a peer and fill him/her in on the specifics of playing the role as the real-life person would.
   C. Practice the situation on videotape until pleased with your performance. Use Table 3.2 to assess your behavior.

7. Identify situations in your past life that have contributed to nonassertiveness.

8. Work with a peer and videotape your responses to criticism using the following nurse responses:

A. acknowledgment	H. content-to-process shift
B. clouding	I. momentary delay
C. probing	J. time out
D. agreeing in part	K. doing nothing
E. agreeing in probability	L. using deflection/humor
F. agreeing in principle	M. joining the attacker
G. broken record	N. standing up for your rights

9. Identify hidden agendas you use; develop a plan for implementing self-instructional statements.

Advanced Level

1. Complete any of # 1–9 that have not been completed previously.
2. Work with a client to help him/her develop empathy using paraphrasing, relevant reading material, and client feedback.
3. Teach a client the difference between assertiveness and aggressiveness/avoidance.
4. Teach a client a relaxation procedure to use prior to attempting assertiveness.
5. Assist a client to audiotape or videotape an assertiveness situation and evaluate the results. Assist the client to devise a plan for practicing the behavior in the real-life situation.
6. Teach a client how to assess his/her level of assertiveness using Table 3.2.
7. Assist a client to identify what prevents him/her from being assertive.
8. Assist a client to deal with criticism using a different situation each time to exemplify:

A. acknowledging the criticism	G. content-to-process shift
B. clouding	H. momentary delay
C. agreeing in part	I. time out
D. agreeing in probability	J. joining and circling the attacker
E. agreeing in principle	K. deflection/humor
F. broken record	L. standing up for one's rights

9. Assist a client to identify hidden agendas.
10. Assist a client who has identified hidden agendas to develop self-instructions for overcoming the agenda(s).

REFERENCES

Carkhuff, R., and Berenson, B. (1976). *Beyond Counseling and Therapy.* New York: Holt, Rinehart and Winston, Inc.

Clark, C.C. (1994). *The Nurse as Group Leader* (3rd ed.) New York: Springer Publishing Company, pp. 30–31.

Dobson, T., and Miller, V. (1978). *Giving In To Get Your Way.* New York: Delacorte.

Dweck, C. (1975). Sex differences in the meaning of negative evaluation in achievement situations: Determinants and consequences. Unpublished paper presented at the Society for Research in Child Development, Denver, CO.

McKay, M., Davis, M., and Fanning, P. (1995). *Messages, The Communication Book.* Oakland. CA: New Harbinger.

Rivers, C., Barnett, R., and Baruch, G. (1979). *Beyond Sugar and Spice: How Women Grow, Learn and Thrive.* New York: Ballantine.

4

STRESS MANAGEMENT

This chapter discusses the following topics:

- Stress: Physiological and Immune System Effects
- Assessing stress symptoms
- Stress management interventions
  - Breathing
  - Biofeedback
  - Use of progressive relaxation as a nursing intervention
  - Self-hypnosis
  - Autogenics
  - Thought stopping
  - Refuting irrational ideas
  - Coping skills procedures
  - Time management
  - Hardiness

STRESS: PHYSIOLOGICAL AND IMMUNE SYSTEM EFFECTS

Stress can be experienced as a result of the interactions of one or more of the wellness dimensions. For example, it is possible to experience stress due to under- or overnutrition, negative interpersonal relationships or nagging thoughts about others or situations, insufficient exercise or ineffective body movement, negative environmental factors or conflicting values or beliefs.

In 1914 Cannon described the *fight or flight response* or "emergency reaction" that prepares the individual to fight or run. Physiological changes include: increase in blood pressure, heart rate, respiration, metabolism, epinephrine, blood glucose, peripheral vascular constriction, dilation of the pupils, and decreased testosterone levels (Benson & Klipper, 1976; Cannon, 1914;

Selye, 1956). If stress is chronic, the immune system weakens, lowering resistance to disease (Zeagans, 1982). With chronic stress, temporary conditions can become permanent, turning transient high blood pressure into hypertension, stomach upset into colitis or ulcers, and so forth. Stress has been related to many diseases and ailments including headaches, peptic ulcers, arthritis, colitis, diarrhea, asthma, cardiac arrhythmias, sexual problems, circulatory problems, muscle tension, and cancer (Davis, McKay, & Eshelman, 1995, p. 6).

A large body of literature has evolved documenting the relationship between stress and illness (Halley, 1991). Evidence points toward stress-induced immunosuppression (Ben-Eliyahu, 1991) though bidirectional effects may be more likely. Knowledge of the relationship between body and mind is rapidly expanding, having spawned the new discipline, *psychoneuroimmunology*. Research suggests that measurable immune system parameters can be influenced by relaxation and imagery techniques, biofeedback, assisted strategies, the use of humor, social support, journalling, therapeutic touch, hypnosis and conditioning (Kiecolt-Glaser, et al., 1986; Acterberg & Rider, 1989; Basmajian, 1989; Levy et al., 1990; Post-White and Johnson, 1991; Houldin, McCorkle, & Lowery, 1993; Quinn & Strelkaukas, 1993).

ASSESSING STRESS SYMPTOMS

It is not possible or even wise to turn off innate fight or flight responses to threats. It is possible and wise to learn to interpret and label experiences differently, thereby lessening negative stressor impact.

The first step in reducing stress is to assess the major sources of stress. The *Holmes "Schedule of Recent Experience"* was developed by Thomas Holmes at the University of Washington School of Medicine in Seattle, Washington. It gives a value for each life event (such as divorce, change in financial state, sexual difficulties, death of a spouse, vacation, etc.) and allows the respondent to obtain a total score. The assumption is that the more change an individual has to adjust to, the more likely he or she is to get sick. Holmes found that 80% of the persons he studied who had a score over 300 were apt to get sick in the near future.

A major controversy about the Holmes scale concerns the idea that some changes are not stressful and may even be pleasant. For example, although Holmes claims that a job change is stressful, it may be less stressful to take a new job in pleasanter surroundings than it is to stay in a job that is dead-end, draining, and results in ongoing resentment. Table 4.1 presents information for assessing and reducing stressful life changes.

Symptom relief can be a powerful motivator for nurses and clients to begin stress management procedures. Table 4.2 offers a Stress Symptom Assessment.

Physical symptoms may have physiological sources, so it is unwise to proceed on the assumption that all symptoms are completely stress-related. Stress management procedures are generally of two types: those that focus on relaxing the body and those that focus on handling stress differently. Often it is useful to use at least one approach from each broad category. For example, breathing exercises and progressive relaxation may be used to calm the body and refuting irrational ideas may be used to reduce perspectives on events that increase stress (Davis, McKay, & Eshelman, 1995).

Table 4.1 Assessing and Reducing Stressful Life Changes

1. Identify sources of stress by listing changes in the following areas in the past 2 years.
   - school
   - work
   - close relationship with friends, family, and significant other people or pets
   - living arrangements or place of residence
   - life style
   - financial matters
   - sudden challenges
   - amount of worry about the future

2. Identify which changes were negative (–) and which were positive (+) by placing a + in front of positive changes and a — in front of negative ones.

3. For the negative changes, decide on a procedure for limiting the effects of unresolved stress.* (See Table 4.2)

Source of Continued Stress	Stress Management Procedure

4. List changes anticipated in the next year and identify at least two procedures to use to reduce the effects of the change on the level of stress.

*Read the rest of this chapter for ideas.

Table 4.2 Stress Symptom Assessment

Rate the stress-related symptom for degree of discomfort on a scale of 1 (slight discomfort) to 10 (extreme discomfort). After ensuring the symptom does not have a purely physiological source, choose the appropriate procedure from list of codes and proceed to use it. After the procedure has been mastered, reevaluate degree of discomfort for each symptom experienced; this will provide a measure of the effectiveness of the procedure.

	Pre-practice degree of discomfort (1–10)	Procedure*	Post-practice degree of discomfort (1–10)
Anxiety in specific situations			___
Test anxiety	___	PR, B, M, I, SH	
Deadline anxiety	___	TS, RII, CS, TM	
Interview anxiety	___		___
Other performance anxiety	___		___
Anxiety in personal relationships		PR, BR, SH, AS	
with spouse/date	___	AF	
with parents	___		___
with children	___		___
other	___		___

Table 4.2 *(continued)*

	Pre-practice degree of discomfort (1–10)	Procedure*	Post-practice degree of discomfort (1–10)
Generalized anxiety	____	PR, BR, M, I, A, TS, RII, CS, E, B, AF	____
Depression	____		
Hopelessness		PR, BR, M, TS, AF	
Powerlessness	____	RII, CS, AS, N, E	____
Low self-esteem	____		
Hostility	____		____
Resentment	____	BR, M, A, RII	____
Anger	____	I, B, N, E	____
Irritability	____		____
Phobias	____	PR, TS, CS	____
Fears	____	I, BR, AF	____
Unwanted thoughts	____	BR, M, TS, I, AF	____
High blood pressure	____	PR, M, A, BN, E I, AF	____
Headaches	____		____
Neckaches	____	PR, ISH, A, B, N, E, AF	____
Backaches	____		____
Indigestion	____		____
Irritable bowel	____	PR, SH, A, B, N	____
Ulcers	____	E, AF	____
Chronic constipation	____		____
Muscle spasms	____	PR, I, SH, B	____
Tics	____	E	____
Tremors	____		____
Fatigue, chronic	____	PR, BR, SH, I, A TS, N, E	____
Insomnia	____	PR, SH, A, TS, B N, E, I, AF	____
Obesity	____	N, E	____
Weakness	____	E, N, I, AF	____

Codes

A	=	Autogenics	CS	= Coping Skills	PR	=	Progressive relaxation
AF	=	Affirmation	E	= Exercise	RII	=	Refusing irrational ideas
AS	=	Assertiveness	I	= Imagery	SH	=	Self-hypnosis
B	=	Biofeedback	M	= Medication	TS	=	Thought stopping
BR	=	Breathing	N	= Nutrition	TM	=	Time management

It is useful to keep a *Stress Awareness Diary* to make note of times that a stressful event occurs and the time a physical or emotional symptom could be related to stress. In time, it is possible to recognize where the body scores muscular tension. With increased awareness, specific procedures for releasing tension in those areas can be practiced. Keeping a record of progress will assist in the change process because it reinforces success and points out what needs further focus.

STRESS MANAGEMENT INTERVENTIONS

Breathing

Breathing is essential for life, yet many breathe in the upper part of the chest, not allowing sufficient blood to reach the lungs, brain, and other tissues. Under stress, many people restrict their breathing even further, increasing fatigue, muscular tension, irritability, and anxiety (Davis, McKay, & Eshelman, 1995).

While breathing exercises can be learned readily, it is important to maintain continued practice of them in a nonstressful, relaxing environment to attain the full benefits. The first step in enhancing breathing is breathing awareness.

Breathing Awareness

Wellness practitioners are best able to teach the client the procedure if they practice it first. The first step is to lie on a rug or blanket on the floor with legs straight and slightly apart and toes pointed comfortably out, with arms at sides, not touching the body, and with palms up and eyes closed.

Attention is brought to breathing and one hand is placed on the spot that seems to rise and fall during inhalation and exhalation. The other hand is placed on the abdomen and breathing is very gently brought to the abdominal area.

The Relaxation Sigh. The relaxing sigh can be used by practitioners prior to approaching a client or can be taught to clients who want to reduce tension levels. The relaxing sigh can be completed in the standing or sitting position. Upon exhalation, a deep sigh is used to let out a sound of deep relief as the air rushes out of the lungs. Inhalation is allowed to occur automatically. The procedure is repeated as necessary, as many times as necessary.

Breathing and Imagery. Breathing can be combined with imagery to provide a powerful healing stimulus. The breath is accomplished in a comfortable position while sitting or lying. The hands are placed on the abdomen; upon inhalation, energy is pictured rushing into the lungs and moving into the solar plexus for storage. Upon exhalation, energy is pictured flowing to all parts of the body. In the case of an injury or illness, energy can be pictured flowing to the injured or ill part.

Alternate Breath. The alternate breath has been found useful for general relaxation and to alleviate tension or sinus headaches (Davis, McKay, & Eshelman, 1995). The procedure is accomplished while sitting in a comfortable position using good posture. The index and second finger of the right hand rest on the forehead, and the right nostril is held closed gently by the thumb. Inhalation occurs through the left nostril. The left nostril is then gently closed with the ring finger and the right thumb is simultaneously removed from the right nostril. Air is exhaled slowly and soundlessly through the right nostril. The cycle is continued in a slow and even manner: inhale through right nostril, close right nostril with thumb and open the left nostril; exhale through the left nostril; inhale through the left nostril. Five cycles are suggested for beginners, slowly working up to 10 or 25 cycles.

Biofeedback

Biofeedback means getting feedback from the body about internal processes. Thus, breathing with awareness, imagery, and any intervention that allows feedback about the body is biofeedback.

More specifically, the term is used to refer to the use of instrumentation to develop the ability to read tension in various body systems. Instruments are especially useful when the client is unable to identify signs of stress, such as decreased hand temperature, increased muscle tension, or increased blood pressure. However, reading the signs of tension is only the first step in reducing stress. Once the clues have been identified, the client will still need assistance in learning to let go of the physical tension.

According to Davis, McKay, and Eshelman (1995), biofeedback works as follows:

> Biofeedback instruments monitor selected body systems that can be picked up by electrodes and transformed into visual or auditory signals. Any internal change instantly triggers an external signal, such as a sound, a flickering light, or readings on a meter.

The following symptoms have been treated with biofeedback: tension headache, migraine, hypertension, insomnia, spastic colon, muscle spasm or pain, epilepsy, anxiety, phobic reactions, asthma, stuttering, and teeth grinding (Davis, McKay, & Eshelman, 1995).

Clients may come to a sophisticated biofeedback center for treatment, or they can purchase inexpensive monitoring equipment for home use. Levels of in-home equipment vary. Sometimes measures are broadly calibrated and may not be completely accurate. Treatment will probably be most effective when the client works with a professional who has high quality equipment and who can assist in overcoming roadblocks that might interrupt progress. A directory of certified biofeedback practitioners is available from The Biofeedback Society of America, 4301 Owen Street, Wheat Ridge, CO 80030.

Progressive Relaxation as a Wellness Measure

Progressive relaxation was developed by Jacobson in 1938 and involves tightening and relaxing the muscle groups of the body, beginning with the hand and moving to the upper and then the lower arm, the forehead, eyes and nose, mouth, neck, upper back, abdomen, buttocks, thigh, calf, and foot for 5 to 7 seconds. The client is encouraged to check for relaxation prior to moving to the next major muscle group. If the practitioner is working directly with the client in a relaxation session, the practitioner and client can agree that if the client is tense, the index finger of the right or left hand will be raised when the practitioner checks for relaxation.

Scandrett and Uecker (1985, p. 33) suggest that a careful assessment of the client is essential prior to employing relaxation techniques. Symptoms need to be identified and an anxiety scale or anxiety symptom checklist may prove useful. Baseline and posttreatment vital sign measures will validate physiological changes associated with relaxation. Essential components of the pretreatment interview include assessing:

- a report of the client's identification of the most bothersome symptom
- onset, duration, and full description of symptoms
- family history of similar complaints
- client interventions and a description of the results
- an investigation of why the client now seeks help for this symptom
- current and recent medications, including over-the-counter drugs
- physical limitations or illnesses
- previous experience with relaxation training
- use of alcohol or mind-altering drugs
- dietary patterns, especially use of caffeine, sugar, and daily alcohol intake
- sleep patterns
- exercise patterns
- overview of daily routine, including stressors
- psychiatric history, including screening for major depressive or psychotic disorders
- willingness to learn and practice at home

Scandrett and Uecker (1985, p. 34) include self-hypnosis, biofeedback, autogenics, and meditation under the rubric of relaxation therapy and suggest the following nursing diagnoses as appropriate for intervention with it: anxiety, sleep disturbance, activity intolerance, powerlessness, ineffective breathing pattern, comfort alterations in pain, ineffectual coping, impaired physical mobility, and fear.

Although progressive relaxation has proven effective in most studies, some precautions for its use include the following (Snyder, 1984, p. 57):

- In persons who are depressed, relaxation may precipitate further withdrawal.
- In persons experiencing hallucinations and delusions, loss-of-reality-contact reactions may occur.
- The toxic effects of medications can be increased by the relaxation state.
- Tightly tensing muscles can increase blood pressure; those with cardiac conditions should use nontensing relaxation exercises.
- Some clients may experience heightened pain by focusing their attention on body functions; for these clients, imagery may be the treatment of choice.

Self-Hypnosis

Hypnosis is a wakeful state of deep relaxation; there is an alteration in the conscious level of thinking and remembering, and an increase in the ability to focus in on a particular situation. Hypnosis is a heightened state of awareness during which people are more open to suggestion; most people have experienced a trance state at one time or another, e.g., while daydreaming, or when concentrating intently on a book, movie, television program, or work project. All hypnosis is really self-hypnosis because no one will accept a suggestion unless he or she really wants to; thus, the "self" is always in control.

When using self-hypnosis as an intervention, the client usually begins by listening to a taped relaxation and suggestion session or works with a health care professional skilled in the maneuver. With practice, clients can learn quite quickly to relax and put themselves in a trance state. Table 4.3 gives basic instructions for self-hypnosis. As with all procedures in the book, the practitioner should try it out first to understand what the experience is like and to anticipate any difficulties clients might have with the procedure.

For hypnosis to be effective, positive suggestions must be used. Suggestions are used all the time by lay and professional people, but often they are in a negative form. Both negative and positive suggestions affect the subconscious mind even when asleep or unconscious. Adverse suggestions, such as "She'll never recover from this," or "It's malignant, the patient doesn't have a chance," or "You can't be helped, you will have to learn to live with the condition" are heard and acted upon by the hearer. The last comment seems innocuous, but taken literally it means the client will die if the symptom is lost (LeCron, 1964).

Table 4.3 Basic Instructions for Self-Hypnosis

1. Sit or lie in a comfortable position. Remind yourself that whenever you want to come out of hypnosis you can.

2. Use a candle, picture, crack in the ceiling, fire in the fireplace, or some other object to encourage eye fixation.

3. While watching the object, suggest your eyes are getting heavier, are beginning to sting, or are starting to flutter (whichever works best) to induce eyelid heaviness.

4. Preselect a word or phrase to use at the moment your eyes close. The words "relax now," or a color or a place that is beautiful and has special meaning to you, can also be used.

5. With eyes closed, begin relaxing all your muscles, starting with forearms and biceps; first tighten, then relax them. Move to the face, neck, shoulders, chest, stomach, lower back, buttocks, thighs, calves, and toes.

6. Picture the top of an escalator with the steps moving down in front of you. As you step on, count back slowly from 10 to 0. Repeat counting back slowly for two more floors.

7. Begin to notice a feeling of heaviness in your right arm (if right-handed, or left arm if left-handed); then notice your arm getting lighter and lighter as if balloons are tied to it, lifting it higher and higher. Soon your hand will begin to move, imperceptively at first, but then it will float, moving closer and closer to your face. When your hand touches your face, you will be in hypnosis.

8. When ready, return from hypnosis, feeling refreshed and relaxed.

Table 4.4 Coaching Clients in Self-Hypnosis

Directions to Give Clients:

1. If uncomfortable with the word "hypnosis," tell the client the experience will increase comfort and relaxation.

2. Encourage the client to practice self-hypnosis regularly; provide praise for a practice attempt; reinforce practice and success and reduce resistance to self-hypnosis by responding with "Good, you are beginning to learn the technique" to whatever they report as effects of their practice.

3. Tell clients they may feel tingling, warmth, or some other sensations, but whatever they experience will be relaxing; this suggestion will reduce resistance and assist clients to integrate transitory reactions.

4. Word suggestions positively and simply; try stating suggestions in a louder, firmer voice.

5. Use rhythm, repetition, and a monotone voice when coaching.

6. If there is a distracting noise during a practice session, give clients the suggestion, "The sounds you hear will tend to deepen your relaxation."

7. Assist the client in setting up a schedule for self-hypnosis practice and agree on a helpful (not nagging) way the practitioner can encourage practice and the client or practitioner can reward success or practice attempts.

Table 4.4 gives suggestions for coaching clients in self-hypnosis.

Suggestions are most effective and wellness-enhancing when phrased in a positive form, e.g., "I will feel comfortable and confident during the interview tomorrow" (as opposed to "I will not feel tension tomorrow"). Formulating suggestions in the becoming mode is often most effective, e.g., "My comfort is gradually increasing" (instead of "I am totally comfortable"). The best results are forthcoming when only one or two suggestions are focused on. Bombarding oneself with numerous suggestions dilutes the force of all of them.

Eighty to 90% of people can be hypnotized, but those who are severely emotionally disturbed, depressed, or suicidal respond more positively to psychotherapy then to hypnosis. Others who may not respond positively to hypnosis include: 1) people with psychosomatic illnesses—who deny any emotional component to their problems—and 2) those who are neurologically impaired or mentally retarded (LeCron, 1964), or who are in crisis (Hadley and Staudacher, 1989).

Clients expected to respond most favorably to hypnosis include those who are highly motivated to learn the technique, are optimistic, willing to try something new, able to concentrate easily, receptive to rather than afraid of hypnosis, and have a good imagination. Clients who do not possess all the above characteristics can learn self-hypnosis if they are willing to practice the technique more frequently.

Some people respond best to permissive suggestions ("I can feel more relaxed and refreshed") while others respond best to commands ("I will feel more relaxed and refreshed"). Experimentation is the best method of determining whether suggestions should be phrased in the permissive or the command mode.

Self-hypnosis can be used to reduce stress related to smoking, drinking, overeating, taking harmful drugs, destructive anger, timidity, anxiety, allergies, itching, asthma, anger, study problems, and pain. The basic self-hypnosis state is induced (see Table 4.4), but the suggestions used differ depending on the stressor. Suggestions can be said aloud, placed on an audiotape, or written and then read to oneself or the client. Bernhardt and Martin (1977, pp. 19–20) suggest the following suggestions be used:

> For my body, not for me, smoking (this harmful drug, destructive anger, anxiety, timidity, head symptom, drinking, overeating) is a poison. I need my body to live, I will protect my body as I would protect (name of loved one).

Suggestions for itching, allergies, and asthma would follow the same format with slight variation (Bernhardt & Martin, 1977, pp. 60–74).

For itching:

Not for me, but for my body, this itch is damaging; it means my body is out of balance. To live comfortably, I need my body in balance. To the point I wish to live in comfort, I will itch when I choose to and at the body location I choose.

For allergies, asthma, or colds, the basic suggestion is used and the following is added:

> If I choose to live this day symptom-free, I can, because I have power over my body. I can tell my nose when to get stuffed up and when not to. I can declare myself master of my body.

Self-hypnosis is also useful in slowing the heart or breathing rate, using the suggestion: "My pulse is slowing down a few beats a minute, and I am relaxing" or "I am beginning to breathe more slowly and comfortably." Clients can be instructed to take their pulse after several minutes until it has slowed sufficiently; at this point, the following suggestion can be used: "This is the heart rate (or pulse) I am comfortable with and want to remain at."

When learning self-hypnosis, some people may not respond well to either muscle relaxation *or* visualization. Poems that use rhythm, repetition, and imagery can be used in that case, or children can be held and rocked rhythmically. Older children (age 4–16 years) can draw a clown face on their preferred thumbnail. They then place a quarter between that thumb and their forefinger while looking at the clown face. Children are told to look only at the clown face and as they do, the coin will slowly become heavy and slip down and fall. When the coin slips, the children are told their eyes will close and they will be very relaxed. Next, the children are told to place their hands on their legs and answer questions by raising their "yes" hand or their "no" hand. (Which hand is which is agreed on prior to the induction technique.) Questions are then asked that pertain to the problem at hand. For example, for bedwetters, the question is asked, "Would you like to have dry beds at night?" Before asking questions about the problem area, children are asked questions of a neutral type such as, "Do you like ice cream?" Those who answer "yes" to the bedwetting question are told they can learn a "trick" but they must practice it very hard every day, and then the "trick" will help them urinate only in the toilet. The children are asked to practice saying the following statement every time the quarter falls out of their hand:

> When I need to urinate, I will wake up all by myself, go to the bathroom all by myself, urinate in the toilet, and return to my nice dry bed. (Bricklin, 1976)

Dr. Karen Olness, Assistant Professor of Medicine at George Washington University, tried this with 20 girls and 20 boys. Within the first month, 20 were "cured" (and had no recurrence of bedwetting 6 months after the study), six others improved, one did not practice, one had a urinary tract operation, and one answered "no" when asked if he wanted a dry bed; this client was referred to psychiatric evaluation (Bricklin, 1976).

Self-Hypnosis and Pain. There are many advantages of using relaxation and self-hypnotic techniques with clients, particularly with those who are immobile due to physical or emotional difficulties. Those who are hospitalized may benefit from this approach because it can replace the sense of mastery and control they have lost due to the process of hospitalization. Being taught self-hypnosis techniques also provides a special experience for them when the health practitioner says, "I understand that you are having a lot of pain (discomfort, trouble, etc.) and I'm going to teach you a special way to feel better."

Often, merely conveying a firm, clear message of intent to help with pain will provide relief. Some comments to use in this regard are: "I am here to help you relieve your pain," or "I want to work with you to reduce your pain." Other types of statements that are helpful are: "What is the pain?" "Describe the pain to me." "What do you do to relieve your pain." This discussion is then followed by a decision by the client (if possible) regarding his or her choice of pain relief measure. Approximately 30 minutes after the choice and implementation, the wellness practitioner discusses the measure if necessary. Assuming clients have pain if they say they have pain, having confidence they can help, using measures other than medication, checking to ensure the relief measure works, finding out which warnings of pain people have and helping them intervene in the pain before it becomes intense are helpful wellness practitioner measures.

Individuals in chronic, ongoing pain tend to take on the pain as part of their identity. They can be encouraged to question, "What meaning does this pain have for me?" "Can I imagine myself without pain?" "Is it worth it to me to give up this pain?" while deeply relaxed in self-hypnosis. Clients with this kind of pain may require self-hypnosis sessions of 15 minutes or more twice a day. Practitioners working with these clients must be willing to spend additional time with them and realize that there may be times when hypnosis does not work.

Clients may experience excruciating pain at meaningful times; for example, one person who had survived a fire that killed her daughter had a great deal of pain (despite hypnosis) at noon, the time the fire had occurred (Zahourek, 1976).

Clients who have ongoing pain begin to ask themselves, "Can I stand this pain indefinitely?" A suggestion to use with these people during self-hypnosis is "No pain lasts forever." Clients who have been through life-threatening situations may come to associate pain with being alive, since the feeling of pain may be the one thing that reassures them they are alive. This idea can remain in their subconscious as a self-given suggestion ("If I did not have this pain, I'd be dead"). These clients will often claim to have pain even while asleep. A suggestion that may be helpful in this case is: "When the other signs of life were missing, the pain was reassuring, but now it is preferable to be alive without this ongoing pain than to be alive with it." According to Ewin (1978), this type of psychic pain can be distinguished from the pain of cancer, arthritis, or fracture in that psychic pain is always present whereas pain from other afflictions is intermittent.

When using self-hypnosis, it is important to involve as many of the senses as possible (smelling odors, feeling ocean spray or warm sun, touching cool water, tasting salty spray, hearing waves on the beach, etc.) A relatively quick way to induce relaxation is to ask the client to picture him- or herself in a quiet, relaxing, comforting place and to hear, smell, taste, feel, and see everything associated with that place. The practitioner can remain with the client and ask that the index finger of the client's right hand be raised to indicate complete relaxation and the index finger of the left hand to indicate lack of relaxation. The practitioner can ask the client to indicate level of relaxation afer a few minutes; if relaxation has not been attained, the practitioner can try progressive relaxation or some other method. For more information regarding the use of self-hypnosis, the reader can consult: Zahourek, Rothlyn P., *Clinical Hypnosis and Therapeutic Suggestion in Patient Care*, Brunner/Mazel, 1990.

Autogenics

Autogenics is a form of self-hypnosis that allows the participant to induce the feeling of warmth and heaviness associated with a trance state. Johannes H. Schultz, a Berlin psychiatrist, combined autosuggestion with some Yoga techniques and developed a system of autogenic training. The system has been found effective in the treatment of disorders of the respiratory tract, the gastrointestinal tract, the circulatory system, the endocrine system, as well as anxiety, irritability, and fatigue. The exercises can be used to increase resistance to stressors, reduce or eliminate sleep disorders, and modify pain reactions.

Autogenic therapy is not recommended for children under 5 years old, or for adults who lack motivation or have severe emotional disorders. Those with diabetes, hypoglycemic conditions, or heart conditions should discuss the use of the method with their physicians. Occasionally, a client may experience a sharp rise or drop in blood pressure when doing the exercises; those with high or low blood pressure should take or have their blood pressure taken to ensure the exercises are useful.

The exercises can be completed in a comfortable sitting or lying position. It may take up to 10 months to master the six exercises. Ninety-second sessions five to eight times a day are recommended for mastery. The client assumes an attitude of passive concentration; initially this will be difficult to attain, but a wandering mind can easily be brought back to concentration. Clients often experience some reactions that are normal but distracting, including a sensation of weight or temperature change, tingling, electric currents, involuntary movements, stiffness, some pain, anxiety, a desire to cry, irritability, headaches, nausea, or hallucinations. These discharges are transitory and will pass as the program is continued.

Each session is ended with a statement to oneself such as, "When I open my eyes I will feel refreshed and alert" and a few deep breaths and stretches until normal awakeness is achieved. Early exercises are focused on heaviness; this cues muscles to relax; the client repeats the following statements, working up from 90 seconds to 4 minutes four to seven times a day. "My right (dominant) arm is heavy." "My left (nondominant) arm is heavy." "Both my arms are heavy." "My right leg is heavy." "My left leg is heavy." "Both my legs are heavy."

Later exercises focus on warmth, which assists in attaining relaxation in blood vessels. The client repeats the following statements working up from 90 seconds to 10 minutes a day: "My right (dominant) arm is warm." "My left (nondominant) arm is warm." "Both my legs are warm." "My right leg is warm." "Both my legs are warm." "My arms and legs are warm."

Next, the client focuses on heartbeat and repeats the following statement: "My heartbeat is calm and regular." Clients who have difficulty becoming aware of their heatbeat can rest their hand over their heart. Those who experience any discomfort are counseled to move to the next three themes and return to the heartbeat theme following the forehead theme.

When focusing on the breathing theme, the client repeats, "It breathes me" or "My breathing is calm and relaxed." The client can picture him- or herself breathing easily to potentiate the effect of slow, deep respiration.

The solar plexus theme is not used for clients who have ulcers, diabetes, or any condition involving bleeding from the abdominal region. The statement that is focused on for other clients is: "My solar plexus (abdomen, stomach, or belly) is warm."

The forehead theme is best repeated while lying on the back since dizziness can result. The client repeats, "My forehead is cool."

Autogenics can also be used for organ-specific work. For example, for blushing, the client can repeat: "My feet are warm" or "My shoulders are warm." For coughs, the statements, "My throat is cool" and "My chest is warm" are helpful. For asthma, clients use, "It breathes me calm and regular."

Additional statements that can be interspersed with standard themes include: "I feel quiet." "My whole body feels quiet, heavy, comfortable and relaxed." "My mind is quiet." "I withdraw my thoughts from the surroundings and I feel serene and still." "My thoughts are turned inward and I am at peace." "I feel an inward quietness." "Deep within my mind, I can visualize and experience myself as relaxed and comfortable and still" (Davis, McKay, & Eshelman, 1995, pp. 81–88).

Thought Stopping

Thought stopping is an approach that is especially useful when nagging, repetitive thoughts interfere with wellness. Unwanted thoughts are interrupted by the client with the command "stop," an image of the letters of the word stop, a loud noise (such as a buzzer or bell), or a negative stimulus, such as wearing a rubber band around the wrist and snapping it when the unwanted thought occurs.

Thought stopping may work because (a) distraction occurs, (b) the interruption behaviors serve as a punishment and what is punished consistently is apt to be inhibited, (c) it is an assertive response and can be followed by reassuring or self-accepting comments, and (d) it interrupts the chain of negative and frightening thoughts leading to negative and frightening feelings, thus reducing stress level.

For effective mastery, regular practice for 3 to 7 days is needed. The client chooses the problematic thought; if necessary, the client can be assisted to prioritize interfering thoughts and focus on the most bothersome one.

Next, the nagging thought is brought to attention. Clients are asked to close their eyes and imagine a situation during which the stressful thought is likely to occur. The next step is to interrupt the nagging thought with an egg timer, alarm clock, snap of the fingers, or an image or verbalization of the word, "STOP."

When clients are able to conjure up and dispense with the nagging thought at will, positive, assertive statements are used to replace the nonconstructive one, e.g.:

- fear of flying: "This is a beautiful view from up here."
- food obsession: "My body is using the food I have eaten to sustain me."
- fear of attack: "I am safe if I use the approaches I have learned to protect myself."
- inability to complete wellness behaviors: "I am confident in my ability to exercise (lose weight, stop smoking, etc.)."

Choosing the best extinguishing behavior and the best replacement statements involves an open discussion with clients; the practitioner enumerates the possible extinguishers and may hint at assertive replacement statements, but clients are encouraged to choose based on their knowledge of what is helpful to them.

Clients who experience failure with the approach can choose a less intrusive thought to begin with; once success is achieved, the more troublesome thought can be attempted. Clients need to know that distressful thoughts may return in the future, especially during times of stress; the procedure discussed above can be repeated in these cases.

Refuting Irrational Ideas

Human beings engage in almost continuous self-talk during their waking hours. *Self-talk* is the internal language we use to describe and interpret the world. When self-talk is accurate and realistic, wellness is enhanced; when irrational and untrue, stress and emotional disturbance occur.

Albert Ellis (*A Guide to Rational Living,* 1961) developed a system to attack irrational ideas or beliefs and replace them with more realistic interpretations and self-talk. At the root of irrational thought is the idea that something is being done *to* the person; rational thought is based on the idea that events occur and people experience these events. Irrational self-talk tends to lead to unpleasant emotions; rational self-talk is more likely to lead to pleasant feelings and a positive interpretation of experiences.

One common form of irrational self-talk is statements that "awfulize" experience by making catastrophic, nightmarish interpretations of events, e.g., interpreting a momentary chest pain as a heart attack, a grumpy word from a supervisor as intent to fire, or silence as negative criticism.

The kinds of statements Ellis considers irrational are:

1. External events cause most human misery—people simply react as events trigger their emotions.
2. Happiness can be achieved by inaction, passivity, and endless leisure.
3. People must be unfailingly competent and perfect in all endeavors.
4. It is easier to avoid than to face life's difficulties and responsibilities.
5. The past determines the present.
6. It is horrible when people and things are not the way they should be.
7. It is a necessity for adults to have love and approval from peers, family, and friends.
8. Unfamiliar or potentially dangerous situations always lead to fear and anxiety.
9. People are helpless and have no control over what they experience or feel.
10. People are fragile and cannot be told the truth.
11. Good relationships are built on sacrifice and giving.
12. Rejection and abandonment are the result if one does not always try to please others.
13. There is a perfect love and a perfect relationship.
14. A person's worth is dependent on achievement and production.
15. Anger is bad and destructive.
16. It is bad and wrong to go after what you want and need.

Goodman (1974) developed several guidelines for turning irrational thinking into rational thought, including:

1. The situation does not do anything to me; I say things to myself that produce anxiety and fear.
2. To say things should be other than they are is to believe in magic.
3. All humans are fallible and make mistakes.
4. It takes two to argue.
5. The original cause of a problem is often lost in antiquity; the best place to focus attention is on the present: what to do about the problem now.
6. People feel the way they think; the interpretation of events leads to emotions, not the events themselves.

Refuting irrational ideas is a skill and requires practice in the following five steps:

1. Write down the facts of the event, including only the observable behaviors.
2. Write down self-talk about the event, including all subjective value judgments, assumptions, beliefs, predictions, and worries.
3. Note which statements are classified by Ellis as irrational; a star or some other symbol can be used.
4. Focus on the emotional response to the event using one or two words, e.g., angry, hopeless, felt worthless, afraid.

5. Select *one* irrational idea to refute.
6. Write down all evidence that the idea is false.
7. Write down the worst thing that could happen if what is feared happens or what is desired is not attained.
8. Write down positive effects that might occur if what is feared happens or if what is desired is not attained.
9. Substitute alternative self-talk.

Table 4.5 provides an example of the use of Ellis's format for refuting irrational ideas.

Table 4.5 Refuting Irrational Ideas

1. *Activating event:* Another employee complained about me to my supervisor.
2. *Rational ideas:* I know she's under a lot of pressure because she's new to the unit.
3. *Irrational ideas:* I can't stand being humiliated in public. Feelings of rage and wanting to kill her are taking over. I'm falling apart.
4. *Main feeling(s):* Rage, anger, humiliation.
5. *Refuting the irrational idea(s):* I'm falling apart.
   a. Being put down in public is not pleasant, but I can handle it.
   b. I'm mislabeling rage and anger as falling apart.
   c. I usually get along O.K. with that employee and once I calm down, I will again.
6. *The worst thing that could happen:* The worst thing that could happen is that I could put down the employee in the future to get back at her.
7. *Good things that could occur as a result of this incident:* I can learn to handle put downs without feeling out of control.
8. *Alternate thoughts:* I'm O.K. It's O.K. to feel anger and rage and know I can still function. I can learn to handle this situation and feel good about myself for doing so.
9. *Alternate emotions:* I'm angry, but feel less out of control. The anger is starting to fade and I am feeling calmer.

Coping Skills Procedure

Coping skills training grew out of relaxation and systematic desensitization procedures that were expanded and refined by Meichenbaum and Cameron (1974). The procedures include a combination of progressive relaxation and stress coping self-statements that are used to replace the defeatist self-talk called forth in stressful situations.

Coping skills procedures can be used to rehearse via the imagination for real-life events deemed stressful. First, a stressful siutation is called forth. Next, progressive relaxation is practiced. Finally, coping skills statements are repeated until the situation can be thoroughly completed in rehearsal without feeling stressed.

The procedures have been shown effective in the reduction of general anxiety and interview, speech, and test anxiety and appear to be effective in the treatment of phobias, especially the fear of heights. Davis, McKay, and Eshelman (1995) report the effects of 2-year follow-ups of hypertense, postcardiac clients showing that 89 percent were still able to achieve general relaxation using coping skills training, 79 percent could still generally control tension, and 79 percent were able to fall asleep sooner and sleep more deeply. According to Davis, McKay, and Eshelman (1995), coping skills procedures can be mastered in approximately 1 week, once progressive relaxation has been learned (1–2 weeks for mastery).

Coping thoughts can be divided into statements useful for different stages of the stressful situation: Preparatory, the situation, and reinforcing success. Examples of statements found effective for each stage follow; clients and practitioners can develop their own list and memorize them and/or carry a copy with them for use in stressful situations.

Preparatory Stage:

* I can handle this.
* There's nothing to worry about.
* I'll jump in and be all right.
* It will be easier once I get started.
* Soon this will be over.

The Situation:

* I will not allow this situation to upset me.
* Take a deep breath and relax.
* I can take it step by step.
* I can do this; I'm handling it now.
* I can keep my mind on the task at hand.
* It doesn't matter what others think; I will do it.
* Deep breathing really works.

Reinforcing Success:

* Situations don't have to overwhelm me anymore.
* I did it!
* I did well.
* I'm going to tell____about my success.
* By stopping thinking about being afraid, I wasn't afraid.

Time Management

According to Davis, McKay, and Eshelman (1995), symptoms of inappropriate time management include: rushing, fatigue, or listlessness with many slack hours of nonproductive activity, chronic vacillation between unpleasant alternatives, chronic missing of deadlines, insufficient time for rest or personal relationships, and the sense of being overwhelmed by demands and details.

Most methods of time management include three steps:

- establishing priorities
- eliminating low priority tasks
- learning to make decisions

Effective time management has been found effective in minimizing deadline anxiety, avoidance anxiety, and job fatigue (McKay, Davis, & Eshelman, 1995).

The first step in time management is exploring how time is currently being spent. An easy way to do this is to divide the day into three segments: waking through lunch, end of lunch through dinner, and end of dinner until bedtime. A small notebook is carried and the number of minutes for each activity engaged in in each time segment is logged. The inventory is kept for 3 days. At the end of the time, the total amount of time spent in each of the following categories is noted: Table 4.6 provides a time management assessment for Eloise Strates, a wellness practitioner. Based on a review of the inventory, she made the following decisions:

1. Put out clothes for the next day prior to going to bed.
2. Get up at the alarm and limit shower to 5 minutes.
3. Make breakfasts that don't require cooking, cut dinner preparation to 30 minutes, and enlist family to do food preparation 3 days/week.
4. Ask for a late lunch to take advantage of most productive work hours (11 a.m. to 2 p.m.).
5. Use thought stopping to limit daydreaming.
6. Stop attending nonmandatory, nonproductive meetings.

Eloise's next step was to set priorities. She began by making a list of things she most wanted to accomplish in the near future and comparing it to how she spent her time. She visualized herself being told she only had 6 months to live and began to imagine how she could best spend the time. She made the list without stopping to evaluate or judge what she wrote and suggested others might also find this the most helpful way to proceed.

Eloise's next step was to make a list of 1-month and 1-year goals she believed she could reasonably accomplish in terms of work, improvement, and recreation. Then she sat back and reflected that she now had long-, medium-, and short- range goals. Next, Eloise prioritized each list by deciding which were the top drawer items (most essential or desired), middle drawer items (can be put off for a while, but still important), and bottom drawer (can easily be put off indefinitely with no harm done).

Table 4.6 Time Management Assessment

Activity	Time (minutes)	Activity	Time (minutes)
Waking through Lunch		After Lunch through Dinner	
Lying in bed and thinking about getting up	20	Working with clients	90
		Daydreaming while staring at paperwork	20
Shower	20		
Decide what to wear and dress	25	Shift report	20
		Socializing	30
Cook breakfast	15	Commute	30
Read paper/eat	30	Shopping	45
Phone friend	15	Phone calls	30
Commute to work	30	Cooking	90
Routine paperwork	30	Eating	30
Daydream	10		
Nonmandatory meeting	60	After Dinner Until Retiring	
Working with clients	120	Phone calls	60
Lunch	45	Television	90
		Study	90
		Prepare for bed/read	30

Eloise then chose two top drawer goals for her liftetime goals, 1-year goals, and 1-month goals to begin working toward.

T-1: Buy a new car (1-year goal).
T-2: Write an article for a journal (lifetime goal to contribute to the profession).
T-3: Have dinner out with husband once a week (1-month goal).
T-4: Investigate ways of becoming a consultant (lifetime goal to communicate wellness knowledge).
T-5: Dance lessons with husband (1-year goal).
T-6: Complete old records pile at work (1-month goal).

Since Eloise was overwhelmed by the six goals, she decided to break each one down into manageable steps. For example, her goal of investigating ways of becoming a nursing consultant was divided into the following steps:

1. Borrow a friend's book on consultation and read a chapter a week.
2. Talk with other practitioners who are currently consultants; ask one or more to be my mentor.
3. Make a list of my wellness knowledge [and combine] to make a list of saleable consulting skills.
4. Purchase stationary, business cards, and brochures detailing my consulting skills.

Eloise found it so difficult to get started even after breaking down her priorities into manageable steps that she developed a daily "To Do" list including everything she wanted to accomplish that day. She rated each item top, middle, or bottom priority and worked only on the top priority items for the day.

This approach helped somewhat, but Eloise still had difficulty until she discovered the rules for making time (McKay, Davis, & Eshelman, 1995):

1. Learn to say "no"; remind yourself this is your life and your time to spend as best befits you. Only when your boss asks should you spend time on bottom priority items. Be prepared to say, "I don't have the time." If necessary, take an assertiveness training course.
2. Build time into your schedule for unscheduled events, interruptions, and unforeseen occurrences.
3. Set aside several time periods during the day for structured relaxation; being relaxed will allow you to use the time you have more efficiently.
4. Keep a list of short, 5-minute tasks that can be done any time you are waiting or are between other tasks.
5. Learn to do two things at once; plan dinner while driving home or organize an important letter or list while waiting in line at the bank.
6. Delegate bottom drawer tasks to sons, daughters, secretaries, or in-laws.
7. Get up 15 to 30 minutes earlier every day.
8. Allow no more than 1 hour of television-watching for yourself daily. Use it as a reward for working on your top drawer times.

Part of time management is the ability to make decisions. Procrastination is the great time robber. Procrastination can often be overcome by (Davis, McKay, & Eshelman, 1995):

1. Recognizing the unpleasantness of making some decisions versus the unpleasantness of putting it off; analyze the costs and risks of delay.
2. Examine the payoffs you receive for procrastinating, e.g., you won't have to face the possibility of failure, you can be taken care of by others, you can gain attention by being chronically unhappy.
3. Join the resistance you have created by exaggerating and intensifying whatever you are doing to put off the decision. Keep it up until you are bored and making the decision seems more attractive than whatever you are doing to procrastinate.
4. Take responsibility for your delaying tactics by writing down how long each delay took.
5. When making unimportant decisions, choose south or east over north or west; pick left over right; smooth over rough; pick the shortest; choose the closest; pick the one that comes first alphabetically.
6. Take small steps toward the decision: if you want to decide to sew on a button, take out the thread and materials and place them by you as a lead-in to the decision to begin.
7. Avoid beginning a new task until you have completed a predecided segment

of the current one; allow yourself to fully experience the reward of finishing something, one of the great payoffs of decision making.

Music

Taped music has been studied and found effective for reducing the stress of anxiety in blood donors (Cameron, 1991), pain after surgery (Slyfield, 1992), and intensive care units (Johnson, 1991).

Hardiness

Dr. Suzanne Ouellette Kobasa has researched the ability of people to survive stress. She found that *psychological "hardiness"* or the ability to survive is composed of three ingredients: 1) Commitment to self, work, family, and other important values; 2) a sense of personal control over one's life; and 3) the ability to see change in one's life as a challenge to master.

Dr. Kobasa tested executives, lawyers, women in gynecologists' offices, telephone foremen, operator supervisors, U.S. Army officers, and college students; the results were the same: biology is not destiny. A hardy personality is more important than a strong constitution. It is possible to come from a family with chronic illness and do better under stress if one is hardy than to come from a "healthy" family but have few inner resources (Kobasa, 1984).

Exercise is a good antidote to stress but may be short-term. Jogging after an argument can help that evening, but the next morning stress levels can rise if the stress-provoking situation is re-encountered. Hardiness skills may be long-term innoculations against stressors.

Three techniques Dr. Kobasa found helpful for increasing hardiness skills are: focusing, restructuring stressful situations, and compensating through self-improvement. Focusing is a technique developed by Eugen Gendlin that can assist in recognizing signals from the body that stress is interfering with comfort. Dr. Kobasa found that executives are so used to pressure in their temples, tightened necks, or stomach knots that they have stopped noticing these signals that something is wrong. A beginning question might be: "Where is my tension located in my body?" Those who have learned to tune out body signals can begin with a progressive relaxation tape; this will assist in identifying body locations of stress and tension. Another step is to make a list of "Things That Are Bothering Me Today." The list is then reviewed and the question, "What is keeping me from feeling terrific today?" can assist in the process. Using an affirmation such as, "This day is getting better and better" may help also.

The second technique (reconstruction of stressful situations) is accomplished by thinking about a recent episode of distress, writing down three ways it could have gone better, and three ways it could have gone worse. This exercise increases the ability to put the situation in perspective, a useful procedure for reducing stress.

The third technique (compensating through self-improvement) works most effectively with stressors that cannot be avoided: an illness, impending divorce, unexpected death or loss of a loved one, etc. The feeling of loss of control that results due to this kind of unexpected event can be balanced by taking on a new challenge. Learning to sew, knit, or scuba dive or teaching someone a skill can reassure that life can still be coped with adequately.

INTEGRATIVE LEARNING EXPERIENCES

Use Table 4.7 for Beginning and Advanced Experiences when called for in this and other chapters. You will note that the "Evaluations" column is divided into "Client Behaviors" and "Practitioner Behaviors." The following guidelines will help you in evaluating the effectiveness of your interventions in each category:

Client Behaviors

- Elicit client evaluative comments, such as:
  "I'm sleeping better."
  "I'm less fatigued."
  "I can listen to criticism without getting mad."
  "You've been very helpful to me with . . . but I expected you to do more . . ."
  "That feels good."
  "I feel whole, peaceful/" (Centering)
  "It's getting easier to do my morning workout."
- Note or record body changes (in bodywork, centering, therapeutic touch, hypnosis, and relaxation procedures—breathing becomes deeper and lower, swallowing may indicate relaxation of throat, skin color changes as circulation improves).

Practitioner Behaviors

Did you:

- Use effective communication skills (initiating, timing, validating, open body posture, consistency of words with gestures/facial expressions/tone of voice, listening, sharing, using "I" or "We" collaborative messages, using clear/concise messages, providing constructive feedback, staying on agreed-upon goal, sharing)?
- Collaborate with client?
- Involve client in decisions?
- Teach client to prioritize wellness needs?
- Assist client to choose wellness goal based on client priorities?
- Assist client to identify blocks to goal attainment?
- Assist client to plan specific measures to overcome blocks to goal attainment?

- Assist client to learn/choose wellness interventions?
- Teach client to evaluate progress toward wellness goal?
- Practice ethically and legally?
- Take steps to ensure client safety?
- Demonstrate interventions correctly without omitting steps?
- Complete interventions within time frame?
- Identify strengths?
- Identify need for further learning/practice?

Table 4.7 Practitioner Process in Promoting Wellness

Assessments	Interventions	Evaluations
(Include teaching or communication problems)	(Include any steps taken by practitioner or client to deal with assessments; include practitioner–client contracts and reinforcement of positive behaviors)	(Evaluate the effectiveness of interventions based on specific observed behaviors; give specific examples for each item; obtain videotape, peer, or faculty feedback regarding effectiveness)

Client Behaviors

Practitioner's (own) Behaviors

Beginning Level

1. Complete the information requested in Table 4.1 with you as client.
2. Complete the information requested in Table 4.2 with you as client.
3. Keep a Stress Awareness Diary for 1 week; summarize your findings.
4. Practice the breathing exercises in this chapter and write a summary using Table 4.7 to organize the information.
5. Practice progressive relaxation to mastery.
6. Practice self-hypnosis (using Table 4.4) to mastery.
7. Practice autogenics to mastery.
8. Practice thought stopping to mastery.
9. Practice refuting one of your irrational ideas using approaches provided in this chapter.
10. Develop coping skills statements for an upcoming situation of your choice.
11. Assess your time management skills, following Eloise's examples.
12. Assess your hardiness and practice skills suggested by Kobasa.

13. Devise interventions for the following clients:

(Give the intervention(s) of choice, *specific* comments you would use to introduce the intervention to a client, and *specific* observations or measurements you would use to evaluate intervention effects.)

A. a student complaining of test anxiety
B. a new graduate complaining of interview anxiety
C. a new employee who fears working with clients
D. a first time parent anxious about bonding with the infant
E. a nursing home resident who feels hopeless
F. a student with low self-esteem
G. an employee resentful that she must return to school for a degree in order to advance in her career
H. a 19-year-old college sophomore who is afraid to leave the dormitory to attend class
I. a 34-year-old secretary who is obsessed with thoughts that she will be raped
J. a 50-year-old executive with hypertension
K. a student with recurring headaches without organic etiology
L. a young executive jogger with backache (no organic etiology)
M. a mother with irritable bowel
N. a student with insomnia
O. an overweight R.N.
P. a victim of an automobile accident who complains of pain despite pain medication
Q. an 84-year-old man diagnosed with terminal cancer
R. a client 2 days postoperative open heart surgery
S. a postoperative client who is scheduled to get out of bed for the first time
T. a cardiac rehabilitation client
U. a client who wishes to quit smoking
V. a client suffering from chronic itching
W. an 8-year-old boy who wets his bed
X. a 28-year-old woman who believes she has no control over what happens to her
Y. a 40-year-old teacher who is always missing deadlines, unable to make decisions, and complains of fatigue and insufficient rest

14. Imagine you are about to teach a client self-hypnosis. What questions or resistances might you anticipate? How would you intervene with each? (Be *specific;* include exact words or actions.)

15. Role play teaching the following to a client; use Table 4.7 to summarize experiences. Discuss the information in *each* column with a peer and get *written* feedback concerning what is omitted, what is well-presented, and hints for further study/practice.

A. Breathing   F. Thought stopping
B. Progressive relaxation   G. Refuting irrational ideas
C. Stress awareness diary   H. Coping skills
D. Self-hypnosis   I. Time management
E. Autogenics   J. Hardiness

Advanced Level

1. Complete any exercises in the beginning level not already completed.
2. Use Table 4.1 with three clients; compare your findings among client with findings of a peer with her clients (sample = 6).
3. Use Table 4.2 with three clients; compare your findings among clients with findings of a peer with her clients (sample = 6).
4. Teach a client how to keep a Stress Awareness Diary, including how to set up the diary, length of recordkeeping, how often progress will be checked and by whom, reinforcement(s), and evaluation procedures. Use Table 4.7 format. Compare your findings with a peer teaching the same procedure.
5. Teach three clients progressive relaxation; be sure to complete a pretreat-interview. Use Table 4.7 format to organize your assessment, interventions, and evaluation. Obtain written feedback from a peer.
6. Teach three clients breathing exercises. Use Table 4.7 format. Obtain written feedback from a peer.
7. Teach three clients self-hypnosis. Use Table 4.4 and Table 4.7 format. Obtain written feedback from a peer.
8. Teach three clients autogenics. Use Table 4.7 format. Obtain written from a peer.
9. Teach three clients thought stopping. Use Table 4.7 format. Obtain written feedback from a peer.
10. Teach three clients how to refute an irrational idea they hold. Use Table 4.7 format. Obtain written feedback from a peer.
11. Teach three clients coping skills. Use Table 4.7 format. Obtain written feedback from a peer.
12. Teach three clients time management skills. Use Table 4.7 format. Obtain written feedback from a peer.
13. Teach three clients hardiness skills. Use Table 4.7 format. Obtain written feedback from a peer.

REFERENCES

Acterberg, J. & Rider, M.S. (1989). Effect of music-assisted imagery on neutrophils and lymphocytes. *Biofeedback and Self-Regulation* 14(3): 247–257.

Basmajian, J.V. (ed.). (1989). Biofeedback: Principles and Practice for Clinicians. 3rd ed. Baltimore: Williams & Wilkins.

Ben-Eliyahu, S., Yirmirya, R, Liebeskind, J.C., Taylor, A.N., and Gale, R.P. (1991). Stress increases metastatic spread of a mammary tumor in rats: Evidence for mediation by the immune system. *Brain, Behavior, and Immunity,* S:193–205.

Benson, H., and Klipper, M. (1976). *The Relaxation Response.* New York: Avon.

Bernhardt, R., and Martin, D. (1977). *Self-Mastery Through Self-Hypnosis.* New York:Signet.

Bricklin, M. (1976). *The Practical Encyclopedia of Natural Healing.* Emmaus, PA: Rodale, pp. 289–290.

Cameron, K. (1991). The effect of music on vasovagal reactions and anxiety among first time blood donors. *Masters Abstracts International*, 31-02: 0758 #71 565.

Cannon, W. (1914). The emergency function of the medulla in pain and the major emotions. *American Journal of Physiology,* 33:356–372.

Davis, M., McKay, M., and Eshelman, E. (1995). *The Relaxation and Stress Reduction Workload,* 2nd ed. Oakland, CA: New Harbinger.

Ellis, A., and Harper, R. (1961). *A Guide to Rational Living.* North Hollywood, CA: Wilshire Books.

Ewin, D. (1978). Relieving suffering and pain with hypnosis. *Geriatrics,* 33(6): 87–89.

Goodman, D. (1974). *Emotional Well-Being Through Rational Behavior Training.* Springfield, IL: Charles C. Thomas.

Hadley, J., and Staudersker, C. (1989). *Hypnosis for Change*: Oakland, CA: New Harbinger Publications.

Halley, F.M. (1991). Self-regulation of the immune system through biobehavioral strategies. *Biofeedback and Self-Regulation,* 16(1):55–73.

Herbert, T.B., and Cohen, S. (1993). Depression and Immunity: A meta-analytic review. *Psychological Bulletin* 113:472–486.

Houldin, A.D., McCorkle, R., and Lowery, B.J. (1993). Relaxation training and psychoimmunological status of bereaved spouses. *Cancer Nursing* 16(2):47–52.

Jacobson, E. (1938). *Progressive Relaxation.* Chicago: University of Chicago Press.

Johnson, N.L. (1991). Physiological and emotional responses to taped music programs in intensive care units. *Masters Abstracts International* 31-02: 0758 # 71762.

Kiecolt-Glaser, J.K., Pennebaker, J.W., and Glaser, R. (1988). Disclosure of traumas and immune function: Health implications for pschotherapy. *Journal of Consulting and Clinical Psychology* 56(2):239–245.

Kobasa, S. (1984). How much stress can you survive? *American Health,* 3(7): 64–77.

LeCron, L. (1964). *Self-Hypnosis.* New York: Signet, pp. 78–92.

Levy, S.M., Huberman, R.B., Whiteside, T.J., Sanzo, K., Lee, J., and Kirkwood, J. (1990). Perceived social support and tumor estrogen/progesterone receptor status as predictors of natural killer cell activity in breast cancer patients. *Psychosomatic Medicine,* 52(1):73–85.

Meichenbaum, D., and Cameron, R. (1974). Modifying what clients say to themselves. In *Self-Control: Power to the Person,* M. Mahoney and R. Cameron, Eds. Monterey, CA: Brooks/Cole.

Post-White, J., and Johnson, M. (1991). Complementary nursing therapies in clinical oncology practice: Relaxation and imagery. *Dimensions in Oncology Nursing,* 5(2):15–20.

Quinn, J.F., and Strelkaukas, A.J. (1993). Psychoimmunologic effects of therapeutic touch on practitioners and recently bereaved recipients: A pilot study. *Advanced Nursing Science,* 15(4): 13–26.

Scandrett, S., and Uecker, S. (1985). Relaxation training. In *Nursing Interventions: Treatments for Nursing Diagnoses,* G. Bulecheck and J. McCloskey, Eds. Philadelphia: W.B. Saunders, pp. 22–48).

Selye, H. (1956). *The Stress of Life.* New York: McGraw-Hill.

Slyfield, C.M. (1992). The effect of music therapy on patient's pain, blood pressure, and heart rate after coronary artery bypass graft surgery. *Masters Abstracts International,* 31-03: 76, #11351497.

Snyder, M. (1984). Progressive relaxation as a nursing intervention: An analysis. *Advances in Nursing Science*, 6(3):47–58.

Zahourek, R. (1978). *Use of relaxation and hypnotic techniques in the care of the difficult patient.* Workshop for nurses at Downstate Medical Center, Brooklyn, NY, November 1, 1978.

Zeagans, L. (1982). Stress and the development of somatic disorders. In *Handbook of Stress: Theoretical and Clinical Aspects,* L. Goldberger and S. Brezwitz, Eds. New York: Free Press.

5

NUTRITIONAL WELLNESS

This chapter discusses the following topics:

- Food and wellness
- Guidelines for reading nutritional information
- Food myths
- Suggested dietary goals
- Vitamins, minerals, and supplements
- Nutrients for prevention
- Drug-nutrient interactions
- Other significant nutrient reactions
- Weight maintenance

FOOD AND WELLNESS

The focus of much funded research has been the study of microbes as the cause of disease, but knowledge is accumulating regarding the preventive and healing aspects of food and the detrimental effects of poor nutrition. As early as 1977, information gathered by the Senate Select Committee on Nutrition and Human Needs associated poor nutrition with 6 of the 10 leading causes of death, "including heart disease, some cancers, stroke and hypertension, arteriosclerosis, diabetes, and cirrhosis of the liver." Table 5.1 identifies signs of balanced eating. Table 5.2 provides one way for assessing what the body needs to be well.

GUIDELINES FOR READING NUTRITIONAL INFORMATION

Some guidelines to keep in mind when reading nutritional information include:

1. Determine the author's background, specificity, and comprehensiveness of references. All authors have biases; be sure you know which ones the author

you are reading has. Many authors do not use complete references, up-to-date references, or only include references supporting their point of view; determine as much as possible which variables are operating.

2.   Go back to the original reference whenever possible to determine unreliable reporting.

3.   Determine the source of funding of the periodical or book; e.g., if food producers are funders, question whether the results or types of research being reported may be biased.

4.   Read as many different kinds of nutritional information as possible in order to get a balanced view of the issues.

5.   When a relatively nonbiased source is found, keep returning to it for information in the future and tell clients about it.

FOOD MYTHS

Be aware of food myths that are held by clients. Some of the most frequently are:

1. *Meat contains more protein than other foods.* Actually, meat contains only about 25% protein and is about in the middle of the protein quantity scale, ranking below soybeans, fish, milk, soybean flour, and eggs.

2. *Large quantities of meat must be eaten to provide sufficient protein to grow and replace body tissues.* Most Americans eat twice the amount of protein their bodies can use; the recommended daily allowance of protein, 50–60 grams, can be reached even when all meat, fish, and poultry are eliminated from the diet. The daily protein requirements of a 170-pound man doing light work is 25 to 30 grams. A bowl of pea or bean soup, a slice of whole grain bread, and a vegetable salad supplies all the protein he needs (Balch & Balch, 1990). For example, by combining wheat and beans, milk and rice, milk and peanuts, or beans and rice, dishes containing all the amino acids necessary for the body can be obtained. Additionally all soybean products such as tofu and tempeh are complete proteins. Fortifying cornmeal with the amino acid, lysine, also results in a complete protein. Strict vegetarians must remember to supplement their intake with vitamin B_{12} which is found only in meat (Balch & Balch, 1990).

3. *Meat offers the highest quality protein available.* Quality of protein refers to amount of protein available that is usable by the body; eggs and milk are more usable by the body than meat is, and soybeans and whole rice are as usable (Lappe, 1975).

4. *Sugar is sugar.* Sugar occurs naturally in milk, fruits, and vegetables; although sugar is being eaten in the food, it is being ingested with fiber, minerals, vitamins, and proteins, thus providing a superior combination of nutrients as compared to processed sugars in candy, sodas, and other sweets.

Table 5.1 Signs of Balanced Eating

One way to ensure your body gets what it needs is to check for signs of balanced eating. Some signs to look for are:

- good endurance and high energy level
- alertness and responsiveness with good attention span
- shiny, lustrous hair
- healthy scalp
- thyroid gland of normal size
- clear, bright eyes
- lack of circles or puffiness around eyes
- moist lips of good color
- pink tongue with papillae present
- pink, firm gums
- clean, straight teeth
- smooth, slightly moist skin
- flat abdomen
- well-developed legs and feet
- lack of tenderness, weakness, or swelling in legs or feet
- normal weight for height, age, and body build
- erect posture with straight back, arms, legs, abdomen in chest slightly out
- well-developed, firm muscles
- feelings of calm
- good appetite and digestion
- easy and regular elimination
- sleeping well

5. *Sugar is a good source of energy.* Refined sugar leads to less energy because the food is digested quickly, and the blood level of sugar (glucose) rises very rapidly. As a result, insulin is released in excess into the blood, and liver reserves of glycogen (stored glucose) are used, leading to fatigue, shakiness, irritability, faintness, and (in some people) violent behavior. Eating refined sugar results in highs and lows, and more coffee (with sugar) or another soda or piece of candy are then used to get a "lift." For high energy, frequent, high-protein meals or complex carbohydrates such as grains or vegetables are recommended.

6. S*tarchy foods put on weight.* Complex carbohydrates such as whole grain pasta, baked potatoes, unrefined rice, and whole grain breads and cereals contain a great deal of fiber that is filling; it is only when butter, margarine, sour cream, or other fillings or toppings are used that calories accrue.

SUGGESTED DIETARY GOALS

The Senate Select Committee on Nutrition of the United States Senate adopted seven dietary goals in 1977 which have been used in *Healthy People 2000* (USDHHS, 1990) as a basis for action:

Table 5.2 What Does Your Body Need?

Because of conflicting opinions and views on nutrition, a useful approach to take at this time is to assume that your body knows what it needs and will begin to tell you when it is not adequately nourished. Some clues your body might give are: ability to sleep after ingesting a particular food, stool the day following eating that food, breath and body odor, and energy level. You might want to begin to chart your body's reactions to one or more foods by asking the following questions:

1. How well does this food seem to go through my digestive system? Does this food seem to be soothing or cleansing or health-promoting?
2. How do I sleep after ingesting this food?
3. What sort of stool is produced the day after I eat this food?
4. How are my breath and body odor the day after I eat this food?
5. How is my energy level the day of and the day after I eat this food?
6. How does what I am eating affect my skin, hair, and fingernails?
7. How does what I am eating affect my body shape and weight?
8. How does what I am eating affect my ability to concentrate?
9. How does what I am eating affect my relationships with others?
10. How does what I am eating affect how I feel about me and my life?

Goal 1. To avoid overweight, consume only as much energy (calories) as expended. Decrease energy intake and increase exercise if overweight. One in three Americans is overweight. The Dietary Goals recommends reducing foods high in fat, refined and processed foods, sugars, and alcohol, and increasing high-fiber foods such as fruits, vegetables, whole grains, and legumes.

Goal 2. Increase consumption of fresh fruits and vegetables and whole grains to 48% of food intake. Complex carbohydrates are satisfying and protect against cardiovascular disease, constipation, cancer, and overweight (Thun, 1992; Ames et al., 1994). To consume 55%–60% of total calories as carbohydrate, meat becomes a condiment, as in Oriental cooking and rice, pasta, potatoes and other starches the main dish. Guidelines for increasing complex carbohydrates and fiber in the diet:

- Choose whole and fresh foods over processed and refined ones; if fresh local foods are not available, choose fresh-frozen ones, avoiding heavy sauces.
- Choose whole wheat products over white, refined flour. The average white flour retains only 76% of the original wheat grain. When refined to white flour, 10-100% of the trace minerals, vitamins, and fiber are lost; only a small minority is replaced in "enriched" products.
- Select whole grain products for breakfast; leftovers from brown rice, bulgar, kasha, or whole grain noodles can be used as cereal. If no leftovers are available, choose hot cereals (avoiding "instant" or "quick cooking" varieties, which imply greater processing) over cold, ready-to-eat cereals made from refined grain products.
- Become creative in increasing complex carbohydrate meals, e.g., chili without beef, salads, soups, sandwich spreads from one or more types of beans and other vegetables, pocket bread sandwiches, vegetable and pasta or rice casseroles.

Goal 3. Reduce consumption of refined and processed sugars to 10% of daily intake. Refined sugars add empty calories that increase weight, rob the body's stores of vitamins and minerals during metabolism, and replace nutritious foods or lead to weight gain. Guidelines for reducing sugar in meal planning are:

- Read labels and avoid foods containing sucrose, raw sugar, glucose, brown sugar, turbinado honey, dextrose, fructose, corn syrup, corn sweetener, and natural sweetener; the closer the sugar is to the beginning of the list of ingredients, the greater the amount of sugar present.
- Substitute fruit juices, nonfat milk, unsweetened tea, mineral water with a slice of lemon, vegetable juice, and water for sugared, fruit-flavored drinks and soft drinks. Although commercial diet soft drinks are low in sugar, they may be high in additives, dyes, phosphates (calcium-robbing), and caffeine.
- Choose fresh fruits or fruits canned in unsweetened juice.
- Choose ready-to-eat cereals with sugar listed as the fourth or lower item on the ingredients list; sweeten cereal with fruit.
- Begin reducing sugar in recipes gradually; use a juice concentrate instead of sugar in recipes.

Goal 4. Reduce fat consumption to 30% of daily intake.

Goal 5. Reduce intake of saturated fat to 10%, and take in 10% of calories in polyunsaturated fats and another 10% in monounsaturated fats.

Goal 6. Reduce cholesterol consumption to 300 grams/day. Saturated fats and cholesterol are strongly associated with increased risk of cardiovascular disease, hypertension, obesity, atherosclerosis, and other degenerative diseases. Polyunsaturated fat is associated with increased risk of cancer. Some guidelines for meeting goals related to dietary fat include:

- Reduce intake of high fat foods: french fries, hamburgers, whole milk, whole milk cheeses, ice cream, bacon, prepared salad dressings, cream, nondairy creamers, hydrogenated oils (available on the grocery shelf and in many prepared foods; read ingredients list on all foods purchased), and whipped cream substitutes.
- Obtain needed essential fatty acids from vegetable oils that are relatively nonprocessed (virgin olive oil; dark, unprocessed oils), unprocessed nuts and seeds, fish, and unprocessed whole grains.
- Reduce dietary cholesterol by lowering intake of eggs, liver, and organ meats, red meats, animal fats (lard and chicken fat or skin), and high-fat dairy products.
- Use low- or nonfat yogurt or cottage cheese as a garnish for baked potatoes.
- Prepare salad dressing from yogurt, nonfat cottage cheese, garlic, onion, spices, vinegar, and lemon juice.
- Select broiled or baked meat, fowl, and fish; remove fat and skin prior to eating.

- Avoid foods implying that fat is used in the preparation, including descriptions such as: refried, creamed, cream sauce, au gratin, parmesan, escalloped, au lait, a la mode, marinated, prime, pot pie, au fromage, stewed, basted, casserole, hollandaise, or crispy.
- Choose foods that are steamed, in broth, in its own juice, poached, roasted, or in tomato or marinara sauce; these imply low-fat preparation.
- Read nutrition information panels prior to purchasing processed foods. Avoid purchasing foods containing: animal fat, egg and egg yolk solids, butter, bacon fat, lard, palm oil, shortening, vegetable fat, hydrogenated or partially hydrogenated oils, whole milk solids, cream and cream sauces, coconut oil, coconut, milk chocolate.
- Elevate meat, fowl, or fish when roasting or broiling; do not baste with drippings; use wine, fruit juice, or broth instead.
- Roast at a low temperature (325–350° F) to enhance flavor and fat removal. High temperatures seal fats into the meat.
- Chill meat or fowl drippings and remove fat prior to preparing sauces or gravies.
- Sauté vegetables in defatted chicken stock.

Goal 7. Limit intake of table salt to 5 grams/day. Use the following guidelines to reduce sodium:

- Read food and medication labels to identify and eliminate foods processed with salt or containing sodium additives, including baking soda, monosodium glutamate (MSG), cough medicines, laxatives, aspirin, sedatives, sodium phosphate, sodium alginate, sodium nitrate, etc.
- Reduce consumption of food processed in brine—olives, sauerkraut, pickles—or soak in water prior to eating.
- Avoid commercial snacks including potato and corn chips, salted peanuts, pretzels, and crackers.
- Avoid salted or smoked meats, sandwich meats, bacon, hot dogs, corned or chipped beef, sausage, and salt pork.
- Reduce or eliminate salted condiments: catsup, mustard, Worcestershire sauce, bouillon cubes, soy sauce, barbeque sauce.
- Limit processed and high salt cheeses; choose the low salt varieties.

Be aware that there still is no solid evidence that lowering salt (NaCl) intake will prevent or control high blood pressure. If it does, only 30 to 40% of adults are salt-sensitive (Muntzell & Drücke, 1992).

VITAMINS AND MINERALS

There are arguments for and against the need for vitamin and mineral supplementation. The American Dietetic Association National Center for Nutrition and Dietetics and the President's Council on Physical Fitness and Sports now recommend using the Food Guide Pyramid including 6–11 daily servings of bread, cereal, rice, and/or pasta; 3–5 daily servings of vegetables; 2–4 daily servings of fruit; 2–3 daily servings of milk, yogurt and/or cheese; 2–3 daily servings of meat, poultry, fish, dry beans, eggs, and/or nuts; and sparing use of fats, oils, and/or sweets (1995).

Loomis (1992) compared fatalities due to vitamin supplements versus prescription and nonprescription, legal drugs to illustrate the safety of vitamin use. For example, in 1990, there was one fatality due to niacin abuse and none for any other vitamin, compared to 487 fatalities due to pharmaceutical drugs. His statistics from 1983–1990 show that vitamins are 2,500 times safer than prescription and nonprescription pharmaceuticals. Some of the reasons cited in favor of proper vitamin supplementation are due to changes in the available food sources.

Justification for Supplementation

- Some soils are depleted and produce crops that are nutritionally inferior.
- Toxic insectides leave harmful residues on food and kill important soil microrganisms and earthworms.
- The increasing use of chemicals in the processing of food has depleted them nutritionally.
- Increasing numbers of people eat vitamin-free sugar as 25% of their daily food intake.
- Chemical additives replace other essential food elements and may also be toxic.
- Numerous life experiences require additional vitamin and mineral stores to reduce stress, including: any difficulty with the digestive tract (diarrhea, colitis, liver or gall bladder disorders); pregnancy; breastfeeding; increased physical activity; infections; the use of antibiotics, aspirin, estrogen, steroids, sulfa drugs, or anticoagulants; inhaling polluted air; drinking polluted water; prolonged emotional stress; smoking or being in a smoke-filled room; fractures; alcohol intake.
- A change in lifestyle in America to a more hectic pace has decreased effective meal planning and led to more "fast-food" meals.

For these reasons, even if it were possible to eat a wide variety of foods, vitamin and mineral supplementation may be necessary. As early as 1943 the Food and Drug Administration (FDA) recognized that food processing was destroying important nutrients. Regulations were passed requiring "enrichment" of processed foods; at the time, the FDA noted that enriched foods were second best to unprocessed ones.

The argument against vitamin and mineral supplementation is that if everyone eats a wide variety of foods, all essential nutrients are available. This argument may be most relevant for the ambulatory, well-informed consumer who is able and willing to eat the wide variety of foods necessary.

Additional information that may be useful as a reference source for practitioner and client appears in the following tables: Vitamin Functions, Deficiency Signs, and Food Sources (Table 5.3), RDAs and Reasons for Supplementation (Table 5.4), Reference to Minerals (Table 5.5), and Wellness-Enhancing Foods (Table 5.6).

NUTRIENTS FOR PREVENTION

Of all cancers in the United States, 35% are estimated to be caused by dietary factors and may be preventable. Diets high in fat or calories are associated with five of the six most common cancers: breast, colorectal, pancreatic, prostatic, and uterine (Shapiro, 1992). There is some dispute whether it is the vitamins per se, or other dietary factors in vegetables and fruits which make the most important preventives (Greenberg et al., 1994).

However, the U.S. Department of Health and Human Services, the U.S. Department of Agriculture, and the National Academy of Science (Eat more fruits and vegetables, 1991), all recommend a diet low in fat and high in fiber, including five servings of fruits and vegetables a day. (One serving is 1/2 cup of fruit, 3/4 cup of juice, 1/2 cup cooked vegetables, 1 cup leafy vegetables, or 1/4 cup dried fruit). Cruciferous vegetables—bok choy, broccoli, brussel sprouts, cabbage, and cauliflower—are specifically recommended and should be eaten several times a week. At least one vitamin A- and C- rich, and high-fiber selection should be eaten daily.

Although nutrients may be effective preventive agents for numerous diseases, the best researched in this regard are cancer and cardiovascular disease. Each category will be considered below. The benefits of a vegetarian food plan for life appear in Table 5.5

Cancer and Preventive Nutrients

Vitamin A, Beta-Carotene and Cancer. As early as 1926, the connection between vitamin A and cancer was made. Laboratory animals deficient in dietary vitamin A developed gastric carcinoma. The two-step model of cancer included an initiation stage and a promotion stage. Plant derived provitamin A (the carotenes) can affect both phases (Garrison & Somer, 1985).

Major dietary studies have found a correlation between the incidence of various types of cancer (lung, mouth, colon, stomach, prostate, and cervical) and beta-carotene intake (Kummet & Meyskens, 1983; Kvale, Bjelke, & Gart, 1982; Malone, 1991; Willett et al., 1993). Foods rich in beta-carotene include carrots, tomatoes, spinach, apricots, peaches, and cantaloupes. Cruciferous vegetables also seem to exert a cancer-protective effect for gastrointestinal and respiratory tract tumors. Examples of cruciferous vegetables include cabbage, broccoli, brussels sprouts, kohlrabi, and cauliflower. Hunter et al. (1993) found that a low intake of vitamin A may increase the risk of breast cancer.

Folate Deficiency and Cancer. Cancer of the cervix ranks as the ninth most common cause of cancer death among women in the United States, and is by far the commonest cancer among women in the developing world. In a case-control study, Butterworth and others (1992) demonstrated that a deficiency of folic acid makes cervical cells more susceptible to the effects of known carcinogens.

Vitamin C and Cancer. Nitrosamines are compounds that have been demonstrated to cause cancer in animals. A variety of foods, cigarette smoke, and food preservatives (nitrates and nitrites) have been linked in animal studies to cancer. Vitamin C has been found useful in inhibiting nitrosamine formation from nitrates and nitrites (Bharucha, Cross, & Rubin, 1980). Vitamin C may also reduce free radical damage (through its antioxidant ability), which is likely significant in the pathophysiology of some cancers, cataract and Parkinson's disease (Ward, 1994). Animal studies also suggest vitamin C reduces immune system damage (Kubova et al., 1993).

When dietary habits of large populations are reviewed, foods rich in vitamin C appear to have a cancer-protective effect (Stahelin, 1991), but these foods are also rich in vitamin A and folic acid. All of these and dietary fiber have been shown to offer some cancer protection (National Academy of Science Committee on Diet, Nutrition, and Cancer, 1982).

Vitamin C has been found useful in blocking the formation of N-nitrosos compounds (which are converted to carcinogens), thus decreasing the risk of bladder cancer (Schlegel, 1975), and may be useful in preventing stomach, pancreatic, liver, and colon cancer (Stahelin, 1991; Nyandieka & Wakkesi, 1993).

Selenium and Cancer. The cancer-protective nature of selenium is supported primarily by epidemiological studies. In the United States and other countries where the soil and forage crops in certain regions are deficient in selenium, the incidence of death from cancer of the digestive organs, lung, breast, and lymph cancer is greater than in those areas that have a high-selenium content in forage crops (Shamberger & Willis, 1971). A comparison of evidence collected from 27 countries revealed that the incidence of cancer was significantly lower in populations with high dietary selenium intake (Schrauzer, White, & Schneider, 1977).

When case-control studies have been conducted on those with cancer, their selenium status was significantly lower than that of a control group for cancer of the breast, gastrointestinal tract, Hodgkin's disease, lymphocytic leukemia, pulmonary carcinoma, otolaryngeal carcinoma, genitourinary carcinoma, and colon and skin cancer (Calautti et al., 1980; McConnell et al., 1980; Willet et al., 1983; Wang, 1992; Han, 1993).

Table 5.3   Vitamin Functions, Deficiency Symptoms, and Food Sources

Vitamin	Functions	Deficiency symptoms or signs	Sources
A and its precursor, beta-carotene	helps fight infection, maintains cell wall strength, and prevents viruses from penetrating and reproducing; blocks production of cancerous tumors	night blindness, itching and burning of eyes, redness of eyelids, drying of mucous membranes, colds or respiratory troubles, dry rough skin, pimples or acne, susceptibility to eye infections, difficulty urinating or performing sexually	carrots, broccoli, kale, turnip greens, watercress, beets, dandelion greens, spinach, eggs, milk fat, papayas, parsley, red peppers, fish liver oils, sweet potatoes, pumpkin, yellow squash, apricots, cantaloupes, organ meats*
B₁ (thiamine)	promotes appetite and good digestion, plays an important role in oxidation, blood and protein metabolism, and growth	tiredness with inability to sleep, swelling legs, loss of appetite, lack of enthusiasm, forgetting things regularly, aching or tender calf muscles, rapid heartbeat, over-reacting to normal stress, constipation, feeling of going crazy	sunflower seeds, brewer's yeast, beef kidney,* whole wheat flour, rolled oats, green peas, soybeans, beef heart, lima beans, crabmeat, brown rice, asparagus, raisins, desiccated liver, wheat germ
B₂ (riboflavin)	contributes to protein and carbohydrate metabolism, tissue repair and formation, growth in infants, proper nitrogen balance in adults, light adaptation	feeling trembly, dizzy, or sluggish, burning feet, chapping lips, tiring easily, being overly nervous, having bloodshot eyes	beef, liver, kidney, or heart,* ham, chicken, hazelnuts, peanuts, hickory nuts, soybeans, soy flour, wheat germ and whole wheat products. spinach, kale, peas, lima beans. brewer's yeast, sunflower seeds, eggs

Table 5.3 (*continued*)

B₃ (niacin)	dilates blood vessels, aids in carbohydrate metabolism and the use of vitamins B₁ and B₂	having cold feet or body numbness, having a swollen bright red tongue or gums, feeling overly anxious, weak, or tired, having memory loss, developing prickly heat rash	wheat germ, wheat bran, brewer's yeast, salmon, prunes, lentils, chicken, peanuts, sunflower seeds, tuna, turkey, rabbit
B₆ (pyridoxine)	activates enzymes, aids in metabolism of fats, carbohydrates, potassium, iron, protein, and formation of hormones, nucleic acids, and antibodies, hemoglobin, and lecithin, dissolves cholesterol and regulates water imbalance, may be useful in fighting off cancer, one form of anemia, and tooth decay	feeling tense, irritable, or nervous, not being able to concentrate or sleep, having tics, tremors, twitches, bad breath, seborrheic dermatitis or eczema, bloating, puffiness, soreness, or cramping in menstruating or menopausal women	brewer's yeast, sunflower seeds, toasted wheat germ, brown rice, soybeans, white beans, liver, chicken, mackerel, salmon, tuna, bananas, walnuts, peanuts, sweet potatoes, cooked cabbage
B₁₂	maintains normal red blood cell formation and nervous system, aids in RNA and DNA manufacture, conversion of folic acid to folinic acid, carbohydrate, fat, and protein metabolism, fertility, and growth and resistance to germs	feeling apathetic, moody, forgetful, suspicious, soreness in arms or legs or having difficulty walking or talking, jerking of arms or legs	organ meats,* raw beef, clams, oysters, sardines, crab, crayfish, mackerel, trout, herring, eggs, some cheeses, nutritional yeast, sea vegetables (kombu, dulse, kelp, wakame), fermented soyfoods (tempeh, natto, and miso)

Table 5.3 (*continued*)

Vitamin	Functions	Deficiency symptoms or signs	Sources
Folic acid	vital to blood formation, cell growth, synthesis of RNA or DNA, resistance to infections and to proper mental functioning	looking pale and wan, feeling "pooped," getting brownish spots on face and hands, panting with slight exertion	asparagus, desiccated or fresh liver,* fresh dark green un-cooked vegetables, wheat bran, turnips, potatoes, orange juice, black-eyed peas, lima beans, watermelon, oysters, cantaloupe
Pantothenic acid	protects against environmental stress and infection, works with pyridoxine and folic acid to create antibodies, assists in production of body energy, protects against side effects of some antibiotics, aids in expelling trapped intestinal gas	having balky bowels, chronic gas or distension, feeling fatigued or not hungry, having constant respiratory infections, strange itching or burning sensations	soy flour, sunflower seeds, dark buckwheat, sesame seeds, brewer's yeast, peanuts, lobster, wheat bran, broccoli, mush-rooms, eggs, oysters, sweet potatoes, cauliflower, organ meats*
Biotin	aids in metabolism of carbohydrates, proteins, and fats, assists in growth, maintenance of skin, hair, nerves, sebaceous glands, bone marrow, and sex glands	having poor appetite, sore mouth and lips, dermatitis, nausea and vomiting, depression, pallor, muscle pains, pains around the heart, tickling sensation in hands and feet	nutritional yeast, liver,* eggs, mushrooms, lima beans, yogurt, and a variety of nuts, fish, and grains

Table 5.3 (*continued*)

Vitamin	Functions	Deficiency symptoms or signs	Sources
Inositol	not clear, but seems to be useful in controlling cholesterol level, hair, growth, fat metabolism	not known	wheat germ, oranges, grapefruit, watermelon, peas, cantaloupes, whole grain breads and cereals, molasses, nuts, brewer's yeast, bulgar wheat, lima beans, oysters, peaches, lettuce, brown rice
Choline	essential to nerve fluid, liver functioning, keeping blood pressure down, increasing body resistance to infection	not known, possibly poor thinking ability	egg yolks, soybeans, liver,* brewer's yeast, fish, peanuts, wheat germ, lecithin
C (ascorbic acid)	contributes to health of blood vessels, gums, teeth, and bones, essential to assimilation of iron, aids body in fighting off infection and cancer-producing substances and in normalizing blood cholesterol level, detoxifies some of the poisons due to smoking, aids in healing process, essential to collagen (body "glue"), slows down aging, and protects against stress, works synergistically with vitamin E	frequent bruises, poor healing, bleeding gums when toothbrushing, frequent infections, feeling run down, having an aching back due to disc lesions	green peppers, honeydew melon, cooked broccoli or brussels sprouts or kale, cantaloupes, strawberries, papaya, cooked cauliflower, oranges, watercress, raspberries, parsley, raw cabbage, grapefruit, blackberries, lemons, onions, sprouts, spinach, tomatoes, rose hip tea or powder

Table 5.3 (*continued*)

Vitamin	Functions	Deficiency symptoms or signs	Sources
D	vital for maintaining health and growth of bones, for using calcium, and for metabolic functions affecting eyes, heart, and nervous system, should be taken with calcium	weakness and generalized bone aches, localized back pain on arising or bending over, pain in areas where spinal vertebrae may have collapsed, brittle bones that break easily, pain in mid- to lower back	fish, liver oil, vitamin D-enriched milk, eggs, salmon, tuna
E	seems to be useful in any condition where there is actual or threatened clotting, decrease in blood supply, increased oxygen need, externally when there are burns, or sores to heal, or to protect against exposure to radiation, body needs zinc to maintain proper levels of vitamin E	not known	nutritional yeast, wheat germ, peanuts, outer leaf of cabbage, leafy portions of broccoli and cauliflower, raw spinach, asparagus, whole grain rice or wheat or oats, cold pressed wheat germ cottonseed, or safflower oil, cornmeal, eggs, sweet potatoes
K	essential to blood clotting	some types of bleeding without clotting	spinach, cabbage, cauliflower, tomatoes, pork liver,* lean meat, peas, carrots, soybeans, potatoes wheat germ, egg yolks

* Remember: Any chemicals ingested by animals concentrate in their organs and especially their livers; if you decide to eat organ meats to ensure adequate intake of vitamins, you might consider taking extra amounts of the vitamins that detoxify your body, such as Vitamin C and pantothenic acid.

Table 5.4 Recommended Amounts of Vitamins for Adults; Reasons Supplementation May Be Needed

Vitamin	RDA	Alternative Recommendations**	Reasons supplementation may be needed
A* or beta-carotene	Adults: 5,000 I.U. daily Nursing mothers: 4,000 I.U. daily Pregnant women: 6,000	10,000 I.U. daily; children require less, based on their weight Pregnant women require more	Americans are eating 30 pounds less fresh fruit and 20 pounds less vegetables per capita per year than in 1950; cooking dramatically decreases the value of the vitamin; widespread use of fertilizers and pesticides interferes with body's ability to convert carotene into vitamin A; high-protein diets require more vitamin A to process; cold temperatures, air pollution require additional amounts of the vitamin.
B_1 (thiamine)	1.2–1.5 mg daily	50 mg	Cereal and rice producers remove thiamine when germ and outer coating are removed; large quantities are lost in cooking water; people who eat little or no organ meats, fresh vegetables, oatmeal, potatoes, and beans may receive little thiamine, as do people who have diarrhea, who eat excess sugars or carbohydrates, drink coffee or alcohol, take antibiotics, or smoke, and those exposed to stress or aging processes.
B_2 (riboflavin)	1.3–1.7 mg daily	50 mg	Supplements are needed by people who eat snack foods, processed desserts, or commercial baked goods; the vitamin is destroyed by cooking or when antibiotics or oral contraceptives are taken; it is destroyed when milk bottles or meat containers are left exposed to light.
B_3	18–20 mg daily	100 mg daily	Heavy intake of highly refined and/or carbohydrate foods requires more B_3 to metabolize; it is lost during cooking; its metabolism is interfered with when taking oral antibiotics; illness and taking alcoholic beverages decreases its absorption.

Table 5.4 (continued)

Vitamin	RDA	Alternative Recommendations**	Reasons supplementation may be needed
B_6 (pyridoxine)	Male adults: 2 mg daily Nursing and pregnant women: 1.6 mg. daily	50 mg daily	Losses of B_6 are due to refining, cooking, processing, storing, and to eating a high-protein diet; there is an increased need when taking steroids (such as cortisone and estrogen), oral contraceptives, or when pregnant or menstruating.
B_{12}	2 micrograms (mcg) daily	300 mcg daily	When eating only vegetarian meals.
Folic acid	400 mcg daily		Needed during pregnancy for an adequate development of fetal nerve cells, when taking oral contraceptives, when growing or aging, when faced with trauma, infection, or chronic daily stress, or when drinking alcoholic beverages; works best when combined with Vitamin B_{12}.
Pantothenic acid (PABA)	4–7 mg daily	25 mg daily	Needed to supplement processed food; greater need when subjected to infection, environmental stress, x-rays, surgery, or antibiotics; helps protect against sunburn.
Biotin	No RDA	30 mcg daily	Needed when eating raw eggs or taking antibiotics or sulfa drugs or when eating beef (cattle are routinely given antibiotics and hormones).
Choline	No RDA	100 mg daily	Infants need it if not breast fed (cow's milk does not contain this vitamin but breast milk does).
Inositol		100 mg daily	Caffeine may rob the body of this nutrient.

Table 5.4 (*continued*)

Vitamin	RDA	Alternative Recommendations**	Reasons supplementation may be needed
C	30–45 mg daily	1000–3000 mg daily	Needed to slow down aging processes, increase healing of infection, disease, or injury; decrease effects of toxic chemicals in the environment; if taking aspirin, more of this vitamin is needed; when smoking or drinking, more is required; soaking vegetables and fresh fruits in water or exposing fruit or juices to air destroys this vitamin.
D*	200–400 I.U. daily		Calcium is not absorbed without sufficient vitamin D; needed at times of insufficient sun exposure in winter, when soot and air pollution filter out sun rays, when spending long hours in offices or indoors; when taking steroids, or when smoking.
E	12–15 I.U. daily	600 I.U. daily	When outer leaves of vegetables are not eaten; when vegetables are placed in vigorously boiling water to cook (rather than bringing the water to a boil); when eating processed foods, exposed to smog, drinking chlorinated water, undertaking strenuous exercise, when exposed to air purifiers, static electricity, sun, x-rays; by those who take oxygen as a therapeutic measure, have had a heart attack or burn.
K	65–80 mcg	100 mcg of alfalfa	People who are elderly, women with prolonged menstruation, people with liver disease, diarrhea, colitis, or who take antibiotics or anticoagulants (blood-thinners).

*Note: Vitamins A and D are the only two vitamins that can be toxic if taken in excess; extra amounts of other vitamins are excreted by the body. If you note symptoms of overdosage in vitamins A or D, discontinue taking it until symptoms disappear, then take a smaller dose. Symptoms of vitamin A overdosage: bone or joint pain that comes and goes, fatigue, insomnia, loss of hair, dryness and fissuring of the lips, loss of appetite, peeling and flaking skin, dizziness. Symptoms of Vitamin D overdosage: nausea, weight loss, loss of appetite, head pain, calcification of bones, and in children a reduction in growth rate. RDAs are based on information provided in *Vitamins and Minerals* by Ellen Moyer, Peoples Medical Society, Allentown, PA, 1993.
** Balch & Balch (1990). *Prescription for Nutritional Healing.* Garden City Park, NY: Avery Publishing Company. The authors suggest working with a health care professional to settle on the appropriate supplements and doses. Individual needs are unique and ever-changing. RDAs were formulated for borderline health, not maximum wellness. Even Balch & Balch agree that nutrition (including supplements) must be combined with exercise and a positive attitude to obtain the best results. Suggested doses are based on the Balchs' extensive study of the literature.

Table 5.5 Reference to Minerals, Recommended Amounts, Functions, Sources, and Factors Leading to Insufficient Intake

Mineral	Functions	Best Sources	Factors leading to insufficient intake
Calcium RDA: 800 mg/day 1.5 g for menopausal women Alternate recommendation*: 1,500 mg/day	Keeps body framework rigid and teeth strong; creates tranquility in nervous system and calms nervousness; necessary for transmission of nerve impulses and for muscle contraction, clotting, some enzymes, "glue" (collagen) that holds body together and cells in place, and to regulate transport of substances in and out of cells	milk, cheese, eggs, green leafy vegetables, fish, butter, tomatoes, whole wheat bread, yogurt, canned sardines, molasses, almonds, soy milk, buttermilk, tofu (Because 1500 mg may be difficult to achieve by eating, supplementation may be necessary, especially for menopausal women. Calcium citrate is the most absorbable, safe form.)	dieting to restrict calories or cholesterol; eating snack foods; drinking soft drinks; having a high protein intake
Chromium RDA: 50–200 mg Alternative Recommendation*: 150 mcg	Helps to keep blood sugar levels in check	brewer's yeast, wheat germ, calf's liver, and animal proteins except fish	refinement of cereal and grain products remove chromium; the elderly and those who are pregnant or protein-calorie malnourished are at risk for deficiency
Copper RDA: 1.5–3 mgm		almonds, avocadoes, barley, beans, dandelion greens, lentils	body levels are reduced by high intake of zinc or vitamin C (and vice versa)
Iodine RDA: 150 mcg		sea vegetables, kelp	depleted soil

113

Table 5.5 (*continued*)

Mineral	Functions	Best Sources	Factors leading to insufficient intake
Iron RDA: 15 mg to age 50 then 10 mg/day Alternative recommendation*: 18 mg/day	Works with copper to produce hemoglobin, an essential substance that carries oxygen to and from the body	organ meats, red meats, kidney beans, molasses, egg yolk, whole-grain breads and cereals	infants remaining on milk for long periods of time or those who are born of women who have low stores of iron; women who are menstruating, pregnant, breastfeeding or post-menopausal
Iodine/Kelp RDA: 130-150 mcg/day Alternative recommendation*: 225 mcg/day	Necessary for normal functioning of thyroid gland; may protect against breast cancer	seafood, brown rice, beans, bananas, green leafy vegetables, kelp	living in areas where soil is low in this mineral (Great Lakes and Rocky Mountain regions)
Magnesium RDA: 250-350 mg/day Alternative recommendations*: 750 mg/day	Works with calcium to ensure good muscle movement and a strong heart beat; seems to prevent blood vessel and heart disease	whole grain breads and cereals, fresh peas, brown rice, soy flour, wheat germ, nuts, swiss chard, figs, green leafy vegetables, citrus fruits, dolomite	having diarrhea, vomiting, taking diuretics, drinking soft water, eating processed foods

Table 5.5 (continued)

Mineral	Functions	Best Sources	Factors leading to insufficient intake
Manganese RDA: 2.5–5mg/day Alternative recommendation*: 2.5–5 mg/day needed	Important to fat metabolism, bone formation, brain function, reproduction, and may protect against cancer of the pancreas	nuts, seeds, whole grains, fruits and vegetables, dry beans and peas, oatmeal	high levels of calcium and phosphorus diminish absorption of manganese
Phosphorus RDA: 800 mg/day	Helps form nucleic acids; a component of cell membranes; aids in metabolism and storage and release of energy; a component of B vitamin coenzymes	liver, yogurt, milk, brown rice, wheat germ, sunflower seeds, brewer's yeast, meat, seafood, nuts, eggs, peas, beans, lentils	people with kidney disease; taking high doses of antacids
Potassium RDA: 1600–2000 mg Alternative recommendation*: 99 mg/day	Works in concert with sodium to move materials through cell walls (osmosis) and maintains acid-base balance; helps muscles contract, heart to beat regularly, nerves to carry impulses properly, and food to be turned into energy	shredded raw cabbage, bananas, turkey, apples, fresh apricots, cooked broccoli, baked potato, wheat germ, spinach, dried fruit, fresh fruits and fruits and vegetables of all kinds	using convenience foods and highly processed foods; profuse sweating; taking certain diuretics (water pills) to lose fluid; taking cardiovascular drugs, steroids, laxatives, enemas; eating licorice candy; breastfeeding, having depression or ulcerative colitis
Selenium RDA: 50–70 mcg/day Alternative recommedation*: 200 mcg/day	Protects against heart disease and cancer; detoxifies the body from effects of pollutants and radiation; important for healthy skin and hair and for production of sperm cells	high protein foods such as meats, seafoods; whole-grain breads and cereals; brewer's yeast; asparagus, garlic, mushrooms	eating beef fed on corn or eating grains grown in selenium-poor soil (northeast, Florida, parts of Washington and Oregon, parts of the Midwest); exposure to industrial pollutants

Table 5.5 (continued)

Mineral	Functions	Best Sources	Factors leading to insufficient intake
Sodium RDA: needed amount not established	Maintains osmotic pressure in the fluid outside the cells	celery, carrots, beets, cucumbers, string beans, asparagus, turnips, strawberries, oatmeal, cheese, eggs, coconut, black figs	some kidney and adrenal diseases; diarrhea; vomiting
Sulfur RDA: needed amount not established	Part of the structure of amino acids, such as keratin, the protein of the hair; component of thiamine and biotin (vitamins); required for many oxidation-reduction reactions and coenzymes; contained in blood and other tissues; detoxifying agent; part of material found in skin, bones, tendons, and cartilage	cabbage, peas, beans, cauliflower brussels sprouts, eggs, horseradish, shrimp, chestnuts, mustard greens, onions, asparagus	no information available
Zinc RDA: 10–15 mg/day Alternative recommendation*: 30 mg/day	Necessary for adequate breathing and digestion; important to taste, hearing, smell, appetite, normal growth and sexual functioning and reproduction, wound healing, healthy hair, good complexion; decreases lead toxicity	oysters, herring, liver, eggs, nuts, wheat germ and red meats	exposure to lead in gasoline, paints, joints in food cans, lead dust, drinking water that comes through lead pipes; eating canned tomatoes in quantity; foods containing phytate (beans, whole grains, and peanut butter) or calcium interfere with zinc absorption; being a vegetarian; regularly eating imitation meats, fast foods, white bread, fried potatoes, and rich desserts; drinking alcohol; being pregnant; having a cold infection, kidney disease, heart problems, cancer, or taking birth control pill.

* Extracted from Balch & Balch (1990), *Prescription for Nutritional Healing,* Garden City Park, NY: Avery Publishing Company, pp. 11-12.

Table 5.6 Wellness-Enhancing Foods

Eat these often	Vitamins provided	Minerals provided	Other advantages
Raw spinach*	A, B$_2$, B$_6$, C, folic acid, E, K	calcium, magnesium, potassium copper, iodine, manganese	provides fiber and complex carbohydrate
Wheat germ (toasted)	B$_1$, B$_2$, B$_3$, B$_{12}$, inositol, choline, E	magnesium, potassium, chromium	high protein
Brewer's** yeast	B$_1$, B$_2$, B$_3$, B$_6$, B$_{12}$, pantothenic acid, biotin, inositol, choline, E, folic acid	selenium, chromium, copper, zinc, magnesium, calcium, potassium	can be sprinkled on foods or in drinks
Kale	A, B$_2$, C	calcium, magnesium, copper, iodine manganese	provides fiber and complex carbohydrate; neutralizes free radicals and is associated with lowering cancer risk
Cantaloupe	A, folic acid, inositol, C	manganese	provides fiber and is a good dessert substitute for "sweets", neutralizes free radicals and lowers cancer risk
Sunflower seeds	B$_1$, B$_2$, B$_3$, B$_6$, pantothenic acid	manganese	easy to carry for a quick snack, provides fiber to lower risk of colon cancer and diverticulitis

* Spinach contains oxalic acid that can decrease the amount of available calcium, so be sure to eat enough calcium from other sources to make up for this.
** Not recommended for people who have yeast infections.

Table 5.6 (continued)

Eat these often	Vitamins provided	Minerals provided	Other advantages
Onions	C, inositol		Reduces cancer risk, lowers cholesterol
Mustard Greens	C, inositol, B_5		Lowers cancer risk
Sweet potatoes/ yams/pumpkins	E, inositol, A		High fiber, lowers cancer risk
Garlic	A		Natural antibiotic action, reduces cholesterol, reduces cancer risk
Parsley	Most nutrient-dense food known		Protects against cancer risk
Rosemary			Inhibits carcinogens or co-carcinogens
Brown rice	B_1, B_6, inositol	magnesium, iodine	Inexpensive, good source of protein when combined with beans, eggs, or milk products
Broccoli	A, folic acid, pantothenic acid, C, E	calcium, magnesium, potassium, copper, iodine, manganese	provides fiber and complex carbohydrate; neutralizes free radicals and protects against cancer risk and diverticulitis

Table 5.6 (continued)

Eat these often	Vitamins provided	Minerals provided	Other advantages
Chicken (no skin)	B_2, B_3, B_6, folic acid	copper, chromium	low fat; very usable protein
Whole grains	B_1, B_2, B_{12}, choline biotin, inositol, E	calcium, magnesium, iron, selenium, manganese, chromium	provides fiber, lowers colon cancer risk, natural laxative, protects against diverticulitis
Cauliflower	pantothenic acid C, E, K	manganese	provides fiber, lowers cancer and diverticulitis risk, complex carbohydrate
Peas	B_2, inositol, K	magnesium, manganese	low calorie, complex carbohydrate, provides fiber, lowers cancer and diverticulitis risk
Lima Beans	folic acid, biotin, inositol, B_2	manganese	complex carbohydrate, provides fiber to lower cancer and diverticulitis risk
Grapefruit (and citrus fruit)	inositol, C, P	magnesium, manganese	lower calorie, complex carbohydrate, corrects acid imbalance; white material beneath the peel contains flavonoids and pectin to reduce pain, lower cholesterol, heal bruises
Soybeans (and other dried beans)	B_1, B_2, B_3, choline K	manganese	inexpensive source of protein, provides fiber. associated with low cancer rate

Table 5.6 (*continued*)

Eat these often	Vitamins provided	Minerals provided	Other advantages
Asparagus	B_1, folic acid, C, E,	manganese	low calorie, complex carbo-hydrates, provides fiber to lower cancer and diverticulitis risk
Cabbage	B_6, C, E, K	potassium	low calorie, complex carbohydrate, provides fiber, lowers cancer and diverticulitis risk
Carrots	A, K	potassium, manganese	low calorie, complex carbohydrate; provides fiber, associated with low cancer rate
Fish (especially salmon, mackerel, and sardines)	B_3, B_6, B_{12}, biotin, choline, co-enzyme Q10	calcium zinc, copper, selenium	low fat, highly usable protein, reduces cancer risk, protects heart
Yogurt (lowfat; plain)	D	calcium	high protein, low fat, provides helpful bacteria
Sprouts	A, B_2, B_3, folic acid pyridoxine, pantothenic acid, E, K	calcium iron, phosphorus, potassium	low calorie, inexpensive, high protein, provides fiber, lowers risk of diverticulitis

Source: Extracted from Simone, C.B., M.D. *Cancer and Nutrition: A Ten-Point Plan to Reduce Your Risk of Getting Cancer.* Garden City Park: Avery Publishing Group, 1992.

Table 5.7 Does Vegetarianism Protect Against Chronic Disease?

Vegetarianism seems to have a lot of advantages and some disadvantages. Let's look at the research and see why a plant-based meal plan may enhance wellness.

Cancer. Vegetarians eat more beans, whole grains, vegetables, and fruits than meat eaters so they take in more fiber, vitamins A and C, and protease inhibitors (anticancer agents). Vegans, who eat no meat, eggs, or dairy products, get a lower percentage of their calories from fat than do nonvegetarians. A low fat diet is clearly related to protection from cancers of the breast, colon, and prostate (R.L. Phillips, et al., Cancer in vegetarians, unpublished research reported in *Nutr. Act* 10 [5]:9, 1983; *N Engl J Med* 307 : 1542, 1982; Am J Epidem 131 : 918, 1989).

Osteoporosis (britttle bone syndrome). It is not clear why vegetarians have less osteoporosis, but they do. One explanation is that meat meals cause the body to excrete excess calcium (*J Am Diet Assoc* 76 : 148, 1980).

Heart Disease. Both types of vegetarians have lower blood cholesterol levels than do nonvegetarians (*J Hum Nutr* 35 : 437, 1981; *Am J Clin Nutr* 23:249, 1970). A new study (unpublished research reported in *Nutr Act* 19(5):9, 1983) shows they also have lower heart attack rates. Twenty-five thousand Seventh Day Adventists (SDA) were monitored for 20 years. Males who ate meat six or more times a week were twice as likely to die of heart disease as vegetarian SDAs if they were 55 or older and ran four times the risk of a fatal heart attack than vegetarian SDAs if they were aged 40–54.

Obesity. Studies show the average lacto-ovo (eats milk products and eggs) vegetarian is slightly leaner than meat eaters and vegans are between 8 and 20 pounds lighter. (*J Hum Nutr* 35:437, 1981; *Am J Med* 36 : 269, 1964; *N Engl J Med* 292 : 1148, 1975; *J Am Diet Assoc* 77 : 655, 1980).

High Blood Pressure. Vegetarianism lowers blood pressure, probably because it helps people lose weight, especially if they omit meat, eggs, and dairy products (*Am J Epidem* 100 : 390, 1974; *Am J Clin Nutr* 48 : 795, 1988).

Diabetes. The vegan diet can assist in weight loss and is very similar to the high-complex carbohydrate, high-fiber plan now being used to treat adult onset diabetes. This raises the question of whether the meal plan may also be preventive.

A vegetarian diet may reduce the risk of *developing* diabetes (Snowden & Phillips, Raghwiam 1985). Specifically, onions (Sharma, 1977), garlic (Sheela and Augusti, 1992), Fenugreek seeds (Sharma, Raghwiam, and Rao, 1990) have been studied. Cow's milk and nicotinamide (a B-vitamin) have been implicated as factors in Type 1 diabetes in children (Knip, 1992).

Vegetarianism offers all these potential benefits, but there are a few disadvantages. Although lacto-ovo vegetarians have no more nutritional deficiencies than meat eaters (*J Am Diet Assoc* 77:61, 1980), vegans, particularly children, may have difficulty obtaining sufficient vitamins D and B-12, calcium, zinc, iron, riboflavin or calories (*Nutr Act* 10 (5):11, 1983).

It appears that the advantages of moving toward a vegetarian meal plan outweigh the disadvantages, especially for adults. And even for children: adding fermented soy products, wheat germ, brewers yeast, cooking with iron cookware, and ensuring adequate sunshine should take care of the disadvantages.

It is believed that selenium prevents cancer by protecting cells from peroxide-induced oxidation (Griffin, 1979). When selenium is given as a supplement, it acts as an immune stiumulant. Organic forms of selenium (methylated and seleonamino acids) and the selenium found naturally in yeast and whole grains are suggested; inorganic forms of selenium supplements and artificially selenized yeasts have potential for mutagenicity (Noda,1979). The recommended daily allowance for adults is 50–200 µg (Helzsouer, 1983).

Vitamin E and Cancer. Vitamin E works as an antioxidant, protecting the unsaturated fatty membranes in the body from the formation of the carcinogens, lipoperoxides. Preliminary studies of tumor growth in animals suggested a potential role for vitamin E in inhibiting the carcinogenic process (Prasad & Edwards-Prasad, 1983), although at least one large prospective study of 89,494 women (Hunter, 1993) provided no evidence of a protective role for vitamin E and breast cancer. Longnecker et al. (1992) did provide evidence of an inverse relationship between serum alpha-tocopheral (vitamin E) and colorectal cancer.

Two large ($s_1 = 3,318$; $s_2 = 29,584$) randomized, double-blind and placebo-controlled nutrition intervention trials in Linxian, China (Li et al., 1993), showed a significant reduction of total mortality (9%), cancer mortality (13%), gastric cancer mortality (20%), and mortality of other cancers (19%) among those receiving beta carotene/vitamin E/selenium supplementation. Tables 5.3 and 5.5 provide information regarding dietary sources of vitamin E and selenium.

Fat, Meat, Fiber, and Cancer. Red meat is a stronger risk factor than total fat for colon cancer (Giovanucci et al., 1994). A diet low in dietary fiber increases the incidence of symptomatic diverticular disease (Aldoori et al., 1994). Red meat was also indicated by Giovanucci and others (1993) for prostrate cancer, as was butter. Fat from dairy products or fish was unrelated to risk.

Other Nutrients and Cancer. Experimental and epidemiological studies have demonstrated that green tea extract and garlic (Dorant et al., 1993; Han, 1993), onions (Belman,1983), licorice root (Wattenberg, 1992); soybean foods (Messina et al.,1994), and olive oil (Martin-Moreno et al., 1994), are also cancer preventives.

Vegetables and fruits are inversely, significantly, and strongly associated with breast cancer risk. There is also evidence that olive oil consumption may reduce the risk of breast cancer, and margarine may increase the risk (Trichopoulou et al., 1995).

Dietary Guidelines for Reducing Cancer Risks

Dietary guidelines for decreasing the risk of cancer were suggested by the American Cancer Society's Medical and Scientific Committee, Nutrition and Cancer. The recommendations and elaborations of them as suggested by Garrison and Somer (1985, pp. 142–144) follow.

1. *Avoid obesity.* Obese people (20% or more above ideal weight) have an increased risk for cancers of the uterus, gallbladder, kidney, stomach, colon, and prostate.

2. *Cut down on total fat intake.* Excessive use of *either* saturated or unsaturated fat increases the risk of developing cancers of the breast, colon, and prostate.

3. *Eat more high fiber foods (whole grains, fruits, and vegetables.)* There is sufficient evidence to warrant the increase of fiber intake and variety of fiber foods eaten. Simply adding bran to a meal plan is not thought to be sufficient.

4. *Include foods rich in vitamin A and/or carotene and vitamin C daily.* (See explanations above regarding these vitamins.)

5. *Include cruciferous vegetables daily.* A component in these vegetables seem to reduce risk of cancer of the gastrointestinal and respiratory tracts.

6. *Be moderate in consumption of alcoholic beverages.* Alcohol increases the risk of cirrhosis, liver cancer, cancer of the oral cavity, larynx, and esophagus. The risk is potentiated in smokers who also abuse alcohol.

7. *Be moderate in consumption of salt-cured, smoked, and nitrite-cured foods.* As mentioned earlier, nitrosamines are cancer precursors. Smoking or barbecuing meats results in the production of procarcinogenic substances.

Cardiovascular Disease and Preventive Nutrients

The likelihood of developing CVD is dependent on the individual's personal decision to avoid or embrace specific risk factors. "Risk factors are any characteristics associated with an above average incidence of a disease" (Garrison & Somer, 1985, p. 149). Risk factors are signals warning that a habit, age, or dietary pattern is associated with disease. If heeded, warning signals can enhance wellness.

In fact, lifestyle changes, including a switch to a low-fat diet plan, have been shown to reverse coronary atherosclerosis, a form of heart disease (Ornish et al., 1989). Likewise, a high intake of fruits and vegetables protects against the development of stroke in men (Gillman et al., 1995) and women (Manson et al., 1994).

Primary Habits Associated with Cardiovascular Disease. The best known cardiovascular disease (CVD) risk factor study is the Framingham study (1948) that identified primary habits associated with CVD (hypertension, cigarette smoking, and elevated cholesterol). Since then, elevated low density lipoprotein-cholesterol has been recognized as the fourth primary risk factor. Secondary risk factors include obesity, diabetes, lack of aerobic exercise, stress, male sex, high serum triglycerides, increasing age, a family history of heart or blood vessel disease, and stress-prone personality type (Garrison & Somer, 1985, p. 149).

Serum Cholesterol. It is well established that serum cholesterol levels are directly related to CVD (Gordon & Verter, 1969; Scott et al., 1972). In countries where serum cholesterol levels are below 160 mg/dl, CVD is nonexistent (Wissler, 1979). Over half of the American people exceed the level suggested by the American Heart Association; when other risk factors such as smoking or obesity are added, a lower serum cholestrol level would be needed to counteract them.

Flaxseed has shown promise for lowering cholesterol. In a 4-week randomized crossover study with 10 healthy subjects, a significant increase in bowel movements and a trend toward lower total cholesterol was observed when participants consumed two flaxseed muffins per day, compared to the control period (Hamadeh, 1992).

Garlic also can reduce cholesterol levels. Compared with a placebo, garlic significantly lowered cholesterol levels by about 9% according to a meta-analysis of all randomized, placebo-controlled trials that tested the effectiveness of oral garlic preparations in which 75% of their participants had initial cholesterol levels exceeding 200 mg/dl (Warshafsky, 1993).

Adding 15 grams of grapefruit pectin (the sticky binding fiber that forms the cell walls of fruits) can reduce cholesterol levels with none of the side effects of cholesterol-lowering medicines. In a study conducted at the University of Florida involving 27 volunteers with high cholesterol, their cholesterol levels were reduced an average of 11% within four weeks after taking grapefruit pectin (Dishong, 1994). Citrus pectin can be obtained by eating the fruit membranes and white portion next to the skin.

High-Density Lipoproteins. High-density lipoproteins (HDL) are heavy and contain the most protein. They collect cholesterol and transport it to the liver; they clear up excess cholesterol lingering in the arteries. (Low-density lipoproteins, or LDL, transport cholesterol from the liver and the tissues; elevated LDL is the primary source of cholesterol and cholesterol esters in plaque; when LDL is high, deposits of cholesterol line the arterial walls.)

HDL can be raised by reducing dietary fat and cholesterol, not smoking, maintaining ideal body weight, and increasing cardiovascular or aerobic exercise. Reduced HDL is primarily caused by obesity and a sedentary lifestyle.

Canadian studies have shown that postmyocardial infarction clients were able to rise their HDL as a result of aerobic exercise. At least 20 km/week of running was required to increase HDL (Kavanaugh, 1983).

Total Fat More Important Than Cholesterol Intake. Total fat in the diet appears to be more important than cholesterol intake. Even in vegetarians, a high fat diet promotes elevated serum lipids, but less so than in nonvegetarians; this is to be expected because vegetarians eat high fiber, fatty acid, and polysaturated foods. There is no correlation between egg consumption (high cholesterol) and plasma lipids (Liebman & Bazzarre, 1983). However, Willet et al., (1994) found an increased risk of myocardial infarct among men with a higher intake of heme iron, mainly from red meat.

The Ratio of Polysaturated to Saturated Fat. The ratio of polyunsaturated to saturated fat must be increased to lower serum cholesterol. Polysaturated acids have a strong antilipogenic ability; they lower liver lipoprotein synthesis and increase lipoprotein removal. Polyunsaturated fatty acids (PUFA) lower cholesterol in another way. Linoleic acid, an essential fatty acid, is available only through diet. Increased intake of oils (e.g., safflower) high in linoleic acid decreases platelet aggregation and decreases serum cholesterol (Bazan et al., 1981; Oliver, 1982; Sacks et al., 1983).

Essential Fatty Acids. "Essential fatty acids may also influence other activities of prostaglandins, including smooth muscle contraction, renal functions and numerous cardiopulmonary functions" (Garrison & Somer, 1985, p. 166).

Although PUFA are beneficient in preventing CVD, increased intakes have been correlated with increased risk of cancer; therefore it is important to reduce the intake of saturated fats and keep the intake of PUFA constant. Oils tend to be high in polyunsaturates and low in saturates. Olive oil has a polyunsaturated to saturated ratio of 0.9 (the closest to a 1 : 1 ratio). Olive oil is used daily in the Mediterranean countries, where coronary artery disease is low compared to the American diet (Garrison & Somer, 1985, p. 168). Monounsaturated fat-based margarines, high in alpha-linolenic acid and omega 3 fatty acids, like the Mediterranean diet, showed benefit in controlling blood fats in a U.S. study (Goldstein, 1994).

Dangers of Hydrogenated Fats. Hydrogenated fats hold special dangers. They supply less PUFA than meats and dairy products. Americans consume 600 million pounds of these frying fats each year in fried and processed foods. A glance at many canned or boxed food items reveals that hydrogenated or partially hydrogenated fats are contained therein. When manufacturers add hydrogens to oils, some of the oils become saturated, others become transfats which raise cholesterol, possibly as much as saturated (animal) fats do (Wooten & Liebman, 1993). The Nurses Health Study (Willett, 1993) has linked transfats (margarine, shortening, cookies, pies, cakes, frosting, chips, crackers, and related foods) to a 50 percent higher risk of heart disease. In another study, (Ascheria et al., 1994), found an intake of margarine significantly associated with myocardial infarction.

There are several dangers lurking in hydrogenated fats. For example, they:

1. increase the need for essential fatty acids such as linoleic acid (Beare-Rogers, Gray, Hollywood, 1979);
2. reduce prostaglandin production and interfere with the conversion of linoleic acid to arachiodonic acid in the formation of prostaglandins (Rutenberg et al., 1983);
3. may elevate serum cholesterol and liver glycerices (Rutenberg et al., 1983);
4. are absorbed, but do not seem to be used readily in cellular energy metabolism, acting more like saturated than unsaturated fats, thereby impairing the cellular function; in heart and smooth muscle this may lead to CVD (McGill, Geer, & Strong, 1965).

It is suggested that food labels be scrutinized and the benefits of a fried or fast food meal be weighed against the disadvantages listed above.

EPA Reduces Risk of Disease. The fatty acid omega-3-eicosapentaenoic acid (EPA), found in cold-water fish, lowers levels of serum cholesterol. Given in supplement form, EPA has produced changes associated with reduced risk of heart disease (Fish oil for prevention of atherosclerosis, 1982). However, EPA supplements do have adverse effects, including thrombocytopenia and hepatotoxicity. Therefore, it is best to obtain EPA naturally in mackerel, salmon, and sardines (Garrison & Somer, 1985, pp. 167–168; Morgan, Raskin, & Rosenstock, 1995).

Phospholipids (Lecithin). The generic term for a phospholipid is lecithin. Lecithin is composed of two phosphatides, phosphatydlcholine (PC) and phosphatylethanolamine (PE). Clinical studies have shown that lecithin can favorably affect the risk of CVD by reducing serum cholesterol (Vroulis et al., 1982).

Both phospholipids increase excretion of neutral sterols resulting in reduction of the entry of dietary cholesterol and "the reentry of endogenous cholesterol into the body" (Garrison & Somer, 1985, p. 169). One study concluded that the ability of PC to emulsify cholesterol may make fat more soluble, thereby less likely to form gallstones (ter Well, van Gent, & Dekker, 1974).

Many cholesterol-rich foods *also* contain their own lecithin; for example, eggs contain eight times as much lecithin as cholesterol. In one study, there was no decrease in serum lipoproteins and liver lipids when rats were fed PC in the form of soybeans, but when they were fed egg yolks (PC and PE), serum cholesterol and apoprotein A-I declined (Murata, Imaizum, & Sugano, 1982). Major sources of licithin include egg yolks, soybeans and soybean products, and lecithin (available in granular form as a supplement).

Blood Pressure and Magnesium. Disturbances in intracellular magnesium (Mg) may contribute to high blood pressure. Resnick et al. (1984) described previous studies showing oral Mg to lower blood pressure. In their study, intracellular free Mg levels were strongly negatively correlated with both systolic and diastolic blood pressures.

Dietary Fiber. Dietary fiber includes nondigestible plant materials free of calories. In addition to preventing CVD, dietary fiber protects against constipation, diarrhea, hemorrhoids, gallstones, hiatus hernia, varicose veins, and appendicitis; in populations in which dietary fiber composes a large percentage of the diet, these diseases are unknown. Fiber normalizes bowel activity, reducing the transit time of food through the intestines (thereby eliminating toxic substances more quickly), influences intestinal flora, and may reduce the formation of intestinal carcinogens (Garrison & Somer, 1985, p. 169). Some types of fiber (excluding wheat bran) appear to lower blood cholestrol and lower the mortality rate from CVD (Allbrink, Davidson, & Newman, 1976).

Pectin is another form of dietary fiber that has LDL-cholesterol lowering effects (Baig & Cera, 1981). It is found in apples and some other fruits, including not completely ripe berries.

Other dietary fibers shown to lower cholesterol include: oat fiber (Anderson et al., 1983), guar and locust bean gums (Zavoral et al., 1983) found in soybean ice-cream substitutes in health food stores, soybeans, chickpeas and peanuts (Malinow et al., 1981), and alfalfa (Malinow et al., 1978).

Although some fiber is beneficial, excessive intake of the substance can bind trace minerals, interfere with their absorption, and irritate the intestinal lining. Thirty-seven g/day of dietary fiber provide the protective effect without producing the negative effects (Garrison & Somer, 1985, p. 170). This amount can be obtained from the following *daily* intake: six servings of *whole grains* (rice, corn, pasta, bread, kasha, etc.); four servings of fresh fruits and vegetables; and one serving of dried beans. It is worthy of note that this reaffirms the wisdom of a primarily vegetarian meal plan for life. Additionally, when planning servings of whole grains, it is imperative to ensure whole grains are used; the best way to do this is to read labels and/or purchase the whole grains and cook them rather than purchasing quick cooking or white enriched products with or without some whole wheat or other flour added.

Unraveling the Complex Interrelationships of CVD. Focusing on one food factor is not a wellness approach to CVD. Since 70–80% of blood cholesterol is manufactured in the body, the building blocks of cholesterol require study. Some of the factors that interact to influence the manufacture and excretion of cholestrol include amino acids, vitamins, minerals, garlic, inositol, aging, and fasting.

Amino Acids in Soybeans Lower Cholesterol. Vegetable-based protein products appear to reduce serum cholestrol levels (Sirtori, Gatti, & Manter, 1979; Kritichevsky et al., 1982) regardless of egg consumption. Soybeans are relatively high in the amino acid arginine and low in lysine—a combination that seems to lower cholesterol (Check, 1982). Taking supplements rather than eating soybeans and soybean products may *not* produce the desired effect; lysine alone may stimulate cholestrol synthesis (Schmeisser et al., 1983). Although it is important to be cautious in extrapolating findings from chicks to human beings, it is wise to remember the principle found here: it is generally safer to obtain nutrients from whole foods rather than supplements whenever possible.

B-Vitamins Important in Lipid Metabolism and CVD. The following B-vitamins are important in lipid metabolism: pantothenic acid, B_2, B_6, and niacin. Substantial amounts of vitamin B_6 are lost in the production of grains and other foods; this is not one of the four nutrients added back when refined foods are "enriched."

Vitamin B$_6$ needs are dependent on protein intake. The American diet, already too high in protein, could aggravate a possible borderline deficiency and lead to CVD.

Vitamin C, Cholesterol, and CVD. Vitamin C is found primarily in fruits and vegetables. An absence of these in the daily food plan has been correlated with increased incidence of CVD (Acheson & Williams, 1983). One explanation for this correlation is that vitamin C is important in the synthesis of collagen, the "glue" that strengthens and supports body tissue. Vitamin C (along with pyridoxine, essential fatty acids, zinc, and possibly niacin) also appears to encourage prostacyclin synthesis, encouraging collateral circulation to ischemic areas of the heart (Garrison & Somer, 1985, pp. 173–174). Studies have demonstrated a direct correlation between vitamin C intake and a reduction in cardiovascular death rates (Knox, 1973).

Low ascorbic acid (vitamin C) levels were found in clients with coronary atherosclerosis in one study (Ramirez & Flowers, 1980). Vitamin C affects the cholesterol content of the blood and positively influences triglyceride and lipoprotein levels. Giving vitamin C supplements to men and women with CVD resulted in a reduction in total serum cholesterol for both groups and a reduction in LDL in men (Horsey, Livesley, & Dickerson, 1981).

MacRury et al. (1992) found a seasonal and climatic variation in cholesterol and vitamin C, but recommended people with blood vessel disease take vitamin C supplements throughout the year. Vitamin C appears to have the most positive effect in HDL in individuals with marginal vitamin C status or cholesterol levels (Simon, 1992).

Vitamin C is most available when food is kept from exposure to air, minimally cooked, not reheated, and when cooking water and juices are eaten. Additional, vitamin C is destroyed when foods are stored; it is best to purchase small amounts of local, fresh produce. Some factors that deplete the body of vitamin C include: cigarette smoke, stress, birth control pills, alcohol, and the consumption of fast foods; the latter tend to be high in fat, salt, and sugar, with little, if any, vitamin C. "Although the potato is a reasonable source of the vitamin, once it has been sliced, stored, fried in hot oil and held under warming lights, little, if any, of the original vitamin C remains" (Garrison & Somer, 1985, p. 174).

The Fat-Soluble Vitamins and CVD. Vitamins A and E play a protective role in CVD because they function as antiperoxidants, antiaggregants, affect oxygen transport and utilization, increase HDL, and enhance hypolipidemic action of niacin (Garrison & Somer, 1985, p. 174; Knekt et al., 1994). On the other hand, vitamin D in excess promotes atherosclerotic lesions, especially when combined with cholesterol (Seelig, 1983).

Vitamin E is a mild antiaggregatory agent, relieves intermittent claudication, and is a powerful antioxidant. Women with a high dietary intake of vitamin E, primarily by supplementation, had a 40% reduced risk of cardiovascular disease (Stampfer et al., 1993) when supplementation exceeded two years. Men showed a similar reduction (Rimm et al., 1993). Supplementation with at least 400 IU a day is recommended for high-risk clients, "those who have had a heart attack at a young age and who do not have other modifiable risk factors" (Swendson, 1995).

Studies in humans and animals have shown optimal intakes of sodium, magnesium, zinc, calcium, iodine, and chromium reduce the risk of CVD (Garrison & Somer, 1985, p. 175.) Calcium has also been shown to reduce risk of high blood pressure by 40% for each 1,000 mg consumed (Dwyer, 1992).

Inositol functions to prevent fatty liver infiltration. It works in concert with folic acid, vitamin B_6, choline, vitamin B_{12}, betaine, and the amino acid methionine to stimulate normal liver management of fats (Gavin, 1941). Dietary sources of inositol include grapefruit juice, cantaloupe, oranges, stone-ground whole wheat bread, cooked beans, grapefruit, limes, and green beans (Garrison & Somer, 1985, p. 177).

Aging affects the body's regulation of cholesterol synthesis; an enzyme crucial to this regulation (hydroxymethylglutaryl CoA) declines with age. Fasting may temporarily lower serum cholesterol levels (Garrison & Somer, 1985, p. 177).

AIDS and Nutrition

Malnutrition is a common consequence of HIV infection. It can be due to decreased intake, malabsorption, altered metabolism, or all three. Early nutritional supplementation may lead to enhanced ability to fight infection.

Selenium deficiency is common in people with HIV positive results (Dworkin, 1994). Chromium picolinate has also been suggested for use with AIDS because of its ability to enhance cellular immunity (McCarty, 1993).

Tang and others (1993) found that the highest levels of total intake (from food and supplements) for participants in the Multicenter AIDS cohort study of vitamins C, B_1 and niacin were associated with a significantly decreased progression rate to AIDS. A high vitamin A intake appeared to decrease progression in some participants and not in others. Zinc was significantly associated with an increased risk of progression to AIDS. Beach and others (1992) found HIV-1-seropositive men had low levels of vitamins A, E, riboflavin, B_6 and B_{12}, together with copper and zinc. Wang and Watson (1994) discussed the important immunoenhancing role vitamin E may play in AIDS, stimulating the immune system.

Tang and others (1993) followed 281 men who tested positive for HIV. The risk of developing AIDS was 40–50% lower for those who consumed either from food or supplements: more than 61 mg of niacin a day, between 9,000 IU and 20,000 IU of vitamin A day, and more than 715 mg of vitamin C a day. The risk started to climb once zinc intake exceeded 12 mg a day.

Pierson (1994) reported that glycyrrhizin (an active phytochemical found in licorice extract) lowered the risk of progression to AIDS, from HIV positive to zero when licorice extract was given to 16 HIV-infected people. Folkers et al. (1993) found coenzyme Q10 and Vitamin B_6 (taken together) enhance immune response.

Cathcart (1984) reported using high doses of oral or intravenous vitamin C, titrated to bowel tolerance, of 50–200 grams/day. A topical vitamin C paste or solution has also been effective for AIDS-related herpes simplex and early Kaposi's lesions.

Calcium Protects

Dietary Calcium and Kidney Stones

In a cohort study of 45,619 men, 40 to 75 years of age, who had no history of kidney stones, Stampfer (1993) found an inverse relationship between calcium and kidney stones. Intake of animal protein was directly related to kidney stones. Potassium and fluid intake were inversely related to kidney stones (Blumberg and Suter, 1991).

Osteoporosis and Calcium. *Osteoporosis* is a degenerative bone disease drastically increasing the probability of bone fracture. It results from dietary imbalances, years of low physical activity, and, for women, hormonal changes of menopause. In approximately 25–30% of postmenopausal women, osteoporosis is a contributor to major orthopedic problems (Avioli, 1981).

If an insufficient amount of calcium is eaten, it will be immobilized from the bones into the bloodstream, leading to bone fragility. Bone loss proceeds gradually; the first sign may be a loss of height, persistent pain in the lower spine area, "dowager's hump," or loss of weight. In some cases, a small trip and subsequent fracture may be the first sign that osteoporosis has occurred. Once bones suffer extensive calcium loss, it is difficult to regain bone strength. The best prevention is to ensure adequate calcium intake.

See Table 5.5 for sources of calcium; although calcium is abundant in many foods, the average woman's diet is low in the mineral. Women over 45 typically consume little more than half the amount recommended; at this level, a loss of 1.5% of total bone mass could occur within a year's time (Avioli, 1981).

Milk is frequently replaced with soft drinks that are usually buffered with phosphoric acid, which can stimulate the release of calcium from the bones. Additional sources of phosphorous include beef and preservatives. A high level of caffeine consumption may increase calcium deficiency (Massey & Wise, 1984).

An intake of 1500 mg of calcium daily will inhibit the age-related bone loss in postmenopausal women (Bonnick, 1994). Table 5.5 provides food sources of the minerals.

To get an idea of the amount of food which must be eaten daily to accumulate 1500 mg of calcium, here are some regular servings of high calcium foods (National Dairy Council, 1990):

1 cup, plain, nonfat yogurt	452 mg
1 cup skim milk	302 mg
1 ounce cheddar cheese	204 mg
1/2 cup tofu with calcium sulfate	434 mg
3 oz. sardines (with bones)	324 mg
1/4 cup almonds	94 mg
1/2 cup turnip greens, fresh, cooked	99 mg
1/2 cup broccoli, fresh, cooked	89 mg
1/2 cup beet greens, fresh, cooked	82 mg

Alzheimer's Disease and the Calcium–Aluminum Relationship

Processed foods, aluminum-containing medications (e.g., antacids), and the use of aluminum cookware has led to an excessive body burden of aluminum. Toxicity due to aluminum is associated with Alzheimer's and other neuromuscular disorders, hyperparathyroidism, and bone loss (Garrison & Somer, 1985, p. 106).

When serum calcium levels are high, aluminum accumulation is reduced (Konig, 1981; Marquis, 1983). Therefore, it is suggested that sufficient calcium intake be guaranteed and that cooking be done in nonaluminum cookware. Perhaps the best cookware is iron because cooking in such containers insures adequate iron intake, protecting against anemia; glass or stainless steel are alternatives. The difficulty with aluminum and the potential protectiveness of iron cookware underline the relevance of wellness theory; environment and nutrition can interact to lead to disease or higher levels of wellness.

Calcium May Protect Against Eclampsia

Fetal losses from eclampsia range from 30 to 35%; about 10% of maternal mortality is due to this complication. A study of Guatemalan women revealed they have a very low incidence of eclampsia despite the presence of other factors (poor prenatal care, poor nutrition, and geography) that are considered high risk for the condition to occur. When the Guatemalan women were compared with Colombian women of a similar socioeconomic level with very high rates of eclampsia, the only difference between the two groups was a high dietary calcium in Guatemala. This finding supports the contention that sufficient calcium intake could be an important preventive measure for eclampsia (Villar, Belizah, & Fischer, 1983).

Premenstrual Tension Reduced With Magnesium, Zinc, Niacin, and Vitamins C, E, and B$_6$ Supplements

A study of serum and red cells of women with premenstrual syndrome found magnesium levels were low. The classical symptoms (headache, dizziness, and craving for sweets) responded well to magnesium, zinc, niacin, and vitamin C supplementation. Breast tenderness responded to vitamin E supplement. Tension anxiety associated with premenstrual syndrome improved with increased doses of vitamins B$_6$ (Abraham, 1983).

Amyotrophic Lateral Sclerosis (ALS) and Aluminum

Young men in Guam have a high rate of amyotrophic lateral sclerosis (ALS or Lou Gehrig's disease) which has been traced to a high level of aluminum and manganese exposure. Following up on this finding, researchers at the Department of Agronomy and Animal Science at the Louisiana Agricultural Experiment Station administered aluminum sulfate and manganese sulfate to animals in varying doses; manganese had no effect on magnesium, but administration of aluminum resulted in symptoms of magnesium deficiency. When the aluminum was removed, the cramping, gastrointestinal complications, and nervous system disorders decreased (Allen, Robinson, & Hembry, 1984). The researchers concluded that aluminum administration can result in magnesium deficiency. This work confirms other studies' findings that a calcium- and magnesium-rich diet offers some protection against aluminum-induced toxicity.

Diabetes, Chromium, Licorice, and Olive Oil

The major role of chromium is that of improved carbohydrate metabolism through facilitation of insulin activity. Long-term ingestion of sugar and other refined carbohydrates is considered a primary factor in chromium deficiency leading to disturbances in the ability to handle sugar. These abnormalitites resemble those of maturity-onset diabetes, including high levels of sugar in the blood and urine and an excessive amount of insulin in the bloodstream (Garrison & Somer, 1985, p. 111).

Several studies have shown that supplemental chromium can benefit elderly diabetics. Brewer's yeast was given to older maturity-onset diabetics; they showed improvement in blood cholesterol levels (Offenbacher, 1980).

Chromium supplementation from brewer's yeast has also been shown to be an effective treatment for abnormal glucose tolerance as well as a protective factor in atherosclerotic disease (Rabinowitz et al., 1983; Saner et al., 1983).

In one study, licorice extract proved effective as an inhibitor of platelet aggregation, implicated in diabetic complications (Tawata et al., 1992). In another, licorice was discussed as a treatment for the low blood pressure caused by the degeneration of the nerves and nervous system in diabetes (Boscaro & Armanini, 1994). Garg et al. (1988) found that high carbohydrate diets controlled blood sugar levels for some people with diabetes, but not for others. Their study substituted olive oil for some of the carbohydrates which resulted in 25% lower triglycerides, lower blood sugar levels and lower daily insulin requirements for most participants. The diet was also more palatable because of the added fat, making it easier to adhere to.

Copper, Zinc, and Immunity

Patients with depressed cell-mediated immunity have been found to have a low serum zinc and elevated serum copper level. In one study when given zinc supplements, they improved. This supports the hypothesis that alterations in zinc and copper metabolism due to dietary imbalance contribute to immunodeficiency (Oleske et al., 1983). However, high zinc intake (300 mg daily) can decrease immune function (Chandra, 1984).

Lead and Behavior

Although lead has been removed from gasoline for a number of years, toxicity still remains a factor due to ingestion of lead from dust and pollution and use of lead sealed canned foods. Decreased IQ, increased fatigue, and loss of concentration have been reported from chronic lead impairment (Marlowe & Errera, 1982).

Lead and Sudden Infant Death Syndrome

Lead levels are significantly higher in infants who die of Sudden Infant Death Syndrome (SIDS) than infants who die of other causes. These findings do not prove a cause and effect relationship but do explain reports linking SIDS to environmental toxins (Erickson et al., 1983).

Fish Oils Slow Kidney Disease

Daily doses of fish oil substantially slows the progress of a form of kidney disease called IgA nephropathy. Special diets and immune-suppressing drugs have not had a positive effect, but 12 one-gram capsules taken daily over a two-year treatment period was effective when compared to a placebo (Donadio, 1994).

Carotenoids, Supplements, and Eye Disease

The Physicians' Health Study provided evidence that men who took multi-vitamin supplements tended to experience a decreased risk for cataract (Seddon et al., 1994). A study conducted at the Massachusetts Eye and Ear Infirmary in Boston provided strong evidence (43% decreased risk for macular degeneration) for eating vegetables containing carotenoids—especially spinach and collard greens (Seddon et al., 1994).

Folic Acid and Neural Tube Defect

Willett (1992) reviewed a series of randomized intervention trials and case-control and cohort studies, women using multivitamins or folic acid supplements during the first 6 weeks of pregnancy (200–400 micrograms per day) experienced three- to fourfold reduction in neural tube defects in their offspring.

OTHER SIGNIFICANT NUTRIENT REACTIONS

Free-Radical Damage

With vitamin supplementation, free-radical damage, which is thought to play a role in aging processes and the development of degenerative disease, decreased in 100 healthy elderly people (aged 60–100 years). Daily supplementation included 400 mg vitamin C and/or 200 mg vitamin E. Peroxide levels progressively declined to as little as 74% of initial values. The researchers suggest that long-term supplementation of elderly people with moderate amounts of vitamins C and E can significantly reduce serum peroxide levels and protect against free-radical damage, and thereby, aging and degenerative diseases (Wartanowicz et al., 1984).

Caffeine and Mineral Loss

The effect of caffeine on mineral excretion was studied in 12 healthy young women who habitually consumed an average of 300 mg of caffeine per day. After an overnight fast, they were given decaffeinated coffee or tea with or without added caffeine. During the 3 hours following a 300 mg dose of caffeine, total urinary excretion of magnesium (Mg) was increased 48% and that of calcium (Ca) and sodium (Na) was increased 142%, while potassium excretion was only slightly increased. Total urinary volume was 35% greater after caffeine than after placebo. Caffeine caused a total excess Mg loss of 4.9 mg which would be more than offset by the Mg contained in coffee (16 mg/8 oz. cup). Calcium losses attributable to 300 mg caffeine averaged 26.6 mg;

coffee contains only 5 mg/cup. A high level of caffeine consumption may increase the risk of calcium deficiency.

Flavonoids

Flavonoids are found in fruits, vegetables, nuts, seeds, grains, and in beverages such as tea, cocoa, and wine. Flavonoids are prominent components of citrus fruits and soybeans. They are known to display a large array of nutritional actions and possess anti-inflammatory, antiallergic, antiviral, anticarcinogenic, antineoplastic, antimicrobial, antihelminthic, liver protective, antithrombotic, and antihormonal activities. They also function as light screens in plants, protecting them from ultraviolet radiation-induced damage. Flavonoids are known to affect a large number of enzyme systems, some of which are critically involved in chronic diseases, including cancer. They reduce the risks of heart disease, cancer, accelerated aging, arthritis, oxidation stress, and many radical-related diseases. They strengthen blood vessels, improve red blood cell flexibility, improve skin health; protect against allergies, fight inflammation and joint inflexibility, reduce pain due to swollen joints, reduce diabetic retinopathy, enhance the immune response, reduce the severity and frequency of colds, help prevent capillary bleeding and floaters in the eye, and act against stomach ulcers and inflammation (Harborne, 1986; Middleton & Kandaswami, 1993).

Some flavonoids, such as those in Pycnogenol, are especially potent antioxidants, metal chealtors and free-radical scavengers. They sequester deleterious oxidant-inducing metals and prevent them from damaging cells. The flavonoids of Pycnogenol also possess vitamin C-sparing activities and promote collagen (the glue that holds ligaments and other body tissues together) production. They improve capillary resistance (important in preventing/healing varicose veins and blood vessel diseases), protect against UV-B solar radiation, and inhibit histamine release in allergy control. Because Pycnogenol is water soluble (while plant sources are not), it is thought to be more readily available for use by the body (Passwater & Kandaswami, 1994).

DRUG-NUTRIENT INTERACTIONS

Research suggests that nutrient losses induced by many over-the-counter and prescription drugs may actually encourage the disease for which the medication was taken (Garrison & Somer, 1985, p. 209).

Some drugs increase appetite and others decrease it; it is the appetite depressants that are of most concern for populations that are already at risk nutritionally, including the elderly, those with a chronic disease, dieters, those who abuse alcohol, cigarette smokers, new mothers, adolescents, and certain ethnic minorities. Table 5.8 displays drug effects on nutrient absorption.

Table 5.8 Drug-Induced Nutrient Malabsorption

achromycin	B_{12} or folic acid
agoral	vitamins A and D
alcohol	folic acid; thiamin; riboflavin; niacin; vitamin C, B_6, B_{12}; magnesium; zinc
aldomet	B_{12} or folic acid
aldoril	B_{12} or folic acid
aluminum hydroxide	aluminum toxicity, vitamin A, folate, calcium
aluminum magnesium	phosphate depletion
antibiotics	vitamins A, K, B_2, B_6, B_{12}, calcium, potassium, iron, folic acid
antihypertensives	B_6
antituberculars	B_6, B_{12}, calcium, magnesium, folic acid, iron, and potassium
apresoline	B_6
aspirin	iron; folic acid; vitamin C
aureomycin	riboflavin; vitamin C, calcium
azulfidine	folic acid
bactrim	B_{12} or folic acid
beta blockers	carotene
biguanides: metformin and phenformin	B_{12}
biscodyl	potassium deficiency
butazolidin	B_{12} or folic acid
chlorpromazine	riboflavin
cholestyramine	fat; vitamins A, K B_{12}, D, beta carotene and iron
cimetidine	vitamin B_{12}
colchicine	fat, carotene, vitamin B_{12}, sodium, potassium, vitamins A, C, B_{12} D, iron
colestid	vitamins D, K and folic acid
cortisone	calcium
deltasone	B_6, B_{12}, or folic acid
depen	B_6
dilantin	vitamin D, folic acid
diphosphonates	calcium
diuretics	B_2, B_6, B_{12}, potassium, calcium, magnesium, zinc and folic acid
donnatal	B_{12} or folic acid, B_6
dyazide	folic acid
dyrenium	folic acid
furosemide	potassium, calcium, magnesium
gluthethimide	calcium
hydralazine	vitamin B_6
indocin	iron
INH	B_6
isoniazid	pyridoxine, niacin
klotrix	B_{12} or folic acid
k-lyte	B_{12} or folic acid
k-tab	B_{12} or folic acid
macrodantin	B_{12} or folic acid
medrol	B_6 and B_{12}
methotrexate	folic acid, vitamin B_{12}
mellaril	riboflavin
micro-k	B_{12}
mineral oil	fat soluble vitamins
mysoline	vitamin K
neomycin	fat, nitrogen, sodium, potassium, calcium, iron, lactose, sucrose, B_{12}
oral contraceptives	A, B_2, B_6, B_{12}, C, folic acid, magnesium, zinc
panmycin	B_2, vitamin C, calcium
para-amino salicyclic acid	fat, folate, B_{12}
percodan	B_{12}

Table 5.8 (*continued*)

phenobarbital	calcium, vitamin D, folic acid, vitamin B_{12}
phenolphthalein	vitamin D, calcium, potassium
phenytoin	folic acid, vitamin D
premarin	B_6, B_{12}
primidone	calcium, folic acid, vitamin K
potassium chloride	B_{12}
prednisone	calcium
questran	vitamin A, D, K, folic acid
ranitidine	vitamin B_{12}
rifamate	B_6, niacin, vitamin D
senna	calcium
septra	B_{12}
serapes	B_6
slow k	B_{12}
soda mint	folic acid
sodium bicarbonate	sodium overload, folate, calcium, copper
stelazine	B_{12}
sulfasalazine	folic acid
sumycin	B_{12}
tagamet	B_{12}
tetracycline	vitamin C, calcium, potassium
thorazine	riboflavin
valproic acid	folic acid, vitamins D, K

Source: Extracted from Drug-Nutrient Interactions, Robert Garrison, 1984–85 *Yearbook of Nutritional Medicine,* New Canaan, CT: Keats Publishing, 1985, pp. 93–112; Pharmacology, Nutrition, and the elderly: interactions and implications. *Geriatric Nutrition* ed. by R. Chernoff. Rockville, MD: Aspen Publishers, Inc., 1991, pp. 337–361; Drug-Induced Nutritional deficiencies, 1994, *The Energy Times* 4(1) : 24–30; *Cancer Nutrition* by Charles B. Simone, M.D., Garden City Park: Avery Publishing, 1992, pp. 86–89.

WEIGHT MAINTENANCE

In the United States 1 out of 4 children is obese. By the age of 3, many American children have fatty deposits in their aortas. By adolescence, deposits are found in their coronary (heart) arteries. Kids Kount Wellness Program at the Ochsner Medical Institution is a family-centered wellness/weight management program for boys and girls ages three through eight who are no more than twice their ideal weight. Emphasis is on nutrition, exercise and development of positive self-esteem. Students and parents have workbooks that include information about all these topics. The children track their daily exercise and keep food diaries, logging what foods they eat, when and why. They learn how to take responsibility for their own health habits, instead of hiding in food. Through play activities and a supportive environment they learn how to build their self-esteem and become realistic about their body image. Their food diaries reveal that many of the children eat hardly any fruits and vegetables and few grains. Kids learn to choose exercise, play, or talk to a friend instead of reaching for ice cream (Cordray, 1993).

Susan Toth, R.N., M.S.N., Carolyn Montgomery, R.N., A.N.P.C.-C., and Judith Bunn, R.D. (1984) summarized studies reporting what helps adults manage their weight.

Stanford University Heart Disease Prevention Program Study

Because personal preferences and learning styles may differentiate who loses and maintains weight, a survey conducted by Stanford tapped these preferences. They found that most people dislike losing weight in a group. Therefore, they developed a mail order extension course that proved successful.

Indiana University School of Medicine Study

At the Indiana University School of Medicine, M. Peri found that buddies are more helpful when it comes to weight loss, unless spouses are overweight and participate in the weight loss program. (This supports the peer facilitation/role model factors found in Clark's study; see pages 326–330.) In the New York study, 70 obese men and women volunteered for training in self-monitoring of foods eaten, nutritional education, and exercise. They were assigned to one of five groups: training only, training supported by a buddy, training supported by a spouse, training supported by both, and a waiting list that received no treatment or training.

After 10 weeks, those who had received training lost an average of 10.5 lb.; those supported by a buddy lost substantially more (14.5 lb.). Those whose spouses had been enlisted for support lost 8.8 lb., less than those who received behavioral training only. The positive effect of a buddy was counteracted by the support of a spouse; those in the buddy/spouse group did less well (9.6 lb. weight loss) than those in the buddy group. Those on the waiting list gained an average of half a pound.

The Georgia Mental Health Institute Study

In a related study in Atlanta, Loveland and Schonitzer found that participation of the spouse in a weight loss program was insignificant unless the spouse was overweight and participated in the weight loss program, too.

The Health Care Plan Medical Center Study

A weight management program at the Health Care Plan Medical Center in West Seneca, NY, helps participants identify situations that promote eating, adjust their eating environment, and make appropriate responses to internal and external cues. Participants receive an 8-week course covering nutrition, body image, assertiveness, appetite control, and stress management. Those who change their behavior are rewarded by receiving up to $30 of their $50 deposit; points are awarded for attending meetings, following the diet, eating breakfast daily, keeping a food diary, exercising three times a week, limiting intake of caffeine, sodium, or cholesterol, submitting tested diet recipes, or reaching the 12-week weight goal. The following activities have also been found successful: (a) Each group member cooks a low-calorie dish which is sampled by the others; (b) a yearly reunion is held in December during the holiday season.

Participants lose an average of 12 lb. in the 12-week program; a 6–12 month follow-up indicated that 35% maintained a weight loss of more than 10 lb. More than two thirds of the participants earn refunds, and participants reported increased feelings of well-being, fewer symptoms of arthritis, and decreased use of medication for diabetes and high blood pressure.

Weight Loss Intervention in Phase 1 of the Trials of Hypertension Prevention

Participants aged 30 to 54 years who had a high normal diastolic blood pressure and were between 115% and 165% of their desirable body weight, were randomly assigned to either an 18-month weight loss intervention (n = 308) or a usual-care condition (n = 256). Intervention consisted of 14 weekly group meetings during which participants learned to alter their lifestyles with behavioral self-management techniques (setting short-term goals, formulating specific action plans, developing reinforcement and social support, keeping food diaries, and graphing their weight). During each meeting smaller groups formed to display their graphs and discuss their self-management efforts. Relapse prevention training included discussing high-risk situations, developing alternative coping strategies, and learning ways to minimize the occurrence of high-risk situations. This program was an effective nonpharmacologic intervention for reducing blood pressure in overweight adults by helping them lose weight (Stevens et al., 1993).

Recommendations for Weight Loss

In a review of factors that help people lose weight, Glantz (1984) found that knowledge about how and what to eat is not sufficient for change; what is needed includes:

- an emphasis on changing behavior through keeping food diaries of types and amount of food eaten, time of eating, location, position, mood, and companions
- a review of the diary with a helping person
- setting specific behavior change goals
- rewards for changing are designated: tokens, money, prizes, participant-identified rewards
- a combination of mass media approaches and one-on-one counseling
- a design for creating ways of keeping participants in the program; less than half of the participants remain in a program long enough to achieve their weight loss goals

- emphasis on the immediate benefits of good nutritional practices such as attractiveness and self-confidence.

The National Center for Health Education in San Francisco (1982) released a report identifying various approaches that have worked with individuals:

- Identify why weight loss is important, listing the reasons in as specific a way as possible.
- Write down the advantages and disadvantages of becoming thinner.
- Record each incident of eating and the circumstances surrounding it for a week.
- Set goals for becoming thinner and formalize them in a contract; have a trusted other person sign it.
- Set up a reward system; praise or other pleasant happening if weight is lost; forfeit money (or another reward) if pledged weight is not lost.
- Find a buddy or a small group of weight losers with whom to discuss the weight loss process and from whom to garner support; keep the support going after desired weight has been reached to avoid slippage.
- Use imagery to picture oneself as fat as currently or as thin as desired.
- Role play with a buddy how to handle pressure from others to eat.
- Learn relaxation techniques and diversionary tactics (drink a glass of water, take a walk, deep breathe) when eating urges overwhelm.
- Get at least one family member involved in the process to offer support and to help change family eating patterns.

Other common weight loss recommendations found helpful by the author in her work with clients include:

- Analyze eating in detail in an individual or group setting, including:
  —Why do I want to change?
  —What are the advantages and disadvantages of changing?
  —Exactly how do I sabotage my eating plan now?
  —What skills do I need to learn to resist pressure from others to maintain old eating patterns? (saying no, refraining from getting defensive)
  —What kind of support do I need from others to attain my goals? (phone calls, or written reminders when I feel I'm slipping)
- Eat only at specified meal times and only while sitting down in the one household spot identified for eating; eating while cooking and eating while watching television increase chances of inappropriate eating.
- Slow down eating pace by putting down the fork after each bite, taking a break during the meal, and concentrating on the taste and texture of food; when food is eaten quickly there is insufficient time for body/mind to identify satiation.
- Never do anything else while eating.
- Set goals guaranteed to bring success; start small and gradually increase expectations as success is achieved.

- Develop an exercise program to increase lean body mass, tone the body, increase fitness, and moderate hunger urges.
- Eat whole foods (e.g., a baked potato rather than french fries) to increase satiety.
- Cut down on appetite stimulants such as coffee, spices, chocolate, sugar, colas, and salt.
- Say or write the following affirmation 25 times each day until it is believed: It is getting easier and easier to eat food that is healthy and that enhances my wellness.
- Stay away from fad diets, monodiets, and other quick loss ideas that end in quick loss and quick weight regain; such a syndrome can result in hypertension, frustration, and reduced wellness.
- To lose body fat, emphasize whole grain cereals, rice, bread and pasta, include plenty of fresh fruits and vegetables and legumes such as dried beans, peas, and lentils. Stick to appetizer-sized portions (three to four ounces) of low or nonfat dairy products, fish, chicken, or turkey, or soy products.
- Use a measuring tape or the way your clothes fit as measures of success. Lost inches are a more tangible sign of a lean body than lost pounds.
- Calories don't always count. You can eat a low-fat diet and unlimited complex carbohydrates. If you're hungry, eat a piece of bread, a rice cracker, an apple or some steamed vegetables topped with lemon and a dash of olive oil. Never allow yourself to feel deprived. Eat something, just be sure it's a grain, legume, fruit or vegetable and you'll still lose weight (Shaw, 1994).
- To add taste to your food, put a thin coat of olive oil in the pan, wipe away the excess, then cook your food.
- Before eating, ask yourself: Do I really want this food? If yes, visualize yourself eating it, savoring the taste, and then picturing how you'll feel one-half hour later. If the experience is positive, eat the food. If not, don't.
- Avoid being negative if you don't follow your plan for a day or two once in a while. Give yourself permission to be human, then resume your program the next day with a positive attitude.

Dr. Roland Weinsier (1985) of the University of Alabama has been investigating another method of weight management called the *"Time Calorie Displacement" (TCD) method.* It features high-bulk, low-calorie foods such as fruits, vegetables, and unrefined starches. These foods take longer to consume than high calories, less bulky foods such as meats, fats and oil, and sugar products. The longer the dieter spends in eating, the greater the satisfaction and the fewer calories consumed. Some of the recommended foods are rice pudding made with small amounts of honey and fiber-rich brown rice and mock pizza sandwiches made with whole wheat English muffins, part skim milk cheese, and tomatoes.

Clinical studies with obese participants at the University of Alabama show that the TCD food plan keeps people satisfied on about 1,500 calories a day, is nutritionally balanced, and is effective in loss of fatty tissue. Thirty-five percent of the participants lost more than 20 lb. and 7% lost more than 40 lb. over an average of 26 weeks. Steady but small weight loss allows participants to establish new eating patterns so that excess weight does not reappear.

Weinsier tested 20 people; 10 were obese and 10 were of normal weight. Given as much food as they wanted, all reached the same degree of fullness while eating half the number of calories from the high-bulk, low-calorie meals as from the high-calorie meals and rated both meal plans as equally enjoyable. A separate study showed that skinfold thickness (a measure of body fat) fell significantly while muscle mass was maintained. Blood levels of all essential vitamins and minerals were also maintained without vitamin supplementation.

Theories concerning weight maintenance have changed radically over the years. Earlier theorists claimed overweight people consumed more food than lean ones; some nutritionists still hold on to this theory, despite research to the contrary (Coll, Meyer, & Stunkard, 1979). The lazy-body hypothesis holds that some become overweight because they are physically less active than others. The sluggish-metabolism theory holds that some people need less energy to keep their bodily processes going and store the excess as fat. All three theories are based on the assumption that overweight is an accident.

A newer explanation, *setpoint theory*, holds that fatness is not an accident of fat. "Each body wants a characteristic quantity of fat and proceeds to balance food intake, physical activity, and metabolic efficiency to maintain that amount" (Bennett & Gurin, 1982, p. 62). It is theorized that fat storage is managed by part of the unconscious brain; cells are believed to release chemical signals telling the brain how much fat they contain and, when necessary, asking for more. According to the theory, the brain synthesizes sensory impressions (taste and smell of rich foods raise the setpoint), amphetamines and nicotine may lower the setting, and physical activity may lower the setpoint, perhaps through hormonal signals.

According to the theory, the body does not know the difference between dieting and starvation. In an effort to protect the individual, the body goes into starvation practices, requiring fewer calories to do the work of the metabolic processes. Thus, when individuals attempt to diet, their setpoint rises and fat is held on to, making weight loss difficult when rich foods, inactivity, and short-term fad diets reign.

Studies of animals under starvation conditions and force fed humans support setpoint theory (Bennett & Gurin, 1982, pp. 64–84).

Recurrent dieting may be an important variable affecting weight gain. Dieting leads to a lower metabolic rate; when "normal" eating is resumed, weight is regained. Repeated dieting may be leading many to weight gain after dieting. Bennett and Gurin (1982) suggest alternatives to dieting; change food plan to reduce intake of fat, sugar, and artifical sweeteners; and increase physical activity.

A number of studies have demonstrated that the setpoint can be countered by physical activity. Working at the University of California at Davis, Judith Stern, a nutritionist, collaborated with two exercise physiologists to study six people placed on a low-calorie food plan. As expected, metabolic rates fell after 2 weeks (starvation reaction). The subjects then began an exercise program and metabolic rates returned to normal in half the dieters; one dieter lost 30 lb. that month.

Basal metabolism decreases at a rate of 2 tp 5% with every decade past the age of 30, so activity may be the only safe way to diminish the accumulation of fat that is normal with aging (Bennett & Gurin, 1982, p. 252). Studies of populations who are vigorously active also end credence to the argument that exercise lowers set point. For example, Norwegian woodcutters do not grow fat with age; they maintain about 15% body fat for 40 years (Skobak-Kaczynski & Andersen, 1975).

If the theory is correct, people should lose weight spontaneously when undertaking an exercise program without dieting. Gwinup worked with a group of obese men and women to test the theory. All participants had been discouraged by repeated failures at dieting. The researcher told the group to forget about what they ate and begin a program of physical activity. Most began with brisk walking for 10 or 15 minutes daily. Although most subjects dropped out, all who reached the point of walking briskly for at least 30 min. 5 days/week lost weight.

The 11 women who stayed with the program chose to increase their activity and within $1^1/_2$ years each lost 22 lb. on the average and continued a steady, slow loss (Gwinup, 1975). The benefits of losing weight in this manner are that there are no negative effects of dieting, including: weakness, increased nervousness, feelings of deprivation, loss of muscle, or quick release of fat-stored toxins into the bloodstream. More than a third of the weight lost during dieting and two thirds lost during a fast reflect loss of muscle, not fat (DeVries, 1974; Oscai, 1973).

Exercise alone is a slow route to weight loss; about one third of a pound is lost per week for the overweight or obese and one tenth of a pound per week for people with ideal weight (Epstein & Wing, 1980). Frequency of exercise is important in weight loss. People who exercise four or five times a week lose weight three times faster than those who exercise 3 days a week; exercising once or twice a week has *no* effect on weight loss (Epstein & Wing, 1980). So much for the weekend athlete syndrome.

A recent study comparing lean to obese men and women found that both groups consumed the same number of calories. What differed was the amount of fat, added sugar and fiber. Obese people derived a greater part of their energy intake from fat, a greater percentage of their sugar intake from added sugar, and a lower intake of fiber than lean people (Miller et al., 1994). Alterations in diet composition rather than number of calories ingested may have been an important weight control strategy for overweight adults.

The type of food eaten, important to weight loss, is even more important to wellness. Combining an exercise program with a very low carbohydrate diet is not wise; carbohydrates are needed to replenish the body's store of glycogen. Short-term, low-carbohydrate diets are incompatible with strenuous exercise; listlessness, dehydration, and acetone-breath are correlates of this kind of regime (Phinney et al., 1980). The following visualization exercise gives information useful for attaining ideal weight.

Table 5.9 Getting to Your Ideal Weight

The idea that your mind controls your body is not new, but how many of us tap our considerable mind power to enhance our wellness? Positive affirmation and visualization can be combined to obtain your ideal weight. Before each meal, try the following exercise:

Step One: Find a quiet, peaceful spot and spend 5 minutes relaxing your body. Keep your eyes closed throughout the exercise.

Step Two: Say, "I see and feel my body as I want it to look and feel." Repeat this sentence 10 times very slowly while picturing your body at your ideal weight.

Step Three: Say, "I am able to move toward my ideal weight with increasing comfort." Repeat this statement 10 times while picturing yourself looking and feeling more comfortable.

Step Four: Say, "I *am* able to move toward higher levels of wellness and positive energy." Repeat this statement slowly five times while visualizing yourself moving to increased states of wellness and becoming filled with positive energy.

Step Five: Slowly open your eyes and prepare to eat, carrying with you the image of yourself at your ideal weight.

Breakfast in the car, fast food for lunch, and a dinner meeting . . . a lifestyle of eating on the go. Here are some tips for healthy habits when you are away from home, from the National Center for Nutrition and Dietetics.

The Choice is Yours
- The type of restaurant you select affects the amount of control you will have over food choices. A full service restaurant offers the most flexibility. Cafeterias allow you to control portion sizes and toppings like gravy, sauce, and salad dressing.
- Do not be afraid to ask questions about how a dish is prepared and whether lower fat substitutions are available.

Less Fat, Still Fast
- Fast food chains are jumping on the low fat bandwagon—look for low fat dairy products and hearty healthy grilled chicken or lean meat entrees.
- Although most chains have converted to all-vegetable fat for frying, fried foods still are among the highest in fat and calories.
- Take a trip to the salad bar for a lower fat sidedish alternative to fries and onion rings. Keep your salad lean by going easy on the bacon bits, croutons, regular salad dressing, and prepared salads, and by choosing low calorie or yogurt-based dressings.

Plan Ahead

- Make up for the extra calories and possible lack of variety in the meal you eat out by having lower calorie, nutrient-rich foods at home. Low or nonfat dairy products, fresh fruits and vegetables, and high fiber breads and cereals provide a lot of the nutrients in shorter supply in meals away from home.
- Healthy choices for snacks at home that you can prepare ahead of time include pita wedges with a cottage cheese and vegetable dip, high fiber muffins, a low fat yogurt parfait made with fruit and dry cereal, or a mixed fruit cup.

Eating on the Road

- Feel like you and your family live in the car? Be sure to take along individually portioned juices, raw vegetables, low fat cheese or peanut butter and whole grain crackers, snack boxes or bags of dried fruits, and seasoned, air-popped popcorn.
- Your best breakfast bets on the road are cereal with milk, waffles or pancakes with fresh fruit toppings, a bagel or toast with preserves, fruits and juices.
- If you are at a convention, buffet, or party, fill up first on raw vegetables and seltzer. Then survey the scene to decide what else to eat.
- Watch out for foods that sound healthier than they are: teriyaki dishes are low in fat but high in sodium, potato skins often are fried and with high fat toppings, pasta primavera can be made with cream, and light menu items may be nothing more than high fat appetizers.

Diabetes and Weight Loss

Although the reason is not completely understood, lowering the body's stores of fat leads to an increased sensitivity to insulin. Therefore, diabetes clients need to reduce their weight. The traditional low carbohydrate diet has been called into question. As long as the overall intake of calories is low enough to produce weight loss and large amounts of refined sugar are excluded, complex carbohydrates, especially whole grain foods, are desirable foods for weight loss plans (Simpson et al., 1981).

In general, whether seeking to prevent a chronic illness (or its complications) or to maintain a lean body, research provides evidence that a primarily vegetarian meal plan is best. Making complex carbohydrates the centerpiece of every meal—loading up on whole grains, fresh fruits and vegetables, and legumes—and decreasing fats and added sugars is the road to nutritional wellness.

INTEGRATIVE LEARNING EXPERIENCES

Beginning Level

1. Scan several books and articles in professional journals and consumer magazines. Use "Guidelines for Reading Nutritional Information" (p. 96) to evaluate what you read; write down your feelings.
2. Role play a response to a client who tells you, "I need a candy bar for energy."
3. Write down a response to a client who says, "I don't eat potatoes or starches anymore; I'm watching my weight."
4. From the guidelines to meet Goal 2 of the Dietary Goals, select one way you plan to meet this goal in the future. (Optional: draw up a contract to do so.)
5. From the guidelines to meet Goal 3 of the Dietary Goals, select one way you can meet this goal in the future. (Optional: draw up a contract to do so.)
6. From the guidelines to reduce dietary fat, select one way you plan to meet this goal in the future. (Optional: draw up a contract to do so.)
7. Make a list of the pros and cons of vitamin and mineral supplementation.
8. Discuss the pros and cons of eating low sodium foods to lower blood pressure.
9. List the nutrients associated with cancer prevention.
10. From the "Dietary Guidelines for Reducing Cancer Risks," devise a plan to lower your cancer risks.
11. Assess which primary habits associated with cardiovascular disease apply to you. (Optional: devise a plan to reduce your risks.)
12. List the preventive nutrients related to cardiovascular disease; assess which apply to you. (Optional: devise a plan to increase the preventive nutrients in your food plans.)
13. Discuss the relationship between calcium, phosphorus, and osteoporosis.
14. Discuss the relationship between calcium, aluminum, and neuromuscular disorders. (Optional: devise a contract based on these relationships.)
15. FOR WOMEN ONLY: Evaluate yourself for premenstrual tension. Devise a plan based on information presented in this chapter.
16. Discuss the setpoint theory and its application to weight maintenance.
17. Write down nutrients for the following client issues based on information presented in this chapter.

A. hypertension	I. heart disease
B. constipation	J. varicose veins
C. infection	K. gallstones
D. cold feet	L. elevated serum cholesterol
E. surgery	M. AIDS
F. pregnancy	N. premenstrual tension
G. diabetes	O. overweight
H. high serum lipids	

Advanced Level

1. Discuss with at least three clients (individually or in a small group) the following issues; record your findings, using Table 4.7, Chapter 4, as a guide.

    A. Guidelines for reading nutritional information
    B. Food myths
    C. Dietary goals
    D. Pros and cons of supplementation
    E. The low salt controversy
    F. Wellness-enhancing foods (Table 5.6)
    G. Nutrients for prevention of cancer
    H. Dietary guidelines for reducing cancer risks
    I. Cardiovascular disease and preventive nutrients
    J. Primary habits associated with cardiovascular disease
    K. AIDS
    L. Osteoporosis and calcium
    M. Alzheimer's disease and the calcium-aluminum relationship
    N. Nutrients and premenstrual tension
    O. Weight maintenance

2. Use Table 5.8 to talk with clients about any medications they take; devise a written plan to reduce the harmful effects of drug-induced nutrient malabsorption.

REFERENCES

Abraham, G. (1983). Nutritional factors in the etiology of the premenstrual tension syndromes. *J. Repr. Med.* 28: 446–461.

Acheson, R., and Williams, D. (1983). Does consumption of fruits and vegetables protect against stroke? *Lancet* 1:1191–1193.

Adori, W.H., Giovannucci, E.L., Remin, E.B., et al. (1994). A Prospective study of diet and risk of symptomatic diverticular disease. *American Journal of Clinical Nutrition.* 60(5): 757-764.

Albrink, M., Davidson, P., and Newman, T. (1976). Lipid-lowering effect of a very high carbohydrate, high fiber diet. *Diabetes* 25:324.

Allen, V., Robinson, D., and Hembry, F. (1984). Effects of ingested aluminum sulfate on serum magnesium and the possible relationship to hypomagnesemic tetany. *Nutr. Rep. Int.* 29:107.

American Dietetic Association (1995). *Ten tips to healthy eating and physical activity for you.* Chicago, IL.

Ames, B. (1993). Oxidants, antioxidants, and the degenerative diseases of aging. *Proc. Natl. Acad. Sci.,* 90: 7915-1922.

Anderson, J., Chen, W., Story, L., and Sieling, B. (1983). Hypocholesterolemic effects of soluble fiber-rich foods for hypercholesteralemic men. *Am. J. Clin. Nutr.* 37:699.

Ascherio, A., Hennekens, C.H., Buring, J.E., et al., (1994). Trans fatty acids intake and risk of myocardial infarction. *Circulation* 891:94-101.

Avoioli, L. (1981). Postmenopausal osteoporosis: Prevention versus cure. *Fed. Proc.* 40: 2418-2422.

Baig, M., and Cerda, J. (1981). Pectin: Its interaction with serum proteins. *Am. J. Clin. Nutr.* 34:50-53.

Balch, J.F., & Balch, P.A. (1990). *Prescription for Nutritional Healing.* Garden City Park, NY: Avery Publishing Company, pp. 12–13.

Bazan, N., Paoletti, R., and Iaconeo, J., Eds. (1981). *New Trends in Nutrition Lipid Research, and Cardiovascular Disease.* New York:Alan R. Liss, Inc.

Beach, R.S., Mantero-Atienza, E., Shor-Posner, G., Javier, J.J., Szapocznik, J., et al. (1992). Specific nutrient abnormalities in asymptomatic HIV-1 infection. *AIDS* 6(7):701-708.

Beare-Rogers, J., Gray, L., and Hollywood, R. (1979). The linoleic acid and trans fatty acids of margarines. *Am. J. Clin. Nutr.* 32:1805-1809.

Belman, S. (1983). Onion and garlic oils inhibit tumor promotion. *Carcinogenesis* 4: 1063-1065.

Bennett, W., and Gurin, J. (1982). *The Dieter's Dilemma: Eating Less and Weighing More.* New York: Basic Books.

Bharuccha, K., Cross, C., and Rubin, M. (1980). Long-chain acetals of ascorbic and erythorbic acids as antinitrosamine agents for bacon. *J. Agric. and Food Chem.* 28:1274-1281.

Bjelke, I. (1974). Epidemiological studies of cancer of the stomach, colon and rectum: With special emphasis on the role of the diet. *Scand. J. Gastr.* 9:1-53.

Bonnick, S.L. (1994). *The Osteoporosis Handbook,* Dallas, TX: Taylor Publishing Co., p. 32

Boscaro, M., Armanini, D. (1994). Licorice ameliorates postural hypertension caused by diabetic automatic neuropathy. *Diabetes Care* 17(11):1356.

Burrows, M., and Farr, W. (1972). The action of mineral on per os the organism. *Proc. Soc Exp. Biol. Med.* 24:719.

Calautti, P. et al. (1980). Serum selenium levels in malignant lympohoproliferation disease. *Scand. J. Haematol.* 24:6366.

Cathcart, R.F. (1984). Vitamin C in the treatment of acquired immune deficiency syndrome (AIDS). *Med. Hypotheses,* 14 : 423–433.

Check, W. Switch to soy protein for boring but healthful diet. *JAMA* 247:3045-3046.

Coll, M., Meyer A., and Stunkard, A. (1979). Obesity and food choices in public places. *Arch. Gen. Psychiat.* 36: 795-797.

Cordray, S. (1993). News from the Ochsner Medical Institutions. New Orleans, LA, March 4.

Dishong, H. (1994). *Florida scientists introduce new pectin rich food powder to help prevent clogged arteries.* Press release, The University of Florida, Gainesville, March 3rd.

Donadio, J.V., Holman, R.T., Johnson, S.B., Bibas, D. & Spencer, D.C. (1994). Essential fatty acid deficiency profiles in idiopathic immunoglobin A nepropathy. *American Journal Kidney Disease* 23(5): 648-654.

Dorant, E. van den Brandt, P.A., Goldbohm, R.A. et al. (1993). Garlic and its significance for the prevention of cancer in humans. *Brit J.Cancer* 67: 424-429.

Dworkin, B.M. (1994). Selenium deficiency in HIV infection and AIDS. *Chem. Bio. Inter.* 91 (2-3): 181-186.

Dwyer, J.H. (1992). *Calcium and reduced hypertension.* Paper presented at the annual meeting of the American Health Association, New Orleans, LA, December 10

Eat more fruits and vegetables: Five a day for better health. (1991). n.a. USDAS, PHS, NIH pub # 92-3248.

Epstein, L., and Wing, R. (1980). Aerobic exercise and weight. *Additive Behaviors* 5:371–388.

Erickson, M. et al. (1983). Tissue mineral levels in victims of sudden infant death syndrome: Toxic metals—lead and cadmium. *Ped. Res.* 17:779.

Federal Food and Drug Administration. Fed. Register, July 1, 1943a.

Fish oil for prevention of atherosclerosis. (1982). *The Med. Letter* 24(622):99–100.

Folkers, K., Morita, M., and McKree, J. (1993). The activities of coenzyme Q 10 and vitamin B_6 for immune response. *Bio. Biophys Res. Commun.* 193(1): 88–92.

Garg, A., Bonanome, M.D., Grundy, S.M. Zu-Jun, Z., and Unger, R.H. (1988). Comparison of a high carbohydrate diet with a high-non-saturated-fat diet in patients with non-insulin-dependent diabetic mellitus. *N.E.J. Med.* 319: 829-834.

Gavin, G., and McHenry, E. (1941). Inositol: A lipotropic factor. *J. Bio Chem* 139 : 485.

Gillman, M., Cupples, A., Gagnon, D. et al, (1995). Protective effect of fruits and vegetables on development of stroke in men. J. *Am. Med. Ass*oc. 273 (14): 1113-1117.

Giovannucci, E., Rimm, E.B., Colditz, G.A. et al. (1993). A prospective study of dietary fat and risk of prostate cancer. *J. Nat'l. Cancer Inst.* 85(19): 1571–1579.

Giovannucci, E., Rimm, E.B., Staupper, M.J., et al (1994). Intake of fat, meat, and fiber in relation to risk of colon cancer in men. *Cancer Research* 54(9): 2390-2397.

Goldstein, M.R. (1994). Mediterranean diet and coronary heart disease. *Lancet* 344:276.

Gordon, R., and Verter, J. (1969). *The Framingham Study: An Epidemiological Investigation of Cardiovascular Disease.* Bethesda, MD: NIH.

Greenberg, E.R., Baron, J.A. Tosteson, T.D., et al. (1994). A Clinical trial of Antioxidants to prevent colorectal adenoma *N.E.J. Med* 331(3): 141-144.

Griffin, A. (1979). Role of selenium in the chemoprevention of cancer. *Adv. Cancer Res.* 29:419–442.

Gwinup, G. (1975). Effect of exercise alone on the weight of obese females. *Arch. Int. Med.* 135:676–680.

Hamodeh, M.J. (1992). The effect of dietary flaxseed on N-3 fatty acids, cholestrol profile, and laxation in the young and institutionalized elderly. *Masters Abstracts International*: (UNM) AAIMM78487, 31–04:1759.

Han, J. (1993). Highlights of the cancer chemo prevention studies in China. *Preventive Medicine* 22(5): 712-722.

Harborne, J.B. (1986). *Plant Flavonoids in Biology and Medicine.* New York: Alan R. Liss.

Horsey, J., Livesley, B., and Dickerson, J/. (1981). Ischemic heart disease and aged patients: Effects of ascorbic acid on lipoproteins. *J. Hum. Nutr.* 35:53-58

Hunter, D.J., Menson, J.E., Colditz, G.A., et al. (1993). A prospective study of the intakes of vitamin C, E, and the Risk of Breast Cancer. *N.E.J.* 329(4): *234-240.*

Kavanaugh, T. et al. (1983). Influences of exercise and lifestyle variables upon high density lipoprotein cholesterol after myocardial infarction. *Arteriosclerosis 3:249-259.*

Knip, M. (1992). Can type-1 diabetes in children be prevented? *Nordic Medicine* 107(8-9) 207-210.

Knox, E. (1973). Ischemic heart disease, mortality, and dietary intake of vitamin C. *Lancet* 1:1465–1467.

Konig, J. (1981). Aluminum pots as a source of dietary aluminum. *NE J. Med.* 304:172.

Kritichevsky, D., et al. (1982). Atherogenicity of animal and vegetable protein. *Atherosclerosis* 41:429–431.

Kubova, J., Thinska, J., Stolcova, E., Mosat'ova, A, and Ginter, E. (1993). The influence of ascorbic acid on selected parameters of cell immunity in guinea pigs exposed to cadmium, *Ernährungswiss.* 32(2): 113-120.

Kummet, T., and Meyskens, L. (1983). Vitamin A: A potential inhibitor of human cancer. *Seminars in Oncol.* 10 : 281.

Kvale, G., Bjelke, E., and Gart, J. (1982). Dietary habits and lung cancer risk. *Proceedings of the Thirteenth International Cancer Congress.* Seattle, WA: International Union Against Cancer, p. 175.

Lappe, F. (1975). *Diet for a small planet.* New York : Ballantine, pp. 62–117.

Li, J. Y., Li, B., Blot, W.J., et al. (1993). Preliminary results of nutrition prevention. *Chung Hua Chung Liu Tsa Chih* 15(3): 165-181.

Longnecker, M.P., Martin-Moreno, J.M., Knecht, P., et al. (1992). Serum alpha tochpherol concentration in relation to subsequent colorectal cancer. *J. Natl. Cancer Inst.* 84(6): 430-435.

Loomis, D. (1992). Which is safer: Drugs or vitamins? *Townsend Letter for Doctors.* April: 219.

MacRury, S.M., Muir M., & Hume, R. (1992) Seasonal and climatic variation in cholesterol and Vitamin C: Effect of vitamin C supplementation. *Scot Med. J.* 37(2): 49-52.

Malinow, M. et al. (1978). Effect of alfalfa meal on shrinkage (regression) of atherosclerotic plaques during cholesterol feeding in monkeys. *Atherosclerosis* 30:27–43.

Malinow, M. et al. (1981). Cholesterol and bile balance in Macaco fascicularis. *J. Clin. Invest.* 67:156–162.

Malone, W.F. (1991). Studies evaluating antioxidant and beta-carotene as chemo preventative. *Am. J. Clin. Nutr.* 53 (suppl.): 305s-313s.

Manson, J.E., Willett, W.C., Stampfer, M.J. et al. (1994) Vegetable and fruit consumption and incidence of stroke in women. *Circulation* 89(2): 678.

Marlowe, M., and Errera, J. (1982). Low lead levels and behavior problems in children. *Behav. Dis.* 7:163.

Martin-Moreno, J.M., Willett, J.C. Gorgojo, L., Banegas, J.R., et al., (1994). Dietary fat, olive oil intake and breast cancer risk. *Int. J. Cancer* 58(6):774–780.

Massey, L.K., and Wise, K.J. (1984). The effect of dietary caffeine on urinary excretion of calcium, magnesium, sodium, and potassium in healthy young females. *Nutr. Res.* 4:43–50.

McCarty, M.F. (1993). Homologous physiological effects of phenoform and chromium picolinate. *Med. Hypothesis* 41(4): 316–324.

McConnell, K. et al. (1980). The relationship of dietary selenium and breast cancer. *J. Surg. Oncol.* 15:67–70.

McGill, H., Geer, J., and Strong, J. (1965). The natural history of atherosclerosis. In *Metabolism of Lipids as Related to Atherosclerosis,* F.A. Kummerow, Ed. Spring field, IL: Charles C Thomas, p. 36.

Messina, M.J., Persky, V., Setchell, K.D., and Barnes, S. (1994). Soy intake and cancer risk. *Nutrition and Cancer* 21: 113-131.

Middleton, E., and Kandaswami, C. (1993). *The Flavonoids.* London: Chapman and Hall.

Miller, W.C., Nicderprucm, M.G., Wallace, J. P., and Lindeman, A.K. (1994). Dietary fat, sugar, and fiber predict body fat content. *J. of the Am. Diet. Assoc.* 94(6): 612-615.

Morgan, W., Raskin, P., and Rosenstock, J. (1995). A comparison of fish oil or corn oil supplements in hyperlipidemic subjects with NIDDM. *Diabetes Care* 18(1): 83-86.

Muntzel, M., and Drüeke, T. (1992). A comprehensive review of the salt and blood pressure relationship. *Am. J. Hypertension* 5(4): 1s-42s

Murata, M., Imaizum, K., and Sugano, M. (1982). Effect of dietary phospholipids and their constituent bases on serum lipids and apolipoproteins in rates. *J. Nutr.* 112:1805–1808.

National Academy of Science Committee on Diet, Nutrition and Cancer. (1982). *Diet, Nutrition, and Cancer.* Washington, D.C.: National Academy Press.

National Dairy Council (1990). *High calcium foods.* Press release.

Noda, M., Takano, T., and Sakuri, H. (1979). Effects of selenium on chemical carcinogens. *Mut. Res.* 66:175.

Nutrition and cancer: Cause and prevention. (1984). *CA-A Cancer J. Clin. Res.* 34(2):121.

Nyandieka, H.S., and Wakhisi, J. (1993). *East African Medical Journal* 70(3): 151–153.

Offenbacher, E. et al. (1980). Beneficial effect of chromium-rich yeast on glucose tolerance and blood lipis in elderly subjects. *Diabetes* 29:919–925.

Oleske, T. et al. (1983). Plasma, zinc and copper in primary and secondary immunodeficiency disorders. *Biol. Tr. El. Res.* 5:189–194.

Oliver, M. (1982). Diet and coronary heart disease. *Hum. Nutr. Clin. Nutr.* 36: 413–427.

Ornish, D.M., Scherwitz, L.W., Brown, S.E., et al. (1989). Adherence to life style changes and reversal of coronary athersclerosis. *Circulation* 80(4): II 57.

Passwater, R.A., and Kanaswami, C. (1994). *Pycnogenol, the super protector nutrient.* New Canaan, CT: Keats Publishing Company, pp. 27, 33–34.

Pierson, H. (1994 May). *The Medicinal Use of Licorice Extract and the HIV Virus.* Paper presented at the Designer Foods III: Phytochemicals in Garlic, Soy, and Licorice. Washington, D.C.

Phinney, S., et al. (1980). Capacity for moderate exercise in obese subjects after adaption to a hypocaloric ketogenic diet. *J. Clin. Investig.* 66:1152–1161.

Pollitt, E. et al. (1982). Behavioral effects of iron deficiency anemia in children. In *Iron Deficiency, Brain Biochemistry, and Behavior,* E. Pollitt and R. Leibel, Eds. New York: Raven Press, pp. 195–208.

Prasad, D., and Edwards-Prasad, J. (1983). Effects of tocopherol (vitamin E) acid succinate on morphological alterations and growth inhibition in melanoma cells in culture. *Canc. Res.* 42:550–555.

Rabinowitz, M. et al. (1983). Effects of chromium and yeast supplements on carbohydrate and lipid metabolism in diabetic men. *Diabet. Care* 6:319.

Ramirez, J., and Flowers, C. (1980). Leukocyte ascorbic and its relationship to coronary artery disease in man. *Am. J. Clin. Nutr.* 33:2079–2087.

Recker, R., Saville, P., and Heaney, R. (1977). Effect of estrogens and calcium carbonate on bone loss in post-menopausal women. *Ann. Int. Med.* 87:649.

Resnick, L.M., Gupta, R.K., and Laragh, J.H. (1984). Intracelluar free magnesium in erthrocytes of essential hypertension. *Proc. Nat'l Acad Sci USA,* 81 : 6511–6515.

Rimm, E.B., Stampfer, M.J., Ascherio, A. Giovannucci, E. Colditz, G.A., and Willett, W.C. (1993). Vitamin E consumption and the risk of coronary disease in men. *N.E.J. Med.* 328(20): 1450-1456.

Roe, D. (1983). *Drug-induced nutritional deficiencies.* Westport, CT: AVI, p. 130.

Rutenberg, H., et al. (1983). Influence of trans unsaturated fats on experimental atherosclerosis in rabbits. *J. Nutr.* 113:835–844.

Sacks, F., et al. (1983). Dietary unsaturated fats affect blood pressures, platelet thromboxane production, and HDL subfractions in normal subjects. *Arterioscl. Councl. Abstr. 3:483A–484A.*

Saner, G., et al. (1983). Alterations of chromium metabolism and effect of chromium supplementation in Turner's syndrome. *Am. J. Clin. Nutr.* 38:574–578.

Schlegel, J. (1975). Proposed uses of scorbic acid in the prevention of bladder carcinoma. *Ann. NY Acad. Sci.* 258:432–437.

Schmeisser, D., et al. (1983). Effect of excess dietary lysine on plasma lipids of the chick. *J. Nutr.* 113:1777–1783.

Schrauzer, G., White, D., and Schneider, C. (1977). Cancer mortality correlation studies. III. Statistical associations with dietary selenium intakes. *Bio Org. Chem* 7:23–34.

Scott, R., et al. (1972). Animal models in atherosclerosis. In *The Pathogensis of Atherosclerosis,* R.W. Wissler and J.C. Geer, Eds. Baltimore: Williams & Wilkins.

Seedon, J.M., Christen, W.G., Manson, J.E., et al. (1994). The use of vitamin supplementation and risk of cataract among U.S. male physicians. *Am. J. Pub. 41th* 84:788–792.

Seedon, J.M., Ajani, U.A., Sperduto, R.D., et al. (1994). Dietary carotenoids, vitamins A, C and E, and advanced age-related macular degeneration. *J. Am. Med. Assoc.* 272: 1413–1420.

Seelig, M. (1983). Vitamin D: risks versus benefit. *J. Am. Col. N.* 2:109–110.

Select Committee on Nutrition and Human Needs. U.S. Senate. (1971). *Dietary Goals for the U.S.* 2nd ed. Washington, DC.: U.S. Govt. Printing Office, p. xxviii

Shamberger, R., and Willis, C. (1971). Selenium distribution and human cancer mortality. *C. Crit. Rev. Clin. Lab. Sci.* 2:211–221.

Shapiro, D.V. (1992). Nutrition and cancer prevention. *Prim. Care* 19(3):481–491

Sharma, K.K. (1977). Antihyperglycemic effect of onion. *Indian J. Med. Res.* 65:4222–429.

Sharma, R.D., Raghwiam, T.C., and Rao, N.S. (1990). Effect of fenugreek seeds on blood glucose. *Eur. J. Clin. Nutr.* 44:301–306.

Shaw, M. et al. (1994). The use of a low-fat diet with moderately obese women. *Am. J. Clin. Nutr.* 59:980.

Sheela, C.G., & Augusti, K.T. (1992). Antidiabetic effects of garlic. *Indian J. Exp. Biol.* 30:523–526.

Simon, J.A. (1992). Vitamin C and cardiovascular disease: a review. *J. Am. Coll. Nutr.* 11:107–125.

Simpson, H., et al. (1981). A high carbohydrate leguminous diet improves all aspects of diabetic control. *Lancet* 1(8210): 1–5.

Sirtori, C., Gatti, E., and Mouter, O. (1979). Clinical experience with the soy bean protein diet. *JAMA* 247:3045–3046.

Skrobak-Kacynski, J., and Andersen, L. (1975). The effect of a high level of habitual physical activity in the regulation of fatness during aging. *Internatl. Arch. Occupt. and Environm. Hlth.* 36:41–46.

Stahelin, H.B. (1991). Beta-carotene and cancer-prevention: the Basel study. *Am. J. Clin. Nutr.* 53: 265s–269s.

Stampfer, M.J. et al. (1993). Vitamin E consumption and the risk of coronary disease in women. *N.E. J. Med.* 328:1444–1449.

Stampler, M.J. (1993). A prospective study of dietary calcium and other nutrients and the risk of sympomatic kidney stones. *N.E. J. Med.* 328(12) : 833–838.

Stevens, V.J. et al. (1993). Weight loss intervention in phase I of the trials of hypertension prevention *Arch. Int. Med.* 153 : 849–858.

Swendsen, S. (1995). High doses of vitamin E reduces risks. *Southwestern Center Times* March: 1,9.

Tang, A.M., Graham, N.M., Kirby, A.J. et al. (1993). Dietary micronutrient intake and risk of progression to AIDS. *Am. J. Epid.* 138(1):937–951.

Tawata, M., Aida., K., Noguchi, T. et al. (1992). Anti-platelet action of isoliquiritigenin, an aldose reductase inhibitor in licorice. *Eur. J. Pharmcol.* 212:87–92.

ter Well, H., van Gent, C., and Dekker, W. (1974). The effect of soy lecithin on serum lipid values in type II hyperlipoprotemia. *Acta. Med. Scan.*195: 267–271.

Thun, M. (1992). The relationship between vegetables, high fiber grains and colon cancer. *J. Nat. Cancer Inst.*84:1461.

Toth, S., Montgomery, C., and Bunn, J. (1984). Weight management: a practical approach. *Pt. Educ. Nslett.* 7(3):3–4.

Trichopoulou, A., Katsouyanni, K., Stuver, S., et al. (1995). Consumption of olive oil. and specific food groups in relation to breast cancer risk in Greece. *J. Nat'l. Cancer Inst.* 87(2):110–116

Villar, J., Belizak, J., and Fisher, P. (1983). Epidemiological observations on the relationship between calcium intake and eclampsia. *Int. J. Gyn. Obst.* 21: 271–278.

Vroulis, G., et al. (1982). Reduction of cholesterol risk factors by lecithin in patients with Alzheimer's disease. *Am. J. Psychiat.* 139: 1633–1634.

Wang, H.Y. (1992). Experimental study of selenium preventing nasophangeal carcinoma. *Chung Hua Yu Fan I Huseh Tsa Chih* 26(5):281–283.

Wang, Y., and Watson, R.P. (1994). Ethanol, immune responses and murine AIDS: The role of vitamin E as an immunostimulant and antioxidant. *Alcohol* 11(2):75–84.

Ward, J. (1994). Free radicals, antioxidants and preventive geriatrics. *Aust. Fam. Physician* 23(7): 1297–1301, 1305.

Warshafsky, S. (1993). A meta-analysis of all randomized, placebo-controlled trials testing the effectiveness of oral garlic preparations. *Ann. Inter. Med.* 119(7):599–605.

Wartanowicz, M. et al. (1984). The effect of alpha-tocopherol and ascorbic acid on serum lipid peroxide level in elderly people. *Ann. Nutr. Metab.*28:186–191.

Watson, L.W. (1992). Resistance to intestinal parasites during murine AIDS. *Parasitology 109:568–574.*

Wattenberg, L.W. (1992). Inhibition of carcinogenesis by minor dietary components. *Cancer Research* 52:2085s–2091s.

Weinsier, R. (1985). News release from Media Relations Director, Manning, Selvage and Lee, 1250 Eye St., N.W., Washington, DC 20005.

Willet, W., et al. (1983). Prediagnostic serum selenium and risk of cancer. *Lancet* 2:130–133.

Willet, W. (1992). The nurses health study. *Lancet* 341:581.

Willet, W. (1992). Folic acid and neural tube defect. *Am. J. Pub. Hlth.*82(5):666–668.

Willett, W., et al. (1993). A case-control study of oral cancer in Beijing. *Eur. J. Oral Oncol.* 29B(1): 45–55.

Willett, W. (1994). Dietary iron intake and risk of coronary disease among men. *Circulation* 89, 3: 969–974.

Wissler, R. (1979). Conference on the health effects of blood lipids, optimal distributions for populations. *Rev. Med. 8:715–732.*

Wootan, M., Liebman, B. (1993). Great transwreck. *Nutr. Action Newsletter* (November): 8–9.

Zavoral, J. et al. (1983). The hypolipidemic effect of locust bean gum products in familial hypochlesterolemic adults. *Am. J. Clin. Nutr.* 38: 285–294.

6

EXERCISE AND MOVEMENT

This chapter discusses the following topics:

- The relationship between fitness, movement, and wellness
- Theoretical frameworks for fitness
- Fitness assessments
- Fitness interventions
- Exercise for special populations
- Overcoming obstacles to exercise
- Body-mind interactions and fitness

Movement is one of the simplest and most effective modes of stress reduction. It also moderates appetite, lowers cholesterol, reduces migraine, and serves a preventive function against aging and some chronic conditions, including coronary heart disease, obesity, joint and spinal disc disease, fatigue, muscular tension, osteoporosis, high blood pressure, stroke, colon cancer, anxiety, breast cancer, and depression. When done correctly, movement and exercise can enhance self-image and self-confidence, reduce joint stiffness, increase circulation, improve posture, reduce depressions, positively affect work performance, decrease blood pressure, enhance ability to relate to others, enhance sleep, decrease the need for stimulants, and enhance breathing ability (The President's Council on Physical Fitness and Sports; National Headache Foundation; Shinton & Sagan, 1993; Pate et al., 1995; Angotti et al., 1994).

Exercise has also been shown to cut the risk of developing non-insulin dependent diabetes in men (Manson et al., 1992), and breast cancer in women (Henderson et al., 1994), and to extend years of life for those over age 70 (Rakowski & Mor, 1992).

Exercisers also file fewer health care claims (Gettman, 1986; Bernacki, 1987). Exercise and fitness programmers in industry also claim exercise programs enhance work performance and productivity (Gettman, 1986; Bernacki, 1984) and reduce absenteeism and turnover (Shephard, 1983).

SOME WELLNESS THEORETICAL FRAMEWORKS
FOR FITNESS

Movement and fitness frameworks that are especially suited to a wellness out-
look are Cohen's and Mills' Developmental Movement Theory, Feldenkrais'
Theory of Awareness Through Movement, and Kurtz and Prestera's Body
Message Theory.

Mills/Cohen Developmental Movement Theory

At the School for Body/Mind Centering in Amherst, Massachusetts, Margret
Mills (a fine arts, movement and theater expert) and Bonnie Bainbridge Cohen
(an occupational therapist, neurodevelopmental therapist, and dance therapist)
developed their theory of developmental movement. The thrust of their theory
is that the body teaches the brain. Through specific movements, the brain is
developed and reshaped, and vice versa.

In Mills' and Cohen's system, evolutionary development is followed through
the course of development of an individual. Infants move in ways similar to
creatures of a lower evolutionary state, such as the worm, fish, etc. As infants
grow, they are capable of movements similar to creatures higher up the evolutionary scale, the rabbit, camel, etc.

Mills and Cohen work with the four basic locomotor movement patterns:
spinal, homologous, homolateral, and contralateral. The more primitive
patterns underlie the more complex ones; thus the spinal patterning must be
mastered or the homologous movements will not exhibit their full range of
balance, strength, mobility, and dynamics. Development also proceeds from
proximal to distal and from push movements to reach and pull movements. In
reading the descriptions of movement below, if it is difficult to understand
what is involved, stop a minute and picture the creature in action, then duplicate the movement.

Spinal movements include an arching of the body in all directions and
flexing and extending the body (concave and convex movements). The fish
represents this movement, which assists the brain in differentiating the front
from the back of the body and the development of the conception of forward-
backward movement.

Homologous movements are those of both upper extremities together and/
or both lower extremities together. The phylogenetic stage illustrating this
pattern is the frog. (Arms push forward, body moves back; legs push, body
moves forward; arms reach, body is pulled forward; legs reach, body moves
back.) This movement pattern underlies the conception of vertical up/down
relationships.

Homolateral movements include an alteration of movement between one
side of the body and the other side. The movements assist in the brain differentiation of the two sides of the body and the right/left discrimination.

The *contralateral* movement pattern is the right upper body and left lower
body moving together and then the left upper body and right lower body

moving together. Movements of the lizard and camel illustrate this pattern, which aids in the diagonal integration of the four quadrants of the body and the relationship of the body in space (3-dimensionality).

If the lower extremities are not developed completely, the trunk will be less stable, and there will be a more static, less mobile support for the extremities. Thus, when walking, kicking, dancing, running, or any movement of the lower extremities is performed, flexibility and strength will be less than is possible (Mills & Cohen, 1979, pp. 1–28).

The pioneering work at the School for Body/Mind Centering connects these movements with the nervous system (alertness, thought, precision, condensation) with the endocrine system (intuition, emotions, automaticity, sense of flow and expansion). Mills and Cohen postulate that specific movements involve the use of the endocrine glands for support and initiation serving to stimulate, activate, and strengthen the endocrine gland involved, thereby influencing posture, energy level, and psychological states.

According to Mills and Cohen (1979, p. 29), the following movements will stimulate, activate, and strengthen the following endocrine glands:

- Spinal push through the head (worm and fish movements): pineal gland
- Spinal push through the tail (worm and fish backward movements): carotid bodies
- Homologous push (frog hop and rocking on all fours): heart, bodies and pancreas
- Homolateral push upper extremities (one side push up, homolateral roll, and diagonal head raising): gonads
- Homolateral push lower extremities (crawling forward, homolateral roll, and hip swing): coccygeal body
- Spinal reach and pull through the head (snake forward and head reaching): mammillary bodies
- Spinal reach and pull through the tail (wagging the tail and tail-leg raising): pituitary
- Homologous reach and pull upper extremities (rabbit hop forward and rope pulling): thyroid
- Homologous reach and pull lower extremities (rabbit hop backward and wall exercise): thymus
- Contralateral reach and pull (forward and backward creep, diagonal roll initiated by the hand or foot, and rope climbing): parathyroids
- Navel radiation (soaring stretch): adrenals
- Breathing (breast stroke and star breathing): thoraco body

Feldenkrais' Awareness Through Movement

Physiologists have found that cells in the motor cortex of the brain assemble into a shape resembling the human body that is called the *homunculus*. This is the motor or movement basis for self-image. Feldenkrais contends everyone's self-image is smaller than it might be and that the combinations and patterning of cells may be more important than their number. For example, people who speak two languages make use of both more cells and more combinations of cells. Some people can speak 30 or more languages; this gives a rough idea of the limitlessness of potential for self-image (Feldenkrais, 1977, pp.14-15).

Everyone has parts of the body for which there is no awareness; for example, it is easy for most people to lie on their back and sense their finger-tips, but it is probably difficult for many to sense the nape of the neck or the space between the ears (Feldenkrais, 1979, p. 21).

Learning to move parts of the body with consciousness will enhance the self-image, according to Feldenkrais.

Some important postulates of Feldenkrais' theory are (1979, pp. 33–62):

1. Awareness and self-image are based on movement.
2. Breathing and movement must be coordinated if movement is to be effective.
3. Movement of the eyes organizes movement of the body.
4. When actions are performed correctly, refreshment and relaxation result; when movements are performed too quickly and without attention to breathing, fatigue may result.
5. The body is constantly fighting against the force of gravity unless it is well organized; without appropriate organization, gravity can pull or push the body and affect movement in a negative manner.
6. Individuals can learn to organize their bodies more effectively by practicing slow, gradual movements while breathing correctly and learning to experience the body sensations associated with effective movement.

Kurtz and Prestera's Body Message Theory

Fixed muscular patterns in the body are central to a person's way of being in the world. They form in response to family and early environment . . . Whatever the feeling, it is also expressed physically, and becomes a way of holding oneself, a fixed muscular pattern and a set attitude toward life . . .These attitudes and fixed muscular patterns reflect, enhance, and sustain one another. (Kurtz & Prestera, 1984, pp. 2–3).

These characteristic patterns inhibit individuals from attaining well-being. When well, the body is:

capable of allowing the free flowing of any feeling. It is efficient and graceful in its movements, aware and responsive to real needs. Such a body has bright eyes, breathes freely, is smooth skinned, and has an elastic muscle tone. It is well proportioned, and the various segments coordinate well with each other. The neck is pliable and the head moves easily. The pelvis swings freely. The entire body is lined up efficiently with respect to gravity; that is, in a standing position, there is no struggle with gravity's downward pull. Pleasure and well-being are characteristic feelings. A person with such a body is emotionally flexible and his or her feelings are spontaneous. (Kurtz & Prestera, 1984, p. 3)

When there is a wholeness to the body/mind/spirit, expression of feelings flows easily; wholeness is disrupted when the flow of energy in the body is disrupted. For example, when an individual experiences anger, but does not express it directly, the breaks in the normally smooth curves of the body can be observed. For example, look at your body right now in the mirror and see if your scapulas are flat and equally so; if not, there is a break in the smooth curve of your back. Likewise, if you look at the front of your body in a mirror, you may see that the right or left side of your chest is more forward, more to the back, wider, longer, or whatever; any of these will look like breaks in the smooth curve of your body. Everyone has some breaks; the difference in magnitude and quantity differentiates all individuals along a continuum from nonmovement and energy blocks to effective movement and energy flow.

In the case of the individual who does not express anger, that unexpressed feeling my be "locked" in a body part; some individuals may lock it in the arms (instead of striking out); others may hold their anger in their abdominal area, leading to digestive upsets and a tight, tense abdomen that may be excessively held in.

Similarly, an infant whose mother constantly grabbed his arm whenever he reached out to explore his environment may turn into an adult with lifeless arms that hang drooping from narrow shoulders; there is no indication of reaching out to life; instead, the infant waits passively for things to come to him.

Infants are born with the capacity for wholeness. Fear can produce blocks. For example, "in blocking the expression of sadness, we tense the jaw, chest, stomach, diaphragm, and some muscles of the throat and face—all the areas which move spontaneously when the feeling is allowed its natural outlets" (Kurtz & Prestera, 1984, pp.8–9).

Blocks impede the normal flow of energy as muscles tense, circulation is constricted, and skin tone and temperature change. Holding in of feelings is manifested as rings of muscle and fascia tension or breaks in the areas between the major segments of the body: neck and upper shoulders, the diaphragm, the lower back between the abdomen and pelvis, the groin, the knees, and the ankles; feet and eyes can also be held. Figure 6.1a shows body areas where holding is common.

Gross changes in function, form, color and development can occur. Hands and feet may be small and cold. The head may be large or the abdomen blown up while the chest is collapsed. As blood supply is reduced due to increased muscular tension, there is a collection of tissue wastes, setting up a mechanism of toxic spasm and stasis. The nervous system responds by firing more signals leading to the pain-spasm-pain-spasm of a headache, backache, or heartache. If this occurs chronically, the tissues harden to splint the area against further attack and structural block develops.

According to Kurtz and Prestera, a backache may be the product of a slipped disc, but the original insult may result in an attempt to hold oneself up or back.

A heart attack may be the end result of blocked impulses to love or be loved that become a block in energy flow, a decrease in circulation, a pooling and thickening of blood, and eventually a physiological blockage. Bear in mind that a wellness view considers all dimensions of wellness, thus, in this view, negative nutritional, fitness, stress management, environmental concerns, and negative relationships are more likely to end in chronic difficulties. On the other hand, this book uses a systems approach; in it, one part of the subsystem, such as an increase in fitness or a change to more effective movement, can affect the entire system's functioning. Thus, by working on the body, the entire body/mind/spirit can be affected.

Harmony with gravity aids in reaching up and out in the world; disharmony leads to attempts by the body to compensate; if the chest is going in and down, the belly may go out and up. "The ideal axis for obtaining the greatest balance is that which connects points at the top of the head, middle of the shoulder, midpoint of the hip joint, center of the knee joint, and center of the ankle joint" (Kurtz & Prestera, 1984, p. 29). Figure 6.1b shows the ideal axis in person 1 and a compensated balance.

Individuals who are out of balance can express it bodily and emotionally; bodies that are bent forward often express feelings of being overburdened; those bending backward experience life as an unending struggle. Figure 6.1c shows a person expressing burden through the way the body is held. In Figure 6.1d, the first figure is bowed back and the second is bowed forward.

Tension and stiffness in the lower half of the body, especially the legs and feet, makes balancing difficult; it is as if the person is bracing against a fall. Tightening up may be to protect against being a "pushover," falling down on the job. In Figure 6.1e, the first figure is falling forward a bit; the second has a locked knee indicating bracing.

Feet can reveal how reality is dealt with by the way the ground is contacted; if one foot goes one way and the other another way, this may indicate confusion. Feet rotated outward put added stress on the ankle and knee joints; feet facing forward reduce this stress, allowing more effective weight transfer through the center of the foot. Locking of the knees could indicate an attempt to hold on, hold oneself up, or stand ground. People with rigid legs have difficulty bending their toes forward or back (an indicator of the condition). Figure 6.1f shows various arrangements for feet.

Limited sexual, anal, and urinary expression is evident in individuals with knees that are quite separate and a space between the thighs terminating in a high peak in the midline, as well as in individuals whose thighs are drawn inward, squeezing the genitals. In the latter case, the chronic contraction of both buttocks and thighs restricts energy flow; if the reader stands up and tries to simultaneously squeeze the muscles in both areas, the degree of tension will be evident. The first person in Figure 6.1g shows high tension in the genital area; the second figure shows a relatively "normal" configuration.

The position of the pelvis also reveals inner feelings; when tucked under, tight buttocks allow for a "dribbling out of emotion and feeling" (Kurtz & Prestera, 1984, p. 60); when retracted, the individual is unable to release and remains "cocked and ready to fire" (Kurtz & Prestera, 1984, p. 61). In Figure 6.1h the first woman has a pelvis squarely under the trunk; the second woman has a retracted pelvis.

Normally the belly wall expands with each breath. In our society where exposing "gut" feelings is not rewarded or encouraged, the closest representative of the natural state is the young child.

> There are three areas in which energy streaming can be cut off: the throat, the diaphragm, and the lower abdomen. In the throat area, tightening occurs every time we are asked by our head center to say something emotionally difficult or phony, i.e., not in tune with our internal instinctual life. The diaphragm tightens whenever our gut feelings are supplanted by our head's ideas. The area across the lower abdomen tightens, freezing the pelvis and cutting off genital feelings whenever our head dictates when, how, and where to have sex without harmonizing the dictates of our belly and heart centers. (Kurtz & Prestera, 1984, p. 68)

An overexpanded chest is held in a tight, inflated position at all times; the heart and heart feelings are kept locked up. Individuals with this condition tend to "stay within" the bounds of rules, schedules, attitudes, and logic, emphasizing success and performance (Prestera, 1984, p. 81). In Figure 6.1i the first man has an overexpanded chest.

The collapsed chest is most closely associated with a basic lack of emotional vitality. The amount of breath taken in is not adequate enough to spark full feeling. In Figure 6.1i person 4 has a collapsing chest. The illustration depicts a progression from person 1 who has stagnant energy in the upper part of his body to person 4 who has stagnant energy in the lower part of her body. To be balanced, energy must flow up with ideas and creativity and down to produce a firm contact with the ground and reality.

ASSESSING FITNESS

The traditional view of fitness focuses on cardiac fitness. A wellness view contends that fitness is more comprehensive. The deaths of a number of world class and other avid runners who were apparently "cardiac fit" provides empirical evidence that a more extensive framework is needed to assess fitness.

When engaging a client from a fitness standpoint, the wellness practitioner involves each individual in self-assessment procedures. Some areas of importance include: developmental assessments, structural assessments, flexibility assessments, and aerobic assessments.

Developmental Assessments

When using Cohen and Mills' developmental movement theory, a number of observations and/or questions can serve as assessments of the client's need to practice developmental patterns that will integrate movement with brain and glandular activity. The wellness practitioner assesses the client's ability to:

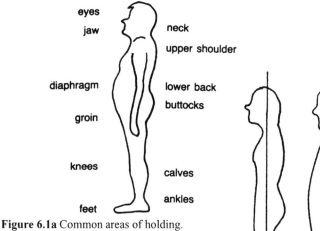

eyes
jaw
neck
upper shoulder
diaphragm
lower back
buttocks
groin
knees
calves
ankles
feet

Figure 6.1a Common areas of holding.

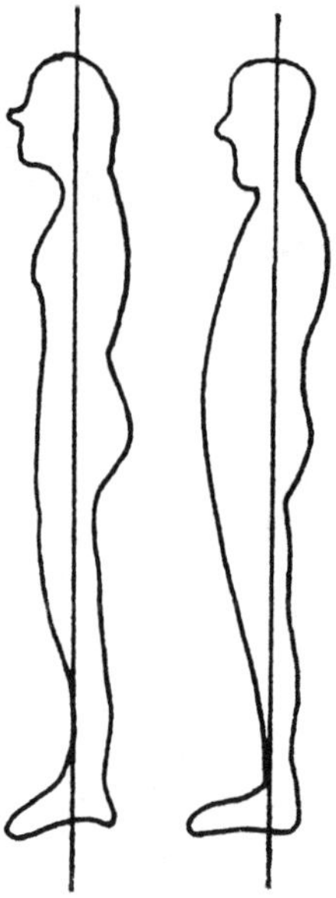

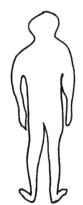

Figure 6.1c An overburdened individual.

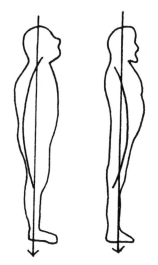

Figure 6.1b The lateral line and compensated balance.

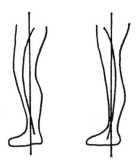

Figure 6.1e Knees.

Figure 6.1d Bowing backward and forward.

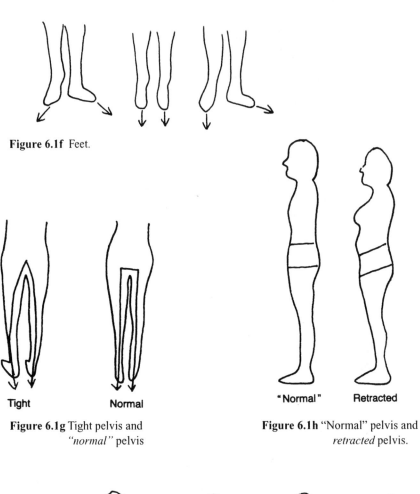

Figure 6.1f Feet.

Tight   **Normal**

Figure 6.1g Tight pelvis and *"normal"* pelvis

"Normal"   **Retracted**

Figure 6.1h "Normal" pelvis and *retracted* pelvis.

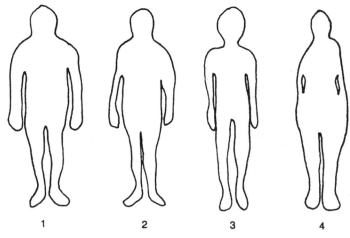

1   2   3   4

Figure 6.1i Progression of top to bottom trapped energy.

- differentiate the front from the back of the body
- move backwards versus moving forward
- move up and down in space
- differentiate the top from the bottom of the body
- use the top versus the bottom of the body
- use right/left discrimination (reversal of letters or numbers) (indicates poor right/left integration)
- differentiate the two sides of the body
- move from side to side
- move the body flexibly and comfortably in space
- diagonally integrate the four quadrants of the body
- use trunk mobility when moving (requires good extremity support, trunk stability, and dynamically mobile trunk support)
- walk upright
- run or jog upright
- coordinate hand-eye movements
- show self-love/self-hatred (ability to integrate coccygeal body with homolateral push, lower extremities: L.E.)
- be creative, give and receive, procreate, be organized, show aggression, passivity, sexuality (integrate gonads with homolateral push, upper extremities: U.E.)
- instinct for survival, fight/flight response, strength of stride in walking, courageousness, life force, separate I/ego sense, pain, rage, fear, anxiety (integrate adrenal glands with navel radiation)
- complete transitional activities, power, spatial awareness, appetite, reaching upward and outward, passion, greed, jealousy, anger, boredom, joviality (integrate pancreas with homologous push, L.E.)
- integrate breathing, align the body, be open, defenselessness (integrate thoraco body with breathing)
- love others, center horizontally, width perception (integrate heart bodies with homologous push, U.E.)
- resist infection/cancers, let go, be irresponsible, show fear, have nightmares and fears (integrate thymus gland with homologous reach and pull, L.E.).
- show commitment/conviction, have a full voice, move energy from lower body to head, have a strong heart, endure (integrate thyroid with homologous reach and pull, U.E.)
- show empathy, express self creatively, balance adrenals, manipulation (integrate parathyroids and contralateral reach and pull, U.E. and L.E.)
- show courage, effortless expression of life force, be artistic, express convictions (integrate carotid bodies with spinal push from the tail)
- show compassion, knowledge, integration of personality, conceptual memory (reading, thinking, studying), linear sequential time consciousness, compulsiveness, racism, paranoia, sexism (integrate pituitary gland with spinal reach and pull through the tail)
- show insight, foresight, and hindsight; hallucinations; undifferentiation of the past, present, and future; psychic ability; schizophrenia; realism (inte-

grate mammillary bodies with spinal reach and pull through the head)
- show integration of all experiences, perfectionisms, lack of self-control (integration of pineal body with spinal push through the head) (Mills & Cohen, 1979, pp. 2–24; Appendix A).

Structural Assessments

Kurtz's and Presera's theory provides the basic material for developing an assessment tool. Table 6.1 provides this tool for use with self and clients. Kurtz and Prestera have not developed interventions; however, Feldenkrais and yoga interventions could be used in many instances.

Table 6.1 Structural Assessments

Front view	Pre	Post
1. Contrast upper body with lower body. Do they appear to fit? Is there a mismatch?		
2. Contrast right side of body with left side for symmetry; is one side more forward or more developed?		
3. Are the eyes of same size and show the same amount of openness?		
4. Is the mouth tight or relaxed?		
5. Is the head titled to one side or the other?		
6. Are the shoulders level or is one higher than the other?		
7. Is one shoulder longer than the other?		
8. Is the chest concave, hyperextended, or relaxed?		
9. Are both the arms the same distance from the body?		
10. Are the hips level or is one higher than the other?		
11. Is the pubic area pulled in toward the center of the body or is the abdomen flat?		
12. Are the knees facing in or out?		
13. Are the knees and lower legs relaxed or tense? The assessor places one hand behind the lower leg and pushes slightly; if knee bends easily leg is relaxed, otherwise it is tense.		
14. Do both feet face forward or does one or the other face out?		
15. Are there any areas where energy appears trapped, that seem over- or underdeveloped? (Look especially at the chest area.)		

Table 6.1 (*continued*)

Side view	Pre	Post
16. Is the head tilted up, down, or level?		
17. Are the shoulders tilted forward or back?		
18. Are the scapula flat and level on both the left and right side?		
19. Is the lower back swayed with the abdomen pushed out or is there a small curve in the small of the back?		
20. Is the pelvis tipped out or back?		
21. Draw an imaginary line through the ear, shoulder, elbow, hip socket, knee, and ankle; where is the line out of line (unaligned)?		

Back view

22. Look for any areas where energy appears trapped, that seem over- or underdeveloped, especially in the upper back and buttocks.

Additional assessment

23. What is the ratio of hip to waist size? (Measure waist and hips with a tape measure; divide waist by hip size. For women the average ratio is about .7. A number above .85 shows a threefold increased risk of diabetes. For middle aged men the average ratio is .9 to .95; potbellied men above this range had more heart disease and strokes and died earlier than those with small stomachs in one study reported in *American Health,* 1984, 3(May): 45.)

Hunches: Look back at the assessment and hold your body as the person you are assessing does, but exaggerate the posture. What current or potential problems might occur to joints, body parts, internal organs, breathing, circulation, digestion, or elimination based on what you have observed? *Write your hunches down here:*

Now check with the person you are assessing and see if he or she has problems in any of the areas you have hunches about. If problems have not yet surfaced, counsel him or her on potential future issues based on your assessment.

Flexibility Assessments

There are two major views of flexibility: momentary and chronic. Momentary flexibility can change due to the emotion of the moment. Breathing rises toward the throat, muscles tighten, and a body "stiffness" is visible. Chronic inflexibility develops from years of not using the body appropriately or may be due to accident, surgery, and/or chronic inhibited emotion.

There are several ways to assess flexibility: observe the body in movement, ask clients which areas of the body "feel" tight or stiff, ask clients to complete range of motion or extension exercises. Asking a client to walk away from and toward the practitioner will reveal aspects of flexibility. Some questions to pose in this regard are:

1. Does this body move as a solid, shuffling block, or does it give the impression of a spring in the step, a lightness and gracefulness, or something in between? Describe what is observed.

2. Are body movements well defined with arms swinging in opposition to leg movement, knees bending, hips moving with legs, neck and chest moveable, or does the body move as a whole, or something in between? Describe what is observed.

3. Is there a difference in the walk when observed from the front and the back in terms of movement, or do both give similar impressions?

4. Does the person slouch forward or hold the head back behind the center of gravity?

5. Does the person lift the body in an exaggerated manner to move forward? Key indicators of this problem are shoulders hunched up, walking on the ball of the foot, and lack of thrusting forward of the hip.

6. Does the person walk duck-footed or pigeon-toed?

7. Does the person favor one leg? A thump-thump sound indicates favoring.

8. Does the person shuffle or scrape the feet?

A "yes" answer to any of the above indicates a loss of flexibility and could indicate a need for stretching or Feldenkrais interventions.

Marshall (1981), a former chief of sports medicine, suggests the following tests for flexibility:

1. Push the tip of your nondominant thumb back toward the forearm; if the angle between the fingers and thumb is more than 70 degrees, better than average flexibility is present; 60–70 degrees is average; and less than 60 degrees indicates less than average flexibility.

2. Measure metacarpal-phalangeal extension by lifting and holding one arm with elbow bent; with the other hand, push back the index finger; estimate the angle formed from the finger extended to the drop in the wrist. More than 115 degress indicates high flexibility; 105–115 degrees average; and less than 105 degrees indicates less than average flexibility (see Figure 6.2).

3. Look at the foot: high arch indicates tight heel cord and tight joints; average arch indicates average flexibility; and flat foot indicates loose joints and extreme flexibility.

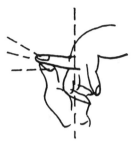

Figure 6.2 Metacarpal-phalangeal extension.

Loose-jointed clients are best suited for endurance activities and patterned movements such as dancing, gymnastics, cycling, swimming, or running. They are prone to ligament problems, partial dislocations, and knee problems. Tight-joint clients are best at explosive activities such as basketball, hockey, tennis, racquetball, and sprinting. These clients are most prone to muscle pulls and tears, torn ligaments and cartilage, lower back pain, tendonitis of the shoulder or elbow, and pinched nerves (Marshall, 1981, p. 63).

These three measures are determined by heredity and cannot be changed; there are four other measures of flexibility that can be improved through exercise:

1. Assess shoulder stretch: while standing, hold two ends of a tape measure, belt rope, or towel; stretch the arms straight out in front with arms and wrists straight; continue to hold the tape and bring it over the head and back out behind as far as comfortable; slide hands apart only as much as needed to accommodate the stretching movement, then bring hands forward again, holding the tape the same distance apart; read the number of inches. Under 30 in. is looser than average, 30–40 in. is average, and more than 40 in. is less flexible than average for clients under 25 years of age; for clients aged 25–45, add 5 in. to each measurement; for clients over 45, add 10 in. to each measurement.

2. Assess thigh stretch: sit on the floor with back straight against the wall; bend knees so bottoms of feet meet and feet are close to groin. Measure distance between knees and floor. For clients under 25 years of age, less than 4 in. is flexible, 4–7 in. is average, and more than 7 in. is tight. For clients 25–45 years add 2 in. to each measurement: for clients over 45 years, add 2 in. more.

3. Assess heel cord flexibility: lie down on a sofa or bed with feet extended from the end and knees straight; flex the ankles to pull toes toward shins; estimate the angle the foot makes to a line extending back through the heel. For all ages, over 105 degrees is flexible, 95–105 is average, and 95 degrees is tight.

4. Assess ability to touch the floor with knees straight and feet together. For clients under 25 years of age, less than 3 in. to touching palms to the floor is flexible, 3–5 in. from palms touching the floor is average, and more than 5 in. is tight. For clients aged 25–45, the measures are less than 4 in., 4–7 in., and more than 7 in.; for clients over 45 years, the measures are less than 5 in., 5–9 in., and more than 9 in. (Marshall, 1981).

Aerobic Assessments

Aerobic exercise involves sustained, rhythmic activity of the large muscle groups. Aerobic exercise uses large amounts of oxygen, causing an increase in heart rate, stroke volume, respiratory rate, and a relaxation of the small blood vessels leading to increased oxygenation. The goal of aerobic exercise is to strengthen the cardiovascular system and increase stamina. Approximately 20 minutes of activity at the appropriate heart rate for each age range produces a training effect without straining the heart unduly.

Aerobic exercise not only conditions the cardiovascular system but can also reduce the amount of body fat. Percentage of body fat can be calculated most easily by pinching the back of the upper middle arm; less than 1/4 in. indicates a below average amount of body fat; 1/4–3/4 in. indicates an average amount of body fat; and more than 3/4 in. indicates a high percentage of body fat. For men, 12% of body weight as fat is desirable; for women, 18%. Other methods of determining body fat (in order of complexity and reliability) are calipers and water displacement. When using calipers, the skinfold sites commonly used are: triceps, subscapula, suprailiac, and thigh.

Calculating a Safe Range for Aerobic Exercise

A safe rate for aerobic exercise can be calculated in the following manner: 220 (maximum heart rate) – age + maximum attainable heart rate - resting heart rate x 0.6 and 0.8 + resting heart rate = safe range.

e.g., $220 - 44 = 176 - 64 = 112 \times 0.6 = 67.2 + 64 = 131.2$
$$112 \times 0.8 = 89.6 + 64 = 153.6$$

In the example, a 44-year-old person with a resting pulse of 64 needs to raise the pulse between 131 and 154 to attain a conditioning effect. The pulse can be taken at intervals during exercise to ensure the safe range is not exceeded (clients can take their pulse for 15 seconds and multiple by 4).

Pros and Cons of Stress Testing Prior to an Exercise Program

Stress testing is most commonly accomplished by placing an individual on a treadmill and using an electrocardiogram to measure the effects of strenuous running on heart activity. Some authorities claim stress testing is a useful way of determining whether a strenuous exercise program can be undertaken. Vickery, a physician, claims that the need has been invented based on an excess of cardiologists and a profit motive. Vickery (1978, pp. 109–111) presents the following information to strengthen his claim:

1. The stress test itself has a greater risk of precipitating a heart attack (a risk level of 30–60%) than does unaccustomed, severe exercise (a risk level of 6 to 12%). Based on this information, Vickery calculates that if people gradually work up to a conditioning level, their risk should drop to less than one fifth the risk of a heart attack than if they have a stress test.
2. The stress test is not a reliable indicator of persons at high risk for heart attack. False positives and false negatives abound. In a study of persons without symptoms of heart disease, 47% who tested "abnormal" on the stress test did not have heart disease; in another study, 62% of those who did have heart disease tested "normal" on the stress test. Based on this low level of accuracy, the use of a stress test is questionable.

There are more reliable indicators that can be used to assess client need for medical supervision prior to beginning an exercise program. Vickery (1978) suggests that a "yes" answer to one or more of the following questions by someone over 35 years of age should result in a visit to the physician; in someone under 35 years old, a call to the physician telling him or her the exercise program planned should be sufficient.

1. Do you have any chest pain when you exert yourself?
2. Do you get short of breath with mild exertion?
3. Do you have pain in your legs when you walk but not when you rest?
4. Do your ankles swell regularly (at times other than when menstruating)?
5. Has a doctor ever told you that you have heart disease?

Even exercise of moderate intensity (30 minutes) or moderately vigorous physical activity accumulated over the course of a day can lower the risks for heart disease, high blood pressure, type II (non-insulin-dependent) diabetes, obesity, colon cancer, arthritis, and bone loss. Regular moderate physical activity also can play a role in managing type I (insulin-dependent) diabetes and can contribute to weight and stress management (Prevention Report, 1994). Common moderate intensity activities, such as walking or cycling, climbing stairs instead of taking the elevator, or walking short distances instead of driving can contribute to the 30 minutes per day that is recommended (Pate et al., 1995).

FITNESS INTERVENTIONS

Developmental Movement Interventions

Crawling, rolling, creeping, hopping, and rocking enhance integration of the lower levels of the brain. Crawling and creeping are especially helpful in integrating the two hemispheres of the brain (Mills & Cohen, 1979, p. xiv). The cross-crawl (a contralateral movement) is especially helpful as a preventive measure for maintaining the normal neurological organization of the brain. Walking with arms swinging freely in opposition to the body, marching in place, crawling on the floor, lying down face up and moving the arms in opposition to the legs, or standing up and doing the dance "the Twist" while touching the right elbow to the left knee all accomplish brain integration (Koenig, 1981). Table 6.2 shows suggested movements for various endocrine developmental difficulties and/or enhancement of movement. The information in Table 6.2 can be used with clients who have organic difficulties (e.g., brain damage, stroke, accident, chronic illness, surgery) as well as with clients who wish to enhance their ability in a sport or activity (e.g., move up and back in tennis more effectively; decrease the possibility of a jogging or running injury; enhance immunity; kicking ability; right/left discrimination when driving; transposed numbers when writing; enhanced breathing; or stimulation of various endocrine organs. To integrate, movement actions should be pictured in the mind while moving through areas described.

Feldenkrais Interventions

Feldenkrais interventions, whether assisted by a practitioner or completed by the client, involve the following principles:

1. Exaggerate the problematic movement first. For example, if the chest is concave, the client exaggerates that situation.
2. Using very small, smooth, slow movements, move the body in the direction of balance with gravity.
3. Breathe in the abdomen while moving.
4. Center the concentration in the moving and breathing.
5. When difficulty in movement is encountered, imagine breathing into that area while moving.

Specific Feldenkrais interventions demonstrate the ease and power of his technique.

Intervention No. 1: Standing while Sitting. Sit in a chair and pay attention to how you stand up; note which part of the body moves first and which other parts follow and with what degree of difficulty, tension, effort. Write down what happened prior to continuing.

Table 6.2 Developmental Movement Interventions*

Issues	Intervention
Differentiate front from back of body; forward/back movement; pineal gland; cartoid body; heart; pancreas gonads; coccygeal body; mammillary bodies; pituitary gland, backward. movement. (Spinal)	Rolling the body as a unit; rolling the body successively from head, through arms, then legs. Roll with arms against chest, head off ground, pushing down the spine through pineal gland and up the spine through the carotid bodies. Lie on stomach, initiate movement through head, reaching through mammillary bodies (in midbrain slightly front and above ear) Wagging the tail and tail-leg raise through pituitary Lie prone, legs extended; head pushes up through pineal and then tail pushes down through carotid (worm) Lie prone, legs extended, full hip and knee extension as legs reach through the thymus (fish)
Stimulate heart, pancreas, thyroid, thymus. (Homologous)	Froghop, rock on all fours, rabbit hop backward, rope pulling (with a real or imaginary rope)
Stimulate gonads, coccygeal body. (Homolateral)	Diagonal head raising through gonads; crawling forward simulating elephant and gorilla movements.
Stimulate parathyroids, balance cerebral hemispheres. (Contralateral)	Forward and backward creep on hands and knees, rope climbing; diagonal roll, head off ground, both hands at right or left side, movement initiated through hands; picture moving each hand and arm through the parathyroid (mid-neck level) as roll is accomplished; hands end up at shoulder level.

*Based on ideas presented by Cohen and Mills (1979) and Koenig (1981). For further information see: Mills, M., and Cohen, B. *Developmental Movement Therapy.* Amherst, MA: The School for Body/Mind Centering, 1979.

Now sit on the edge of a chair, and let your body rock forward and backward without any sudden increase in effort. Make no attempt to get up. As you continue the movement, grasp the hair at the top of your head so any tensing of the cervical spine can be felt. When tension in the cervical area exists, increase the movement of your head forward and upward by moving your hip joints until the buttocks rise from the chair.

Note the difference in effort in rising when the chest muscles, ribs, and chest are relaxed. Repeat the second part of the exercise, making sure to breathe during it. Summarize your findings.

Intervention No. 2: Increasing Range of Motion in the Neck. Sit in a chair. Turn the head slowly and easily to the left as far as is comfortable. Note a spot on the wall or ceiling that marks that spot, then return the head to face front. Remember to keep breathing as you complete the exercise. Next, turn the head slowly and easily to the left while keeping the eyes looking forward; return the head to face front. Now turn the eyes *and* the head slowly and easily to the left again. Note how far the head turned this time and compare it with the first time you turned the head to the left.

Almost everyone reports an increase in range of neck motion as a result of this simple exercise. It supports Feldenkrais' theory: use small, slow movements; breathe and concentrate on the movement and its results; break the movement into its component parts and then reconstruct it to attain more efficient movement.

Intervention No. 3: Using Imagery and Movement. Sit comfortably in the chair, breathing in your lower abdomen. When ready, keep your head facing forward, but *picture* your head turning slowly and comfortably as far as possible to the left and then returning to the front facing position. Breathe comfortably and slowly turn your head to the left as far as comfortable to do so. Note the spot on the wall or ceiling and compare it with your other efforts.

Results from this intervention are frequently astounding. Using this series with thousands of participants, the author has found nearly everybody greatly increases their range of motion with this final exercise. This supports Feldenkrais' (1977) theory that imagery can affect movement in a positive manner.

Intervention No. 4: Improving Movements of the Lower Back. This intervention is effective for tightness in the lower back, tension, and for improving efficient use of the lower back. Lie on the floor with knees bent and feet flat on the floor. Cross the right leg over the left knee as if sitting in a chair with the legs crossed. Extend arms out at shoulder level and let them relax. Continue breathing easily while very slowly and smoothly letting the legs drop to the left toward the floor as far as is possible comfortably. Continue breathing and using one slow, continuous movement, return the legs to center and let them drop to the right toward the floor. Continue breathing and repeat the exercise, allowing the legs to move slowly to the right side of the floor and then to the left side of the floor. Then with legs facing front, slowly place legs flat on the floor and observe the sensations in the lower back, pelvis, and legs. Lie still, breathing, and noting changes and sensations.

Intervention No. 5: Increasing Movement in the Shoulders and Upper Back. This exercise is especially useful for people who sit reading or writing for long periods of time or for those who carry their tension in the upper part of their chest or back. Complete all parts of the exercise as if doing so in slow motion.

Lie on the floor, knees bent and feet flat on the floor. With arms extended, and palms meeting one another in front, breathe comfortably and gradually allow the two arms to move toward the left at the level of the shoulder; move as far toward the floor as is easily accomplished. Continue breathing and gradually, and in one continuous movement, allow the arms to move in an arc over the body, directly over the nose and then toward the right side of the body at shoulder level. Continue breathing as the arms sweep to the left side and then return to the right side of the body; use a *very* slow, continuous movement; pay attention to points of resistance, relaxation, tension, etc. Note differences in ability to carry out the movement on each repetition. When relaxation is attained, stop the movement and lie flat on the back breathing easily and noting the effect on the body.

When ready, gradually turn onto the left side of the body with the left leg on the bottom, slightly bent, and the right leg bent at a 75–90 degree angle to the trunk; find the angle of comfort. Continue breathing and slowly bend the right arm and move it across the body easing (but not in any way forcing) the arm with the left palm on the right elbow moving to the right shoulder as movement continues. Hold the position of easy stretch and breathe easily; continue holding the right arm and picture breathing into the shoulder as if there are tiny lungs located in the shoulder inhaling and exhaling as you inhale and exhale. Continue to *gradually* stretch the right arm (using the left arm to support and assist in the stretch). Holding the right hand in the left gradually (in one slow, continuous movement) move the right arm to the right side of the body and then back to the left side of the body; continue breathing easily throughout. Lie flat on the floor on the back and note sensations in the upper and lower body as a result of the exercise.

Turn to lie on the left side of the body as before. Turn the right shoulder to the left side of the body (assisting with the right arm gradually and continuously while breathing). Hold the shoulder at the point of stretched comfort and move the left hand to the right shoulder. Hold the hand there and breathe into it, moving the left palm after several breaths to another spot on the shoulder when warmth is felt emanating from the shoulder. Closing the eyes and imagining energy and warmth being generated in the shoulder will help to accomplish this feat. After several moments, lie flat on the back and note the effect. Repeat all portions of the exercise using the right side of the body and the left shoulder.

This series can also be completed while sitting in a straight chair. The opposite shoulder/arm is cradled in the other arm. A final component can be added while sitting. Place the left palm on the front of the right shoulder and gradually and firmly place the shoulder back as far as is comfortable while breathing deeply in and out. Hold in the extended position and picture tiny lungs breathing in and out at the point of pressure. Relax and note body sensations. Repeat with that arm several times and then repeat with the other shoulder. For further informations see: Feldkrais, M. *Awareness through Movement.* New York: Harper and Row, 1977.

Table 6.3 Choosing a Shoe for Running or Walking

Five Features to Look for in a Good Running Shoe

1. 1/4"–1/2" heel lift or wedge; the shoe should be thicker and softer in the heel than an ordinary sneaker.
2. The middle area of the sole should be considerably softer than the outer sole to absorb the shock of running on a hard surface.
3. The outer sole should be very flexible at the ball of the foot; test by compressing it with the thumb.
4. The toe should be rounded to allow sufficient room for toe nails and reduce the chance of blisters.
5. The shoes should feel comfortable from the first moment they are tried on, allow at least 1/4" room in front and to the side of the toes when standing, and the heels should not slip unduly.

Seven Features to Look for in a Good Walking Shoe

1. The toe area should have sufficient room for toes to wiggle and spread out.
2. The sole should flex at the ball of the foot; bend the shoe and see what force it takes to bend it; that force is equal to the amount needed for the foot to flex the shoe when walking. *A good shoe should not have to be broken in.*
3. The shoe should have a cushioned sole; this is mandatory for walking long distances.
4. The shoe should have an arch support; if it does not, cut out a piece of foam rubber to support the arch.
5. The upper part of the shoe should be made of a material that allows the shoe to breathe; leather and nylon mesh is a good combination. Shoes with laces allow for the best fit.
6. The shoe should be lightweight.
7. The shoe should have a curved sole to facilitate the rolling heel–toe action of correct walking.

Adapted from S. Hoag, 1981, *Choosing a running shoe;* and G. Yanker, 1983, *The Complete Book of Exercise Walking.*

Deciding on an Appropriate Aerobic Exercise Regime

According to the National Exercise for Life Institute, there are several factors to consider when choosing an aerobic exercise.

1. Is the exercise weight-bearing? Only weight-bearing exercise can prevent osteoporosis.
2. Is the exercise safe? Avoid exercise that puts undue strain or impact on the back, knees, or other joints. Immediate or delayed pain is a sign the exercise is not the right type.
3. Is the exercise for the total body? Using both arms and legs is the best for a cardiovascular benefit.

The aerobic exercises discussed in this section include: running, jogging, walking, swimming, aquadynamics and aerobic dance. Although running and jogging are efficient, inexpensive approaches to increasing cardiovascular fitness can be begun in stages at any age and by those who have been ill and require rehabilitation, injuries of the ankle, knee, and lower back are common. Some can be prevented by improving posture (see Feldenkrais & Cohen), using appropriate shoes (see Table 6.3), and strengthening the abdominal muscles (see Table 6.4). It might also be wise to consider another form of aerobic exercise if low back pain, previous injury, or poor jogging posture already exists.

Pender (1987, p. 260) suggests that a walk-jog program be completed prior to continuous jogging, as follows:

1. Work up to 12 sets for 3 consecutive days of 30 seconds of walking, followed by 30 seconds of jogging.
2. Work up to 12 sets for 3 consecutive days of 30 seconds of walking followed by 1 minute of jogging.

Although jogging and running are popular, walking is still superior in several ways: fewer injuries are reported and walking is better for losing weight *if brisk walking* is maintained. A study at the U.S. Olympic Training Center found that brisk walking burned calories at the rate of 1,012 per hour while running burned only 782 calories per hour. The best way to differentiate brisk walking from jogging is that in walking the feet are always on the ground, never in flight (Clark, 1984).

Yanker (1983, pp. 36–64) recommends the following for achieving proper walking technique:

Table 6.4 Keeping Your Back Fit

Low back pain affects 80% of the population at some time in their lives. Here are some tips for avoiding the affliction; you can also use them if you have back pain as a way to reduce discomfort.

• Strengthen your lower back

1. Bring your knees to chest while lying on your back, keeping your head on the floor.
2. Kneel on all fours; alternately raise your head and then arch back like a lazy cat.
3. While lying on the floor, press your pelvis to the floor, holding for 5 seconds. Repeat 5–25 times. For soreness or stiffness, touch each point of your pelvis to the floor for each hour of the clock position from 3 p.m. all the way around to 2 p.m.
4. Sit on the floor with one leg straight and the other bent. Move the flexed knee to the side and bend forward. Hold for 10 seconds to one minute. Repeat with other leg straight.

5. While seated on a chair, press your buttocks together. Hold for 6 seconds. Relax and repeat. Gradually build up to 20 repetitions a day.

6. Stand with your back against a wall with feet shoulder width apart. Slide down to a crouch with knees bent to about 90 degrees. Count to five and slide back up the wall. Work up to five times.

7. Lie on your stomach with your hands under your shoulders, elbows bent. Raise the top half of your body, keeping hips and legs on the floor. Hold position for 1–2 seconds. Repeat up to 10 times, several times a day.

8. Lie on your back with knees bent and feet flat on the floor (or legs at 90 degree angle). Reach with your head, shoulders and hands toward (or past) your knees until you feel your abdominal muscles tighten. 5–100 times.

9. Stand behind a chair with your hands on back of the chair. Lift one legback and up while keeping that knee straight. Return slowly, 5 times each leg.

10. For pain on one side of the lower back: Lie on back on the floor or bed and bring the knee to the chest on the sore side and hold with both hands behind knee. Keep the other leg straight and raised off the floor or bed, several inches, then slowly swing leg out to the side to a 45 degree angle, then drop it to the floor or bed, raise it up and return to a straight position. Repeat 1–5 times.

11. Sit upright in a chair with your legs straight. Lift one leg waist high and return it to the floor. 5 times each leg.

12. For backache or spasm: Stand in door frame with your toes about 12" back from the floor line of it. Bend your knees, keep rib cage and pelvis vertical, grasp door frame with thumbs, lean back slightly as if going to sit down. Stretch and hold.

- Avoid jogging, biking, paddling, rowing, baseball, and softball as regular activities; they all put added strain on your back.
- Check your posture whenever you pass a mirror; look to see if your knees are slightly bent, your head is not bent forward, your shoulders are not rounded, and your abdomen or buttocks do not hang out, giving you an exaggerated forward curve to your lower back.
- Enhance your posture by completing the following movements:

1. Stand in a comfortable position and move your shoulders forward as if trying to get them to touch, then to a middle position, and then to the neck as if trying to touch your shoulder blades together. Return to the middle, front, and back several times more.

2. Sit in a straight-backed chair without arms. Hold your arms at shoulder height with your arms bent at elbows. Twist your body gently to the left and then to the right. Repeat several times.

3. Get on the floor on your knees; shift your weight back toward your feet. Place your hands out in front of you and walk your arms, using your fingertips, out from your body. This should look as if you're playing a vertical piano keyboard.

Table 6.4 (*continued*)

4. Stand with a chair in front of you. With knees bent and stomach muscles tight, keep your shoulders and lower back still while you stick your buttocks out and in and then tilt your pelvis forward. Repeat in a slow continuous movement 8–30 times.

• When bending over from the waist to brush your teeth or pick up an object always bend your knees slightly.

• When getting up off a chair or the toilet, bring your feet under you, hold your abdomen in, and straighten up; this lets the legs, not your back, do the work.

• When doing tasks that require long standing, place a foot on a low stool or bench to release back pressure; also move around occasionally and do a few movements such as making circles with your shoulders; tilting your pelvis forward and back while contracting your abdominal muscles; and stand while inhaling as you stretch up on your toes as far upward as you can, then exhale fully as you bend over and let your head move toward the floor.

• Cut back on sugary and fatty foods; being overweight can put added strain on your back.

• Eat sufficient calcium; it can help keep you limber, your spine supple, and can ward off the effects of aging. Be sure to include more or at least some of the following in your meal plan: sardines, salmon, sunflower seed, tofu, milk, or milk products, dried beans, and green vegetables. Reduce your intake of foods that contain oxalic acid (chocolate, rhubarb), fat, and phytic acid (grains) since they prevent calcium absorption.

• Get enough vitamin C since it seems to aid in calcium mobilization and bone growth. The best natural sources are berries, citrus fruits, green and leafy vegetables, tomatoes, cauliflower, potatoes, and sweet potatoes.

• Learn to relax. Tense muscles can bring on back problems. Purchase or record your own relaxation tape and listen to it twice daily.

• Use mental imagery to picture your back as strong, supple, and relaxed. Conjure up this picture several times each day.

• Think positive thoughts about your body in general and your back in particular. Write these on a 3 ¥ 5 card and carry them with you; be sure to read them several times a day. Some affirmations to use might be: My back is becoming stronger and more relaxed; it's getting easier and easier to keep my back well and strong.

• If you sit most of the day, devise a system to remind yourself to get up once an hour and walk around, stretch, and take a few deep breaths.

(For additional ideas see: *Goodbye Back Pain* by Leonard Faye (Tale Weaver, 1990).

• To improve walking posture:

1. Hold head and back erect, tighten abdominal muscles, tuck buttocks under, and walk tall (image of a golden cord attached and pulling up from the upper chest may help with posture).

2. Point toes in direction of travel, reaching out with hip, knee, and heel.
3. Plant the back edge of the heel of the forward moving foot at a 40-degree angle to the ground, setting the ankle slightly to the outside, leg and foot at a 90-degree angle.
4. Pull forward with the leading leg while pushing back with the back leg.
5. Hold hands loosely clenched, arms at a 90-degree angle, just brushing the side; forward movement high as the chest, move backward near shoulder level. Inhale on left-arm swing, exhale on right-arm swing. Right arm forward with left leg and vice versa.
6. Focus eyes 10–15 feet ahead.
7. Check out nonparallel leg movements by walking in the snow or sand and observing. For a duck-footed walk, walk with a wider stance and practice the heel walk. To correct pigeon-toed walking, exaggerate pointing the toes before the heel strikes; picture the toes pointing straight. To correct favored-leg walking, concentrate the forward flow of the legs.

Based on the flexibility/tightness assessment, appropriate exercises can be chosen (see Table 6.5). Swimming is an excellent conditioner if bearing weight on the lower joints is contraindicated. However, Diamond (1990) has found that swimming the breaststroke, a homologous movement, weakens the thymus.

Besides choosing an aerobic workout that is useful, it is also wise to choose one that is fun, or it will not be continued on a lifelong basis. A variant of swimming is aquadynamics or water exercise. The President's Council on Physical Fitness has produced a booklet detailing the basics and various programs from mild toning to conditioning.

Aerobic dancing is a popular conditioning method. However, there are pitfalls to be aware of. Jones (*The Wellness Newsletter,* 1985), a dance instructor, describes some. Even with an excellent teacher, the student may misread instructor movements and create injuries, overemphasize gross body movement, use the limbs inefficiently, and not take advantage of the neuromuscular enhancement available.

EXERCISE FOR SPECIAL POPULATIONS

Even nursing home populations can benefit form exercise. Fiatarone (1994) showed that exercise training and multinutrient supplementation was beneficial for residents in a nursing home whose average age was 87.1 years.

Probably the best exercise for clients of all ages and conditions is walking. Exercises for bedridden clients are presented in Table 6.6.

Most of the above exercises can be adapted for use in a wheel chair or armchair. Even those severely debilitated can approximate some of the exercises or at least rotate the wrists and ankles, flex and stretch wrists and feet, rotate the head in clockwise and counterclockwise directions, and exercise the face by exaggeratedly saying the vowels (A E I O U).

Table 6.5 Flexibility Exercises

1–3 Reach left hand over shoulder and clasp right hand for 30 seconds and then switch arms.

4 Stand with feet 3 feet apart, and fingers laced behind back, palms up. Slowly lift arms up and over head while lowering the head gently towards the floor.

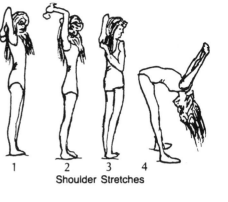

Shoulder Stretches

1–2 With legs wide apart, and palms on the floor, shift hips to the left, bending the left knee; then shift weight to the right, bending the right knee. Repeat 10 times each side in a slow, controlled motion.

3–4 Sit on the floor with soles of feet together; press with hands on the inside of the knees and hold for 30 seconds, then relax. Repeat 20 times.

Thigh Stretches

Place hands and feet on the floor, backside up; bend left knee and press right heel to the floor and hold, feeling the pull in the calf. Straighten left leg and bend right knee and press left heel to the floor and hold. Do 20 repetitions each side.

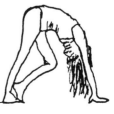

Heel Cord Stretches

Table 6.5 (*continued*)

1–2 Squat with palms on the floor directly under shoulders with head to knee; straighten legs, keeping palms and heels on the floor, then lower. Repeat 10 times.	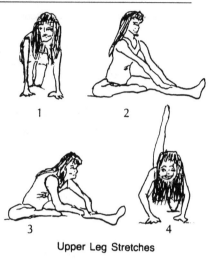
3–4 Sit on the floor, one leg bent into opposite thigh, other leg straight out with foot flexed. Reach arms down the straight leg, lowering chest toward it. Bob very gently 15 times and then switch legs and repeat.	

Upper Leg Stretches

Note. It is recommended that flexibility exercises of this type be completed *prior to and following* any exercise session.

Feldenkrais' movements can be used with the elderly to enhance leg and hip movement. Masters and Houston (1978, pp. 160–167) suggest the following series.

1. Sit halfway forward in a straight-back chair, legs spread a little wider than usual, knees bent, and feet parallel. Rest hands on the chair seat or side, not on the legs.
2. While breathing, let the right leg begin to drop slowly to the right, then bring it back to the middle, paying attention to the sensation in the hip joint.
3. Extend the right leg out in front, resting the heel on the floor. Let the foot fall to the right, keeping the leg straight. Try it again, this time with the knee slightly bent. Repeat 20–25 times while breathing. Rest and observe the sensations in the lower body.
4. Extend the right leg in front, resting on the heel. Let the foot fall easily to the left, keeping the leg straight. Let it gradually return to the middle. Repeat as in no. 3 above.
5. While continuing to breathe throughout, extend the right leg and push the foot along the floor, keeping the leg straight, pushing off and back with the heel. Let the right side of the body follow the movement; hold the side of the chair for balance. As the movement is repeated (20–25 times), notice how the left shoulder goes back as the right shoulder moves forward.
6. Spread the feet and legs a little farther apart. Continue breathing regularly while letting the right leg fall toward the other leg. Pay attention to the hip joint and right buttock as the leg falls. Put the right leg out a little further in front and continue breathing and dropping the right leg toward the left leg and returning it to center. Watch as the leg moves and feel what happens in

the hip joint and buttock.

7. Turn the right foot toward the left leg and then away from it; notice the pressure on the left buttock when turning the right leg away from the left leg. Let the whole body shift with the foot movement and pay attention to the body sensations. Repeat the movement while breathing for 20–25 times. Rest.

8. Place the right foot parallel to the left foot and let the right leg flop from the left to right. As the leg flops to the right, the foot will tilt on its right side; as the leg flops to the left, the foot will tilt on its left side. Experiment with different positions until the point where the leg moves the most freely is found. Rest and breathe.

9. Shift the body weight onto the left buttock slightly so the right buttock rises a little off the chair. Sink into the right buttock and observe the left buttock rising off the chair. Repeat right buttock, left buttock, noticing what happens in the hip joint during the movement and breathing on each movement.

10. Extend the right leg, foot off the floor an inch or so, sitting way back in the chair. Make circles with your foot, keeping the leg stiff, and breathing. Make a few in the other direction, continuing to breathe throughout. Experiment with small circles, large circles, fast and slow circles. Rest.

11. Sit back in the chair with right leg extended and foot off the floor a few inches. While breathing, move the foot and leg as a piece from left to right several times. Continue to breathe and flop the foot left and right, keeping the leg straight. Rest.

12. Lean forward and extend the right leg, placing the heel on the floor. Slide the foot backward and forward along the floor, keeping the knee straight. Note how differently the hip joint is being used now. Let the whole body move as the foot slides forward and back. Place the right hand on the right hip and feel the movement as the right foot and leg are moved to the right and to the left. Sense where the socket is that connects the leg into the hip and notice what is happening to the left side of the rib cage. Rest.

13. Place the two feet side by side with the legs bent. Move the right knee from left to right and see how it moves. Breathe in as the right knee is moved from left to right. Do the same movements while breathing out. Note which movement is easier. Repeat the movement using the breathing that is easiest. Rest.

14. Extend both legs and lift the right leg several times and then the left one. Note which feels lighter. Get up and walk around. Turn to the right and then to the left. Note in which direction it is easier to turn.

15. Lift the right leg in front and then the left leg; note which leg made the larger movement. Rest and note the sensations in both sides of your hip, and in both legs.

16. After a rest, or the next day, repeat nos. 1–15 above using the left leg. Continue doing the exercise daily, alternating legs.

Those with diabetes can benefit greatly from exercise. Exercise increases

Table 6.6 Exercises for Bedridden Clients

NOTE: Ask client to breathe throughout all exercises.

1. Raise the head from pillow as far as possible; add one raise of the head a week to a maximum of 10 repetitions.

2. Turn the head slowly to the left and then to the right; add one turn of the head per week to a maximum of 10 repetitions.

3. Shrug the shoulders up and back toward the ears as far as possible; add one repetition per week to a total of 10 repetitions.

4. Rotate the shoulders

5. Bring the right arm (fully extended) over the head, left arm at side; bring down right arm to the side of the body and bring the left arm (fully extended) over the head. Work up to a maximum of 10 repetitions.

6. Cross the wrists at the abdomen and circle both arms at the same time, first clockwise and then counterclockwise; work up to 10 repetitions.

7. Clench the fists tightly and hold for several seconds, then extend the fingers and reach up as far as possible; work up to 10 repetitions.

8. Extend the arms forward and spread the fingers as far as possible; work up to 10 repetitions.

9. Make a fist and rotate the thumbs clockwise and then counterclockwise; work up to 10 repetitions.

10. Raise the right leg up as far as possible and return it to the bed; keep the leg as straight as possible without straining the lower back; work up to 10 repetitions each leg.

11. Grasp the right knee with both hands and very slowly pull it toward the chest while slowly moving the head toward the knee; work up to 5 repetitions with each knee.

12. Grasp both knees with both hands and very slowly pull them toward the chest while slowly moving the head toward the knees; work up to 10 repetitions.

13. With arms at sides of the body, slowly raise the head, shoulders, and legs several inches; hold, then return to lie flat; work up to 3 repetitions.

14. Extend both ankles toward the bottom of the bed; hold, then flex them toward the shins, hold, then relax. Work up to 10 repetitions.

15. Bicycle both legs slowly, completing up to 10 circles.

16. Lie on the stomach with chin resting on hands. Put heels apart and big toes together; squeeze the buttocks together as though trying to prevent a bowel movement; while squeezing, bring the heels slowly together and hold for 2–3 seconds, then relax on the bed. Work up to 5 repetitions.

17. Lie on the left side in a straight line and raise the left leg as high as possible over the other other leg; hold, then return it to the bed. Work up to 10 repetitions. Turn on right side and raise left leg up to 10 repetitions.

18. Raise hips 5"–6" off the bed, keeping arms at sides; hold several seconds, the relax into the bed. Work up to 5 repetitions.

Those with diabetes can benefit greatly from exercise. Exercise increases insulin sensitivity. "The effect is most pronounced in muscles, which are a major customer for the circulating blood sugar. As muscles are conditioned, they seek to increase their stores of glycogen, and . . . call for more sugar from the bloodstream. After about of exercise, insulin and glucose levels fall for a day or so, and can be seen before any loss of weight or fat" (Brownell & Stunkard, 1980).

Those who participate in a regular exercise program show enhanced insulin action and reduced plasma glucose levels. The relationship between degree of physical conditioning and ability to metabolize glucose holds despite differences in age, sex, or ratio of body fat to total body weight. Elevated levels of blood glucose may be associated with many of the physical problems experienced by people with diabetes. Thus, exercise may ward off problems and enhance wellness for them.

Studies conducted in Sweden by Dr. Ralph A. DeFronzo of Yale University support the beneficial effect of exercise. The researcher found that 85% of body glucose uptake occurs in the skeletal muscles. This explains why people with diabetes show improved control over their disease when they participate in physically conditioning exercise (*Research Resources Reporter,* 1983).

Exercise is beneficial to those with arthritis, too. Researchers at the University of Michigan Medical School in Ann Arbor asked women with the affliction to pedal on a stationary bicycle from 15 to 35 minutes 3 times a week. After 12 weeks the women reported higher energy levels, less pain and swelling, increased ease in doing household chores, and heightened interest in social activities. Those who pedaled for 15 minutes showed more improvement than those who pedaled for 35 minutes.

Exercise can have a positive effect on bone mineral loss. Smith reported studying a group of 30 elderly women for 3 years. Eighteen did nothing special in terms of exercise, while 12 participated in a 40–45 minute exercise program 3 days a week. They did exercises from the sitting position in a straight-backed chair. At the end of 3 years, the control group had a 3.2% loss in bone mineral measurements while the physically active group showed a 2.29% increase. Physical activity plays an important role in preventing loss of flexibility and bone mass. Thus effects of aging need not include bone aging.

Overly vigorous exercise is not needed. In fact, female marathon runners showed a decrease in bone mass in a study conducted at the University of California in San Francisco. Most had stopped menstruating, yet their estrogen levels were not different enough from nonrunners to explain the loss in bone mass. Thus, marathon running, at least for women, may not ward off the effects of bone aging as well as chair exercises.

Memory loss effects of aging can also be warded off with exercise. Researchers at the University of Utah divided volunteers (average age 61) into three groups: one that exercised aerobically, walking up to a target pulse of 120 beats per minute for 40 minutes; a group that did pushups and lifted weights; and another that remained inactive. After 4 months of training, the aerobic group improved their oxygen intake by 25% and showed improvement in six of eight mental tests; the weight lifting group improved their oxygen intake by 9% and improved in only one of eight mental tests; the inactive control group remained the same in oxygen intake and mental agility. An English study by psychologist Patrick Rabbit corroborates this study; he found that of 1,200 elderly people, the 10% who showed no memory loss at all had intact cardiovascular systems. His findings support the idea that good memories need sufficient oxygen. Exercise is probably the best way to ensure that sufficient oxygen reaches the brain to keep the mind active (Clark, 1983).

Children, too, can benefit from exercise, but certain kinds may reduce their level of wellness. According to Bob Arnot, M.D., Sports Medicine Specialist, football, weight lifting, running, or jogging can be bad for children who have not reached adolescence yet. They can damage growth plates and may incur physical and emotional damage in these activities if pushed too hard. Ballet is not a good exercise either because feet can be deformed by walking on pointed toe too frequently.

On the other hand, lacrosse, gentle stretching, situps, side-to-side hopping, soccer, and swimming are good, especially if properly supervised. The International Athletic Association Federation echoes the refrain. They discourage intensive competition and strenuous training in puberty and prepuberty age groups because separation of growth plates may occur in the pelvis, knee, or ankle. Although these separations can heal with rest, it is not known whether harmful effects might turn up later. The Medical Committee of IAAF suggests that up to the age of 12 children should not run more than 800 meters in competition. Russell Pate at the University of South Carolina is researching the topic of marathon running for children (The Department of Physical Education, Columbia, SC).

Following myocardial infarct or bypass surgery, significant reductions in health care costs have been attributed to exercise programs (Ades et al., 1992). Exercise for people with coronary artery disease is based on the traditional prescription for developing a training effect in healthy persons, including mode (e.g., walking, bicycling, swimming, etc.), frequency (usually 3 nonconsecutive days a week), duration (usually a warm-up and cool-down period of at least 10 minutes combined with 20–40 minutes of cardiovascular activity), intensity (usually moderate and comfortable intensity at 55–90% maximal heart rate), and progression (usually gradual). Wellness practitioners may be involved as observers and monitors of heart rate and rhythm and as teachers of clients to monitor their own progress. The American College of Sports Medicine recommends that exercise programs for people with coronary heart disease include a comprehensive pre-exercise medical evaluation and an individualized exercise prescription (American College of Sports Medicine, 1994).

OVERCOMING OBSTACLES TO EXERCISE

Attrition in exercise programs is a major problem (Jordan-March, 1985). Davis, McKay, and Eshelman (1995) contend there are two major obstacles to overcome in undertaking and keeping at an exercise program: making exercise part of a lifestyle and avoiding injury. Suggestions for making exercise a safe part of a lifestyle include:

1. Start small and keep it fun.
2. Keep records of daily and weekly progress; include both subjective reactions and objective measures: weight, blood pressure, pulse.
3. Focus on the rewards of exercise; keep a record of moods and compare differences in relaxation, energy, concentration, and sleep patterns.
4. Post goals, mottos, pictures of the ideal self, affirmations, and notes of encouragement.
5. Use visualization daily to picture successful attainment of exercise benefit, e.g., looking toned, radiant, graceful.
6. Work with a peer facilitator or join a structured exercise class, running club, or fitness center. Spend more time with people dedicated to wellness.
7. Reward and congratulate yourself for working toward exercise goals as well as attaining them. For example, after a month in an exercise program, buy a new pair of running shoes or treat yourself to a meal out.
8. Use proper equipment and clothing when exercising.
9. Include at least 10 minutes of warm-up and cool-down exercises in an exercise program. Avoid running up to the front door, going inside, and sitting down; complete stretching exercises, shower, and change to dry clothes.
10. Stop exercising or at least slow down and consult with a practitioner if any unusual, unexplainable symptoms occur.
11. Avoid exercising for 2 hours after a large meal and eating for 1 hour after exercising.
12. Vary exercise regimes to counter boredom.
13. Walk or dance during lunch break and find other ways to work exercise into the daily calendar.

BODY/MIND INTERACTIONS AND FITNESS

A number of investigators have examined the relationship of exercise to mood. Roth et al. (1994) found that adults with epilepsy who exercised regularly reduced depression. In a series of four studies, Thayer et al. (1994) found that exercise was the most effective mood elevator, but the best general strategy to change a bad mood was a combination of relaxation, stress management, cognitive and exercise techniques.

Although many of the studies use small samples, they all point in the direction of the positive effect of exercise in anxiety, depression, and/or self-esteem (Bradley, 1994; Braden et al., 1993; Brown et al., 1992; Davis, Raglin et al., 1993; deSouza et al., 1992) Dua & Hargraves, 1992; Jin, 1992; Koniak-Griffin, 1994), Norris et al., 1992; Norvell & Belles, 1993; O'Connor & Davis, 1992; O'Connor et al., 1993; Rabichaud-Ekstrand,1992; Rejeski et al.,1992; Steege & Blumenthal, 1993).

When using exercise as a treatment for anxiety or depression, the following practical considerations should be kept in mind:

1. Use a slow, graduated exercise program. It fosters a sense of mastery; a new, positive self-image; and cathartic relief.
2. Run with a companion who runs at about the same speed and is not competitive. (An indicant of noncompetitiveness is the ability to make complimentary comments regardless of fitness level.)
3. Monitor pace with the talk test (never exerting beyond the capacity to maintain a conversation with one's peer). Keep moving even if fatigue necessitates a slow walk.
4. Keep a log of activity for self-motivation, reinforcement of the activity, and to chronicle progress.
5. Make a contract with a peer or practitioner providing a substantial bonus for success and a meaningful penalty for failure.
6. Teach clients to synchronize breathing with movement. (Feldenkrais and yoga (see Chapter 7) are possible interventions to combine with an exercise program.)

7. Provide more extrinsic rewards for novice runners; in time, runners get intrinsic reward from running. Until then, reinforcement for running may need to be provided by a peer or practitioner.

INTEGRATIVE LEARNING EXPERIENCES

Beginning Level

1. Assess yourself using the following measures:
   A. Cohen/Mills developmental movement theory
   B. Kurtz and Prestera's structural assessments
   C. Aerobic conditioning (calculate safe ranges)
   D. Marshall's flexibility tests
2. Develop and try out appropriate interventions based on the above assessments.
3. Calculate your safe aerobic exercise range and cross check yours with a peer.
4. Role play responses to the following client responses using assertiveness criteria to evaluate your efforts:

   A. "Cancer is due to a virus. What good can thinking or imagining do?"
   B. "I don't want to exercise; I'm too depressed."
   C. "I have diabetes and I have to take it easy or I'll need more insulin."

Advanced Level

1. Complete an assessment of one child, one young adult, and one senior client using assessments based on the frameworks of: Cohen/Mills, Kurtz/ Prestera, aerobic conditioning, Marshall's flexibility criteria.
2. Develop appropriate interventions for the three clients assessed: organize the information gathered using Table 4.7, p 91.

REFERENCES

Ades, P.A., Huang, D., and Weaver, O. (1992). Cardiac rehabilitation and participation predicts lower rehospitalization costs. *Am Heart J* 123:916-921.

American College of Sports Medicine Position Stand. (1994). Exercise for patients with coronary artery disease. *Med Sci Sports Exerc* 26(3): i-v.

Angotti, C., Levine, M.S. (1994). Review of 5 years of a combined dietary and physical fitness intervention for control of serum cholesterol. *J Am Diet Assoc.* 94: 634–638.

Bernacki, E. (1987). Can corporate fitness programs be justified? *Fitness in Business* 1:173-179.

Bernstein, L. et al., (1994). Physical exercise and reduced risk of breast cancer in young women. *J Nat Cancer Inst.* 86(18) 1403-1407.

Braden, C. J., McGlone, K., and Pennington, F. (1993). Specific psychosocial and behavioral outcomes form the systemic lupus orythematisis self-help course. *Health Ed. O* . 20(1): 29-41.

Bradley, M.B. (1994). The effect of participating in a functional electrical stimulation exercise program on affect in people with spinal cord injuries. *Arch Phys Med Rehab* 7(6): 676-679.

Brown. R., Ramirex, D., and Taub, J. (1978). The prescription of exercise for depression. *Physician Sports Med* 6:34–49.

Brown, S.W., Welch, M.C., Labbe, F.E., et al. (1992). Aerobic exercise in the psychological treatment of adolescents. *Perceptual Motor Skills* 74(2): 555-560.

Brownell, K., and Stunkard, A. (1980). Physical activity in the development and control of obesity. In *Obesity,* A. Stunkard, Ed. Philadelphia, PA: W.B. Saunders, pp. 330–324.

Cathcart, R.F. (1984). Vitamin C in the treatment of acquired immune deficiency syndrome (AIDS). *Med Hypothesis* 14: 423-433.

Chandra, R.K. (1984). Excessive intake of zinc impairs immune responses. *JAMA.* 252:1443-1446.

Clark, C. (1983). Exercise—the way to keep young and pain free. *The Wellness News.* 4(3):2.

Clark, C. (1984). Walking better than jogging for losing weight. *The Wellness News.* 5(2):1–2..

Davis, J. (1963). Review of scientific information on the effects of ionized air on human beings and animals. *J. Aerospace Med* 34(1):1.

Davis, M., McKay, M., and Eshelman, E. (1995). *The Relaxation and Stress Reduction Workbook,* 3rd ed. Oakland, CA: New Harbinger Publications, p. 201.

de Souza, V., Maun, A., & Sargeant, A. (1992). Aerobic exercise in the adjunctive treatment of depression: A randomized controlled trial. *J R Soc. Med.* 85(9): 541-544.

Diamond, J. (1990) *Life Energy.* New York: Paragon House Publishers.

Dua, J., & Hargraves, L. (1992). Effect of aerobic exercise on negative stress, and depression. *Precept Mot Skills* 75(2): 355-361.

Even some exercise offers health benefits (1994). *Prevention Report* (October/November): 1.

Feldenkrais, M. (1977). *Awareness Through Movement.* New York: Harper and Row.

Fiatarone, M. (1994). Exercise training and nutritional supplementation in very elderly people. *N.E. J. Med,* 330(25): 1769–1775

Gettman, L. (1986). Cost benefit analysis of a corporate fitness program. *Fitness in Business 1: 11-17.*

Henderson, B.E., Hanisch, R., Sullivan-Halley, J., and Ross, R.K. (1994). Physical exercise and reduced risk of breast cancer in young women. *J. Nat'l. Cancer Inst.* 86:1403-1408.

Hoag, S. (1981). Choosing a running shoe. *The Minn Wellness J* (July), pp. 1, 4.

Jin, P. (1992). Efficacy of Tai Chi, brisk walking, meditation, and reading in reducing mental and emotional stress. *J of Psychosomatic Res* 36)4): 361-370.

Jones, D. (1985). What's missing in aerobic dance? *The Wellness Newsl.* 6(3):2.

Jordan-Marsh, M. (1985). Development of a tool for diagnosing changes in concern about exercise: A means of enhancing compliance. *Nur Res* 34(2): 103–107.

Koniak-Griffin, D. (1994). Aerobic exercise, psychological well-being, and physical discomfort during adolescent pregnancy. *Res Nsg Health* 17(4): 253–263.

Kurtz, R., and Prestera, H. (1984). *The Body Reveals.* New York: Harper and Row.

Manson, J.E., Nathan, D.M., Krolewski, A.S., Stampfer, M.J., Willett, W.C., and Hennekens, C.H. (1992). A prospective study of exercise and incidence of diabetes among U.S. male physicians. *JAMA* 268(1): 63–67.

Marshall, J. (1981). How to get good looks, top performance and staying power for your body. *Self* (March), 56–72.

Masters, R., and Houston, J. (1978). *Listening to the Body.* New York: Delta.

Mills, M., and Cohen, B. (1979). *Developmental Movement Therapy.* Amherst, MA: The School for Body/Mind Centering.

National Headache Foundation (1995). Exercise your headache away. *Let's Live* February: 81

Norsis, R., Carroll, D., and Cochrane, R. (1992). The effects of physical activity and exercise training on psychological stress and well-being in an adolescent population. *J Psychosom Res* 36(1): 55-65.

Norvell, N., and Belles, D., (1993). Psychological and physical benefits of circuit weight training in law enforcement personnel. *J Consul Clini Psycho* 61(3): 520-527.

O'Connor, P.J., Bryant, C.X., Vetri, J.P., et al., (1993). State anxiety and ambulatory blood pressure following resistance training *Med Sci Sports Exer* 25(4): 516-521.

O'Connor, P.J., and Davis, J.C. (1992). Psychobiological responses to exercise. *Med Sci Sports Exercise* 24(6): 714-719.

Pate, R.R., Rate, M., Blair, S.N., et al. (1995). Physical activity and public health: A recommendation from the Centers for Disease Control and the American College of Sports Medicine. *JAMA* 273: 402-407.

Pender, N. (1987). *Health Promotion in Nursing Practice.* E. Norwalk, CT: Appleton-Century-Crofts.

President's Council on Physical Fitness and Sports. (n.a.). *An Introduction to Running: One Step at a Time.* Washington, D.C.: National Institute of Health, n.p.

President's Council on Physical Fitness and Sports. (1983). *Aquadynamics.* Washington, D.C.

Raglin, J.S., Turner, P.E., and Eksten, F. (1993). State anxiety and blood pressure following 30 minutes of leg ergometry or weight training. *Med Sci Sports Exec* 25(9): 1044-1048.

Rakowski, W., and Mor, V. (1992). The association of physical activity with mortality among older adults in the Longitudinal Study of Aging (1984–1988). *J. Gerontol* 47(4): M122–M129.

Rejeski, W.J., Thompson, A., Bruaker, P.H., et al. (1992). Acute exercise: Buffering psychosocial stress responses in women. *Health Psychol* 11(6): 355-362.

Research Resources Reporter. (1983). Washington, D.C.: National Institute of Health, n.p.

Resnick, L.M. et al. (1984). Intercellular free magnesium in erythrocytes of essential hypertension: relationship to blood pressure. *Proc Nat'l Acad Sci* 81: 6511–6515.

Robichaud-Ekstrand, S. (1992). The anti-depressive effects of post-infarct exercise. *Canad Nurse* 88(6): 41-44.

Roth, D.L., Goode, K.T., Williams, V.L. and Faughtly, E. (1994). Physical exercise, stressful life experience, and depression in adults with epilepsy. *Epilepsia* 35(6): 1248–1255.

Shephard, R. (1983). Employee health and fitness: The state of the art. *Preventive Medicine* 12: 644-653.

Shinton, R., and Sagar, G. (1993) Lifelong exercise and stroke. *Brit Med J* 307: 231-234.

Sime, W. (1982). A new look at the association /dissociation in long distance running. *Running Psychol* (May), 5–6.

Steege, J.F., and Blumenthal, J.A. (1993). The effects of aerobic exercise on premenstrual symptoms in middle-aged women. *J Psychosom Res* 37(2): 127-133.

Thayer, R.E., Newman, J.R., and McClain, T.M. (1994). Self-regulation of mood: Strategies for changing a bad mood, raising energy and reducing tension. *J Pers Soc Psychol* 67(5) 910–925.

Vickery, D. (1978). *Life Plan for Your Health.* Reading MA: Addison-Wesley, pp. 10–11.

Willer, J., Dehen, H., and Cambier, J. (1981). Stress induced analgesia in humans: endogenous opioids and naloxone reversible depression of pain reflexes. *Science* 212: 689–691.

Yanker, G. (1983). *The Complete Book of Exercisewalking.* Chicago, IL: Contemporary Books.

7

SELF-CARE, TOUCH,
AND WELLNESS

This chapter discusses the following topics:

- Theoretical frameworks for touch and healing
- Self-care assessments
- Touch and healing assignments
- Smoking cessation: an example of a self-care intervention
- Touch and healing interventions
- Other self-care measures

This chapter is closely related to Chapter 6; both deal with aspects of the wellness dimension of fitness. This chapter is focused on self-care and touch and their relationship to wellness. Theories, assessments, and interventions for behavioral kinesiology, therapeutic touch, yoga, massage, acupressure, reflexology and psychoneuroimmunology are provided. Additionally, information and skills to enhance self-care skills are presented.

THEORETICAL FRAMEWORKS FOR TOUCH
AND HEALING

Diamond's Theory of Behavioral Kinesiology

I have come to believe that all illness starts as a problem on the energy level, a problem that may exist for many years before it manifests itself in physical disease. It appears that a generalized reduction of body energy leads to energy imbalances in particular parts of the body. If we become aware of these energy imbalances when they first occur, we have a long grace period in which to correct them. We will then be practicing primary prevention. (Diamond, 1979, p. 2)

Diamond developed his theory after years of working as a traditional psychiatrist, investing huge amounts of his own energy to bolster up the clients who were not really interested in changing. "I could never get it through to them that their well-being was really their responsibility" (Diamond, 1979, p. 4).

Noting that the longer his clients remained in therapy, the more depressed therapist and client became, he searched for a broader framework from which to practice—one that included nutrition and various physical and postural therapies. Diamond's *Behavioral Kinesiology*

> uses the basic testing techniques of Applied Kinesiology, but focuses on the factors in the . . . surroundings and life-style that are raising and lowering body energy. Many of the factors that lower energy are products of the technological revolution: the poisons and noises in our environment, the overrefined and unnatural foods we find on the supermarket shelves, the synthetic fabrics from which so many of our clothes are made. Other factors are individual habits or tendencies, such as posture, ability to handle stress, and human relationships. (Diamond, 1979, p. 7)

The thymus gland is of great import in Diamond's work. He points out that until recently (most prevalent around the period from the 1920s to the 1950s), the thymus gland was irradiated (to make it smaller) and thought to have no function in adult life. It is now known that the thymus gland is crucial to the immunity mechanism in the body. Hormones in the thymus influence lymphocytes to mature and give rise to lymphocytes called T (thymus-derived) cells that protect the body from foreign cells by the process of immunological surveillance. Thus the thymus is a true endocrine gland. During severe stress, injury, or sudden illness, the thymus shrinks to half its size as millions of lymphocytes are destroyed (Diamond, 1979, pp. 8–13).

Diamond has developed a muscle test using the deltoid muscle as an indicator of the body's energy supply. "A device that measures muscle strength, called a kinesiometer, shows that strong muscles can withstand up to 40 pounds of pressure, whereas a muscle that is weak can resist a pressure of about 15 pounds" (Diamond, 1979, p. 17). His research suggests that it is the thymus that is being tested by having subjects who test weak chew a tablet of thymus extract and upon retest the indicator muscle becomes strong.

Chi is the term used by the Chinese to describe energy. They developed an ancient and accepted treatment in the United States called acupuncture. In this system of thought, energy is believed to flow along pathways called meridians that do not appear to follow any *known* anatomical pathway. Behavioral Kinesiology is not testing "the mechanical strength of the muscle, but rather the energy in the meridian associated with that muscle and the ability of the body to replenish energy" (Diamond, 1979, pp. 27–28). In Diamond's theory, the thymus gland monitors and regulates energy flow in the meridian system.

According to Diamond, if the thymus monitors and balances energy, well-being occurs; if not, physical damage and ultimately organic disease occur. Various stressors have been found to decrease muscle strength in the indicator muscle, indicating impairment of thymus function and a lack of balance in the left (rational, logical) and right (holistic, creative) hemispheres of the brain, including thoughts and actions. Negative attitudes which persist yield energy imbalances which can ultimately lead to illness (Diamond, 1985).

Krieger's Theory of Therapeutic Touch

Dolores Krieger, R.N. Ph.D., theorizes that *prana* (Sanskrit term for energy) is transferred in the healing act. She draws upon Eastern literature, finding apt analogies in Western thought. For example, the source of prana in Eastern thinking is the sun; likewise, the source of energy for photosynthesis is the sun. Eastern thinking contends that well people have an excess of prana; Western physiology texts state there is a great deal of redundancy in the human body. Krieger pictures the healer as a person with excess prana or energy who has a strong sense of commitment and intention to help people. Healing is described as "the conscious full engagement of your energies in the interest of helping another" (Krieger, 1993, pp. 17–18). Healers do not become depleted of energy because they are in a constant state of energy input-throughput-output. Healers become depleted of energy only if they become too closely identified with the process or try to draw on their own energy (rather than being a channel for energy).

A body of research is accumulating to back up the usefulness of therapeutic touch for anxiety (Heidt,1979; Quinn,1982; Hale,1986), stress reduction (Kramer, 1990), pain (Meehan, 1985), and wound healing (Wirth, 1990).

According to Krieger, Therapeutic Touch works well with all stress-related diseases, having a significant effect on the autonomic nervous system, thereby influencing nausea, dyspnea, tachycardia, pallor, and peristalsis. Her report of one day's work at a clinic included seeing people with the following diagnoses: low back and shoulder pain, rheumatoid arthritis, post-abdominal surgery, cancer of the uterus, cancer of the breast, panic attack, TMJ, HIV+, multiple sclerosis, and peptic ulcer (Krieger, 1993, pp. 136–137). Therapeutic Touch has also been used during birth and delivery for post-episiotomy or cesarean healing, for colic, PMS, irritability, fatigue, elevated temperature, vomiting, diarrhea, AIDS symptoms, chemotherapy, radiation sickness, and the dying process (Krieger, 1993, pp. 136–164.)

Signs that Therapeutic Touch has occurred in the client include a deepening of voice level; slowing and deepening of respirations; a sigh, deepened breathing, or comments such as "I feel relaxed"; peripheral flush or pinking of the skin due to dilation of peripheral blood vessels, first noticed in the face.

The healer centers and uses the hands (placed 2–3 inches from the client's skin) to move quickly over the body, reading signals of congestion or blockage of energy flow. The feeling of pressure sensed in the hands when congestion or blockage is present can be explained biophysically; as the healer moves the hands over the body, positive ions are picked up; this pressure sensation is related to atoms that have lost an electron. Positive ions are associated with feelings of lethargy, headache, irritability, and inflammations of the mucosal tissues; negative ions have been noted in areas that may induce a feeling of well-being, such as waterfalls and mountains (Davis, 1963; Robinson & Dirnfeld, 1967).

Krieger refers to the pressure as a "ruffling in the field"; the healer can remove the positive ions by shaking or wiping the hands. When the healer's hands are placed in the area of a "ruffle"and then the hands are moved away from the body in a sweeping gesture, the pressure is reduced and the feeling of energy flow is sensed; this is called *"unruffling the field"* (1979, p. 54). The unruffling motion can be used to soothe babies or reduce pain and tension. A 2- to 3- minute treatment is sufficient for children or the debilitated. With others the healer stops when the body feels balanced.

The object of Therapeutic Touch is to balance the healee's "field" so that symmetry of energy flow is restored. With practice the hands begin to move toward areas of unbalanced energy flow as they become more sensitive to changes in the field of another person's body.

Krieger reports that prana can be transferred to objects, especially cotton. By holding a piece of cotton in one hand and placing the other hand above the cotton and imagining reaching down to the hand under the cotton, energy can be transferred. In this way energy can be stored to be used at a later date when less energized or to prepare for clients' use when they feel fatigued (Krieger, 1979, pp. 28–29).

Yoga

The word *yoga* means to unite, implying the balance or harmony that can exist within the individual. Yoga is an Indian philosophical system that emphasizes the practice of special techniques to attain the highest degrees of physical, emotional, and spiritual integration. Hatha yoga is the branch that emphasizes physical postures (asanas) and breathing practices (pranayama) to attain body/ mind balance.

Studies of the effects of hatha yoga have shown it especially beneficial to optimal functioning of the endocrine, circulatory, musculoskeletal, respiratory, and nervous systems (Iyengar, 1966; Udupa, Singh, & Settiwar, 1971). Yoga has been demonstrated to reduce blood pressure, lower pulse rate, reduce serum cholesterol, regulate menstrual flow and thyroid function, increase range of motion in joints, reduce joint pain, and increase feeling of well-being (Berger & Owen, 1993; Lasater, 1984, p. 296).

Massage

Touch is one of the major reasons people seek complementary therapists. Massage is an easy, everyday skill that can be learned by almost anyone. There are some cultures where massage is taught to children the same way we teach ours to brush their teeth (Harrold, 1992, p. 7).

Massage is the oldest known healing art. The Orientals were using massage at least three thousand years before the birth of Christ. In China, it was one of the four classical forms of medical treatment, along with acupuncture, moxabustion (heat energy) and herbalism. In the East, massage remains an integral part of family life (Harrold, 1992, p. 8).

The effects of massage are psychological, mechanical, physiological, and reflexive. Massage is an art (a unique way of communicating without words and showing caring) and a science; systematic manipulation of the body tissue produces beneficial effects on the nervous and muscular systems, local and general circulation, the skin, viscera, and metabolism (Knaster, 1984, p. 247).

During massage, "the hands stimulate the sensory receptors of the skin and subcutaneous tissues, causing a series of reflex effects . . . some of these effects are capillary vasodilation or constriction, relaxation or stimulation of voluntary muscle contraction, and possible sedation or stimulation of pain in an area remote from the area being touched" (Tappan, 1984, p. 262).

Ruth Rice (1975), a wellness practitioner/psychologist and specialist in early child development, has researched sensorimotor stimulation of premature infants. She developed a specific stroking and massage technique. Her research demonstrated that touching, movement, and sound stimulate the nerve pathways and increase myelination (speeding up neurological growth), increase the release of the growth hormone somatrophin (leading to faster weight gain), and increase the output of the hypothalamus (general arousal center) leading to increased cell activity and endocrine functioning.

Acupressure

Acupressure is the predecessor of acupuncture. It grew from the instinctual response of massaging sore muscles by pressing sore spots on the body and noting the positive effects. Currently, the term is applied to a number of techniques of applying pressure to stimulate acupuncture points on the body.

Acupressure releases tension and relieves pain. It is a preventive treatment used to balance energy. Chinese medicine contends that the vital force, *chi*, that controls the functioning of the body systems permeates living tissue circulating along clearly defined pathways called meridians. There are 12 organ meridians; each one takes its name from the organ to which it is connected. Energy is believed to flow through each of the 12 meridians, flowing into one another, forming a continuous pathway for energy. When energy is blocked, it can be balanced by applying pressure to specific points.

Theory of Reflexology

Reflexology is based on the premise that body organs have corresponding reflex points on other parts of the body. The reflex points are believed to be up to 20 times more sensitive than the corresponding organs. The foot is viewed as one of the scanner screens that records body functions. Working the reflexes in the feet helps rebalance organs that are functioning properly by releasing blocks that impede the smooth flow of body energy. Reflex points also influence functional relationships to that organ. For example, stimulating the heart reflex on the foot helps balance energy flow to the heart as well as the rest of the circulatory system (blood vessels, lymphatics, etc.). There are other areas with reflex points (wrist, hand, ear, neck, abdomen, face, head, arms, legs, nose, and iris), but the feet are the most effective because:

1. They link with energy from the earth and are strong energy poles of the body.
2. Working on feet is relatively nonthreatening and noninvasive.
3. Feet accumulate deposits of acids and tensions (due to the effect of gravity pressure, and the normal wear and tear of walking upright), causing tissue degeneration which can easily be felt, seen, and treated.
4. Touching the feet is a soothing gesture that can deeply affect others; for example, agitated children can be calmed by rubbing their feet.
5. Clearly charted representation of the body organs on the foot are available.
6. Because feet are usually covered with shoes and socks, they remain tender to the touch and more sensitive than some other reflex points. Additionally, there is less body musculature that might interfere with assessment and intervention than in most other parts of the body.
7. Feet are a symbolic representation of the infinite energy in the universe. Jesus washed the feet of his disciples, linking, cleansing, protecting, and blessing their whole being (Berkson, 1977, pp. 1–2).

Berkson has developed the Integrated Treatment from her study of reflexology, nutrition (she has a master's degree in the subject), acupressure (she is a certified shiatsu therapist), yoga, massage, and polarity. Her method combines diet, exercise, and healing visualization and affirmations to broach the physical, mental, spiritual, and artistic. Blocks are released and deposits are thrown off, increasing vitality of the whole person and increasing relaxation and activity potential (physical). The act of reflexology is a giving and receiving, a sharing of communication resulting in confidence and calming (mental). Together, healer and healee call upon the healing energy of the universe to surround, uplift, and permeate; the use of affirmations and the projection of a positive healing environment is a spiritual act of being of service to others (spiritual). The Integrated Treatment calls for knowledge, skills, and a personalized interaction between healer and healee to produce healing (art) (Berkson, 1977, pp. 7–8).

Theory of Psychoneuroimmunology

The new field of *psychoneuroimmunology* focuses on the links between the mind, brain, and immune system. The latter is a very complex system consisting of about one trillion cells called *lymphocytes* and about one hundred million trillion molecules called *antibodies*. The immune system has a special capability that allows it to patrol the body and guard its identity. Many immune functions may be impossible to understand if the classical scientific method is used—reducing the system to its simplest elements and attempting to predict the behavior of the whole from its parts (Institute of Noetic Sciences, 1984).

A number of studies by David McClelland at Harvard University examined the role of correlation between the levels of one immune substance in saliva (Immunoglobulin A or IgA, a measure of defense against respiratory infection) for individuals with different motivational styles. He found those driven by an inhibited power motivation had lower IgA levels than those concerned with forming warm, close relationships (1985).

In an interview with Joan Borysenko (1985), McClelland revealed the findings of his latest research. Working with movies of healers such as Mother Teresa, McClelland found that although not everyone reacted the same *consciously* to caring and loving, all their bodies reacted by secreting more IgA. At the conscious level, some reported intense dislike for religiosity, discounted the healers' ability to help, and/or described the movie as phony in written stories about the film. The subjects' opinions of the movie had no correlation to whether their immune function improved. Salivary IgA increased even in people who intensely disliked Mother Teresa. McClelland states these findings support the premise that it is not necessary to believe in the healer (placebo effect) in order to benefit. "At the conscious level, a person may not believe at all, but at the unconscious level, something in the person may still respond to the healer" (Borysenko, 1985, p. 36).

To examine the differences between those watching the films whose immune function improved and those whose did not, McClelland coded the watchers' thoughts and fantasy patterns to find what correlated with increased salivary IgA secretion. He found the most positive correlation with a "kind of affiliative connection in which a person is doing something positive involving another person, trying to help someone, or to establish a love relationship, or a friendly relationship; the curious part of it is the person is not invested in the outcome . . . on the goal of the activity" (Borysenko, 1985, p. 36).

McClelland describes the concept of unconditional love that has relevance for practitioners; when using a wellness framework it is important for practitioners to ensure they are acting based on true caring, not on a need to have power over others.

> People with the need for power often express it by helping others, even when it isn't required. In that case, giving help isn't motivated by a true expression of caring but is used as a means to achieve importance or control . . . noninvolved striving is the highest level of activity, because if you are concerned about the outcome, that's your ego. In a way it correlates with self-love, with self-esteem, in the sense that the state of being egoless comes from recognizing that you're okay within yourself. You don't have to prove that you are worthwhile by looking for reflections of your goodness in the activities that you pursue. (Borysenko, 1985, p. 37)

In the interview with Borysenko (1985, pp. 37–38), McClelland reports a study of students who were developing colds and were sent to a local healer. With one of the groups, the healer actively spent time, touching them and telling them how wonderful they were. The second group (control group) was told by the healer to see someone else to whom he had given his power. Among those the healer attended to, 11 of the 13 did not come down with a cold; in the control group, 11 of the 13 did. Students who did not show cold symptoms had a much higher concentration of IgA. Some of the strategies the healer used were: comment on their positive physical attributes, use testimonials (e.g., show people letters from somebody just like them who had persevered and done well). "Studies tell us that's important—just to know that someone else has succeeded in whatever it is you want to do. It supports choice, and that freedom counteracts helplessness" (Borysenko, 1985, p. 38).

> Type A behavior and the inhibited power motive syndrome are connected with the increased secretion of catecholamines, which suppress some aspects of the immune function . . . too much of the catecholamine norepinephrine is associated with decline in immunoglobulin A, which thereby makes the body less able to fight off certain viruses. (Borysenko, 1985, p. 38)

Studies done two decades ago demonstrate that hypnotic suggestion can alter some aspects of immunity. Other studies have shown that warts (virus-induced) can be removed by hearing or repeating a suggestion specific to removing warts while in a deeply relaxed, hypnotic state. As holism and wellness become more accepted approaches, these findings may be applied with the same enthusiasms and scientific sanction that some surgical and chemical treatments are receiving today.

At Georgetown University, Nicholas Hall, a biochemist examined the physiological basis for imagery's effect on immunity. Focusing on the hormone thymosin, he demonstrated a correlation between use of imagery and an increase in thymosin and white blood cell count (an immune system measure).

Psychoneuroimmunology provides a first step toward an "affirmative science" that makes quality of life as important as traditional science's attempts to achieve "value-free" inquiry. This shift in emphasis raises new kinds of questions, including (Institute of Noetic Sciences, 1984):

* What changes occur in the body as a result of being given a nontreatment (placebo)?
* What are the physical changes that take place when positive emotions occur?
* When there is a buildup of positive emotion, does well-being occur?
* Is human touch vital to the will to live?
* Can the ability to enhance the immune system be learned, thereby eliminating the need for medication and surgical treatment?

McClelland cautions against the use of drug short cuts to enhance immunity:

A second possible pitfall is that people will look for short cuts. They will look particularly for drug short cuts, because if we find that certain psychological conditions do something to the hormones, people will say, why go to all this trouble to change psychological characteristics, you can just give a pill that will produce the same hormonal effect . . . I think you almost always run into side effects when you do things that way . . . When people go through programs in which they learn how to use meditiation-based therapies and realize why they have their individual approaches to things and discover different choices, not only does all that frequently make their immediate symptoms go away, it also leads to larger life changes. They have learned something fundamental about themselves—and of course, you don't learn that from a pill. (Borysenko, 1985, p. 39)

SELF-CARE ASSESSMENTS

A wellness view engages the client in self-assessment and in learning to examine family members and determine when professional assistance is needed and when it is not. Such a view not only demystifies the process, but leaves the practitioner free to teach, discuss outcomes with clients, and enhance independence.

Tables 7.1–7.7 present information that can be used to teach clients self-assessment procedures relevant to prevention and self-knowledge. Additionally, the practitioner can teach the client vital sign procedures. Studies have shown that when clients take their own blood pressure at home the findings are more reliable than when a professional takes it in a physician's office; the factor of anxiety probably interferes to lower reliability.

Table 7.1 Directions for Breast Self-Examination

1.	Examine your breasts by looking in the mirror at them. First, place your arms at your sides, then place both your arms over your head. The breasts should look about the same, although many women have one breast that is a little larger than the other. Look especially for dimpling of the skin, bulges in one breast, or any *change* in size or shape.
2.	Examine your breasts while lying flat. Examine each breast with the hand from the opposite side of the body. Press the breast tissue gently against the chest wall, using the inner fingertips. Roll the tissue between your fingers and the chest wall, moving your fingers in a circular massage motion. Do not pinch the tissue, because all breast tissue feels lumpy then. Examine the inner half of each breast while holding the same-side arm over the head. Examine the outer portion of each breast while holding the same-side arm down at your side. Examine underneath the nipples and over to and including the armpit.

Note:Use imagery, nutrition and environmental safeguards to keep breast-well.

Screening as a Preventive Measure

Screening for a disease does not provide primary prevention; it may prevent further complications once an illness is present. Screening can also create problems by stigmatizing those tested; for example, children labeled as having heart murmurs became psychologically damaged while they grew out of the condition physically (Abrams, 1979; Bergman, 1977; Napodano, 1977).

The use of screening is currently being reevaluated. Physicians who used to recommend yearly checkups are now saying they are no longer needed. The American Cancer Society (ACS) has revised its recommendations for screenings, finding that there is no correlation between checkups and survival for several cancers; instead, prevention is being recommended for lung cancer, including smoking cessation. Examination of the breast by a physician is now recommended every 3 years (instead of yearly) until age 40, when yearly exams are recommended. (Since women can learn to examine their own breasts, it is not clear why physician examinations are needed for those properly prepared. It is possible to envision a future where women practice preventive measures and screening becomes totally obsolescent.) Table 7.6 presents detection tests and prevention measures for major illnesses; Table 7.7 lists questionable screening procedures.

Table 7.2 Directions for Examining Some of the Lymph Nodes

Neck Glands
1. Relax jaw and neck muscles.
2. Place the first three fingers of each hand immediately below the ears, and move the fingers in a smooth circular motion.
3. Move the fingers down a short distance and a little to the side, and repeat the circular motion.
4. Continue moving the fingers down and toward the front of the jaw little by little, until the fingers of one hand are very close to the fingers of the other hand.
5. Note enlarged glands.

Underarm glands
1. Drop one arm to the side and relax it.
2. Use the opposite arm to feel for gland under the arm, with the thumb on the chest and the fingers using a circular movement under the arm, including high into the underarm region.
3. Note enlarged glands.

Groin glands
1. Place fingertips in the groin area, and move the fingertips from side to side, using firm pressure.
2. Move fingertips downward toward the thigh.
3. Note any enlargement.

Table 7.3 Directions for Examining the Abdomen of Another Person

1. Make sure the room temperature is warm enough.
2. Ask the other person to lie on his or her back on a firm surface such as a mat on the floor.
3. Have the person remove any clothing that covers the area from their chest to the hair line of their pelvis, and to place both arms comfortably at the sides of the body or at the back of the head.
4. Ask the other person to bend his or her knees slightly, to take a few deep breaths, and to concentrate on relaxing the abdominal area.
5. Place one hand on top of the other, both palms down, and fingertips touching. Use the top hand to provide pressure, and the bottom hand to feel the abdomen.
6. Move your hands over the entire abdomen, pressing lightly. Ask the other person to signal whenever pain is felt.
7. Note when the person tenses up when you examine an area and ask, "What did you feel?"
8. If the other person complains of being tickled, use slightly firmer pressure.
9. Note and record any areas of tenderness or areas that are rigid to the touch.

Table 7.4 Communicating About Our Sexual Experiences

Directions:

Ask yourself the questions in the left-hand column and your partner those in the right-hand one. Share the information you gain and use it to enhance your sexual relationship.

Questions to ask self	*Questions to ask my partner*
"How can I tell you when I want to make love and when I want to cuddle or hug?"	"How can I tell when you want to make love and when you want to cuddle or hug?"
"How can I help you tell me you're interested in sex so I don't feel threatened, forced, or used?"	"How can I tell you I'm interested in sex without threatening or forcing you?"
"How can we work it out when I want sex and you don't?"	"How can we work it out when you want sex and I don't?"
"What pleases me sexually?" "How can I let you know this?"	"How can I best tell you when what you do pleases me sexually?"
"How could I guide you or tell you so you know how to please me sexually?"	"How can I guide you or tell you so you know how to please me sexually?"
"What do I know about what pleases you sexually?"	"What can you tell me about what pleases you sexually?"
"What is sexual turn-off for me?"	"How can I tell you about what turns me off sexually?"
"What method of birth control do I think we should use?"	"How can I talk to you about birth control methods we plan to use in a way that enhances our sexual relationship?"
"How pleased am I with the method of birth-control we are currently using?"	

Table 7.4 (*continued*)

"Do you think about sex as if performance is the most important or as if pleasure is?"	"Do you think about sex as if performance is the most important or as if pleasure is?"
"How can I focus more of my attention on pleasure than on performance?"	"How can I help you to focus more on pleasure than on performance?"
"Do I want to introduce some new experiences or position into our sexual relationship?"	"Do you want to introduce some new experience or position into our sexual relationship?"
What interferes with me letting go and enjoying a sexual experience?"	"What interferes with your letting go and enjoying a sexual experience?"

Table 7.5 Vaginal Self-Examination

One of the areas least accessible to women is their vagina; many women have never seen what their vagina looks like. Learning to examine one's own vagina is not a substitute for a pelvic exam, but it can help integrate the vagina into self-image, alert the owner to potential problems, check birth control equipment and natural birth control methods (cervical texture, color, os, mucus, and shape change indicate ovulation; adequacy of diaphragm coverage and correct placement of an IUD can be assessed), fertility (mucus is liquid and thin when close to or at time of ovulation), and pregnancy (blueing or purpling and softening of the cervix and increased vaginal secretions).

Before Beginning
1. Purchase a plastic speculum or, during your next pelvic exam, ask for the one used.
2. Find a flashlight with a high-intensity light.
3. Find a hand mirror; a self-supporting one is best because it leaves one hand free.
4. Find a firm surface to lie on and a private place for your exam.
5. Make sure you have time so you won't have to rush.
6. *Optional:* Have some K-Y jelly handy to make insertion of the speculum easier. Vaseline is not recommended; it closes vaginal pores and isn't sterile.
7. Practice using the speculum with one hand, holding it upside down. (Hold the speculum with the bill pointed away; thumb on level which opens the blades; push level in and up to lock the speculum; pull down to close the blades for entry and withdrawal.)

Examining the Vagina
1. Get into a reclining position with equipment nearby.
2. Put K-Y jelly on the bill of the speculum (*optional*).
3. Hold the speculum in the right hand (if right-handed) and spread the labia with the fingers of the left hand.
4. Take a few deep breaths and wait until you are comfortable prior to proceeding; if anxiety is encountered, use imagery or a relaxation exercise to become calm. Use the measure at any time during the examination that discomfort or anxiety is experienced. Ensure a pleasant, meaningful exploration.
5. Gently insert the speculum to the base of the blades and turn it so handle is up; open the blades and lock them open.
6. Reach for mirror and flashlight and look for the ridges of the vaginal walls and on the back wall, a smooth, pink, muscular ring that is the cervix. (If the cervix is not readily visible, bear down for a moment.) The color of the walls should look like the inside of the mouth (pink, not red); look for any sores, reddened irritated areas, unusual discharge or bleeding, and growths or bumps on the walls.

Note: For further information on vaginal self-exam and interpreting vaginal discharges, see nurse practitioner Carol Berry's "Doing Your Own Vaginal Self-Exam," *Medical Self-Care.* 1980, pp. 281-284.

Table 7.6 Detection Tests and Preventive Measures for Major Illnesses

Illness	Detection tests	Preventive measures
Heart disease	blood pressure checked at least once per year have infants age 1–6 months examined for heart malformations	have a throat culture when you have a *very* painful sore throat that lasts longer than a few days; if culture is positive, take antibiotic to reduce chance of rheumatic heart disease
		stop smoking; use stress reduction measures* and positive imagery and self-talk; exercise regularly
		lose weight or maintain ideal weight; take 100 I.U. of vitamin E a day; cut down on fat, sugar, and highly processed foods
		eat more whole fresh fruits and vegetables, whole grains and fish
Cancer	self-examination of breasts by women; self-examination of the thyroid (for women over 18 years of age who are sexually active) obtain a Pap smear yearly until 2 negative results are obtained, then obtain smears every 3 years to age 35 and every 5 years from age 35–60 examination of the skin for changes–for example, increase in size, number, or look of moles self-examination of the testicles by men	do not get an x-ray without questioning why it is necessary; refuse those that seem unnecessary stop smoking and being near smokers
		do not participate in sexual activity at an early age and/or with many different partners know environmental chemicals that are cancer-producing, and work to eliminate them and your exposure to them limit drinking alcohol exercise regularly

*In one study (Kawachi et al., 1994) risk of fatal heart disease increased with levels of phobic anxiety.

Table 7.6 (*continued*)

Illness	Detection tests	Preventive measures
Cancer (cont'd)		limit exposure to the sun and/or use PABA cream to block exposure increase fiber intake try to eat foods not sprayed with dangerous pesticides increase intake of fresh whole fruits and vegetables and whole grains
Stroke	none, except some strokes are preceded by temporary clumsiness and numbness in hand or foot, temporary blindness in one eye or slurring of speech: these should be immediately brought to the attention of a physician	same as for heart disease
Diabetes	self-test for sugar in the urine, using Tes-Tape, Clinistix, Clinitest Tabs, Diastix, or similar products available in pharmacies; especially useful for juveniles who have extreme thirst, frequent urination, and weight loss	lose weight increase exercise low-fat, high fiber, high fruit and vegetable meals to date it is not known that anything can be done to prevent juvenile diabetes, but there are some links to cow's milk
Tuberculosis	PPD or Tine Skin Test every year or two for ten years after exposure to tuberculosis	avoid exposure to people who have it; keep immune system well through high intake of fresh whole fruits and vegetables, exercise and stress reduction measures
HIV/AIDS	Have blood test	avoid contact with infected sexual partners, sharing used needles and blood transfusions* use condoms; use discretion in choice of sexual partner eat a diet centered around whole fresh fruits and vegetables, practice stress reduction measures and use supplements to boost immune function

* Although blood is screened for HIV, the virus may not show up in tests if recently contracted.

Table7.6 (*continued*)

Illness	Detection tests	Preventive measures
Arthritis	none, except for ankylosing spondylitis; in this case, you should check with a physician if you answer yes to four or five of the following: Have you had back pain for three months or more? Has your back been stiff in the morning? Did the problem start before you were 40? Did the pain and stiffness begin slowly? Does the problem improve with exercise?	some experts suggest doing weight-bearing exercise daily and taking calcium and magnesium supplements will ward off osteoarthritis keep stress managed and eat well—the onset is often associated with physical or emotional stress or bacterial infection
Gout*	possibly uric acid blood test in middle-aged, overweight men with a family history of gout	avoid gravies, rich foods (cakes, pies, etc.) and meat (high in uric acid); control weight and /or lose weight gradually to decrease uric acid levels avoid alcoholic drinks use stress reduction measures
Veneral disease (VD)	having a culture made from the cervix (opening) to the uterus or penis is useful only for people who have large numbers of sexual partners having a blood test (VDRL, FTA) one to three months after exposure	avoid contact with infected persons use condoms use discretion in choice of sexual partner
Glaucoma	having the eye pressure measured with an instrument called a Schiotz Tonometer once every four years after the age of 40, or once a year after age 30 if anyone in your family has glaucoma	use stress reduction measures; avoid prolonged eye strain use exercise to reduce stress and enhance circulation eat a diet centered around whole fresh fruits and vegetables and foods or supplements rich in vitamins B, C and E to enhance eye health

*Gout occurs when there is too much uric acid in blood and tissue. Uric acid crystals in the joints cause swelling and pain. Meat has high amounts of uric acid. Alcohol increases the production of uric acid.

Table 7.6 (continued)

Illness	Detection tests	Preventive measures
Anemia	an occasional microhematocrit (not a complete blood count) is reasonable for *children* especially if they are *not* eating an adequate diet	a balanced diet that includes vitamins and iron
Thyroid problems	self-examination for small lump to the side of the Adam's apple	refuse x-rays to the head or neck for acne, ringworm, enlarged tonsils, or adenoids
	those who *have* had radiation treatments for acne or ringworm to the head or neck or for enlarged tonsils or adenoids should have their thyroid examined yearly and learn to do a self-examination of the thyroid	
Mental retardation	if you are pregnant and know of a genetic disease that causes mental retardation in your family, see a genetic counselor, think about getting amniocentesis (test of fluid from uterus or womb); likewise, if you are over 40	if there is genetic illness in your family, get genetic counseling prior to marriage
	If there is phenylketonuria (PKU) in your family, have your baby tested immediately after birth and start him or her on the special PKU diet	
Kidney/bladder disease	urine test for pregnant women	avoid drugs or medications with adverse kidney effects; avoid high protein diet; obtain protein from peas, beans, lentils, mushrooms and asparagus Women who suffer from recurrent bladder infections should avoid tampons and nylon underwear or pantyhose. Dandelion root or extract aids in excretion of kidney waste products Obtain sufficient vitamins and minerals by a diet focused on whole fresh fruits and vegetables

Sources: Material is extracted from *Prescription for Nutritional Healing,* Balch & Balch, Avery, 1990; Tang, AM et al. Dietary micronutrient intake and risk of progression to AIDS in HIV-1-infected homosexual men. *AMJ Epidemiology* 1993, 138 (11);937-51.

Table 7.7 Questionable Screening Procedures

1. rectal exams
2. xeromammography (x-ray) of the breast (unless you are over age 40 and your sister or mother has breast cancer)
3. proctosigmoidoscopy (looking into the rectum and lower bowel through a tube) prior to age 50
4. x-ray to detect lung cancer
5. test for hidden blood in the stool prior to age 40
6. glucose tolerance test if elderly (77 to 100% will test positive for diabetes when they may not have the illness)
7. coronary arteriograms (they are very complex and have a significant chance of causing disability or death)
8. electrocardiograph stress tests (findings are inconclusive unless you have symptoms of heart disease; the test itself may be disabling)
9. screening for heart murmurs in children (the vast majority of murmurs do not indicate disease; children and parents' reactions may cause them to act *as if* there is a disease when there is not)
10. screening for high levels of uric acid for gout (unless you are a middle-aged, overweight man, with a family history of gout)
11. tests to determine whether you have a high cholesterol level (there is no definitive study to show that lowering the cholesterol level will prevent artherosclerosis or coronary heart disease)
12. tests to determine abnormalities through such procedures as chest x-rays, rectal, gastrophy, urine and sputum cytology
13. x-ray examinations to evaluate lower-back pain
14. tests to identify carriers of sickle cell anemia
15. abdominal x-ray to judge liver size or gastrointestinal bleeding
16. x-ray to detect ankle sprain
17. routine barium enemas for hernia
18. urograms and arteriograms for people with high blood pressure
19. daily (portable) x-rays of all patients in coronary care units (CCUs)
20. bone survey x-rays of people with hyperparathyroidism
21. preemployment x-rays of the chest and spine
22. use of CAT scan or MRI in inappropriate situations*
23. and x-rays during pregnancy

* In one study (Jensen et al., *New Eng. J. of Medicine*, July 1994), physicians ordered expensive MRI scans of the lumbar spine in 98 men and women who had no back pain. 64% were found to have disk abnormalities in their spines. 38% had abnormalities of more than one disk. Given the high percentage of bulges and protrusions in people with no back pain, the authors concluded that MRI detection of disk problems in people without back pain may be just coincidental, and the resultant surgery, unnecessary.

NOTE: It is important to keep in mind that besides questioning screening procedures, laboratory tests are also at question due to the large percentage of false positives and false negatives that occur. No test is 100% sensitive or able to distinguish between those who have the condition and those who do not (Galen, 1974). Additionally, laboratory testing has been found to be up to 50% inaccurate by the Centers for Disease Control that monitors and regulates testing (Mendelsohn, 1979). Finally, a large number of tests may be performed at teaching hospitals because residents must perform a minimum number in order to have a residency program approved; this increases the likelihood of performing tests when they may not be warranted. These factors interact to produce unreliable results. Probably the best protection is to obtain as much information as possible from qualitative procedures rather than relying on laboratory tests. Observing the client and asking pertinent questions is certainly more humanistic and can provide more useful information if the practitioner is well prepared in observation and communication skills.

TOUCH AND HEALING ASSESSMENTS

Behavioral Kinesiology Assessments

Diamond's behavioral testing technique requires two people: the assessor stands facing the client, who is asked to stand erect with the right arm relaxed at the side and the left arm held straight out to the side. The assessor places his or her left hand on the right shoulder and the right hand on the client's wrist. The client is then asked to resist as the assessor pushes his or her arm down. Neither smiles during the procedure as this can affect the outcome. The assessor is measuring the spring of the muscle and does not push to muscle fatigue. Clients whose thymus is weakened by stress will not be able to hold their arm up.

Clients are then instructed to thump the sternomandibular joint 10–12 times (on the skin over the point where the second rib joins the breastbone), and the assessor retests. Diamond's research shows the client will now test strong and be able to hold the arm with a great deal more resistance than prior to tapping over the gland.

Clients who test strong are called "centered" by Diamond: "his energies are centered and he is invulnerable to stress" (1979, p. 32). The centering effect has a physiological analog in the concept of right-brain (holistic, creative) and left-brain (rational, logical). Diamond has developed a test for cerebral imbalance that tests magnetic, not electroencephalographic, activity. The client and assessor stand as before, but this time the client bends the right elbow, holding the right palm to the side of the head at ear level (not touching the head or hair and keeping the head straight) at the left side of the head. If the client is cerebrally balanced, the indicator muscle will remain strong when the assessor pushes down on the wrist; the client will also test strong when the right hand is placed at the right side of the head.

Muscle testing an be used to determine whether a food, supplement, herb, item of clothing or whatever engenders a strong or weak response. Establish a base reading by asking the client to hold the extended arm "strong," then have client hold the item over the thymus and compare arm strength to base reading. Items that test weak should not be used or consumed then. Re-test at a later time.

Therapeutic Touch Assessments

Krieger suggests that both telereceptive and personal field assessments be completed by the practitioner (1979, pp. 23–51). Prior to approaching a client, the practitioner centers to ensure a fully integrated, unified, focused assessment. Centering also protects the practitioner from picking up negative energy from the client and/or bringing his or her negative energy into the assessment process. Although Krieger does not suggest it, the practitioner can use imagery to place a shield of light (or some other substance) around the practitioner that allows energy to be picked up and sensed, but not to personally affect the practitioner.

Telereceptive assessments include:

- What do clients' voices tell me about their emotional level?
- What do clients' gaits tell me about their locomotion, guarding of body parts, hesitancy, tension level?
- What do clients' facial expressions tell me about their level of involvement with me?

Human field assessments are completed standing, facing clients, moving from the head quickly to the feet while holding the hands 2–3 inches away from their bodies. The back of the body is assessed while standing behind clients and moving in the same manner over the area until an assessment is completed. The practitioner does not hesitate in a spot, but continues moving the hands; if sensations are unclear, the practitioner moves body and hands to the side or away from clients and repeats the downward movement until an assessment is clear. The practitioner searches for differences in energy flow and uses the following questions to assess blocks:

- What does the area around clients tell me about them?
- Which areas of the body "feel" hot, cold, like shocks, pressure, tingling, pulsating, or dead to me?
- What sensations can be picked up on my hands on the right side of the body vs. the left, top vs. bottom, and back vs. front?

Clients can also be assessed while they are sitting in a chair or on the floor. The practitioner stands, kneels, or sits, depending on which position allows for the most complete assessment of the client.

In preparing to assess a client, the practitioner first enhances hand sensitivity by rubbing the palms together and gradually separating them until energy flow between the hands is noted. By experimenting, the distance between the two palms at which sensations are most evident is probably the distance from the client's body at which the practitioner's hands should be placed during assessment.

Yoga Assessments

An assessment for the utilization of yoga postures includes a determination of whether the following conditions responsive to specific movements exist:

- low back pain
- nausea
- indigestion
- tension/worry
- pregnancy

- morning sickness
- pelvic congestion
- menstrual cramps
- osteoarthritis
- spinal disc problems
- thyroid dysfunction
- prolapsed uterus
- varicose veins
- depression
- upper respiratory conditions

Massage Assessments

An assessment for the use of massage includes a determination of whether the following conditions or needs exist that are believed to be responsive to the approach:

- parent/infant bonding
- muscle spasm/soreness
- headache
- buildup of toxins and wastes
- inadequate healing
- fatigue
- tension
- premature infant development

Acupressure Assessments

An assessment for the use of acupressure includes identifying the existence of the following conditions or needs that have been found to respond to the technique:

- headache
- arthritis
- back tension and lower back pain
- menstrual discomfort
- labor and delivery
- morning sickness
- deficient lactation or mastitis
- overall balance
- appetite balance
- circulation balance
- digestion balance
- elimination balance
- fainting
- fracture healing
- inflammation
- motion balance
- muscle balance
- pain control
- sciatic relief
- substance abuse
- throat
- strains, sprains, and their prevention

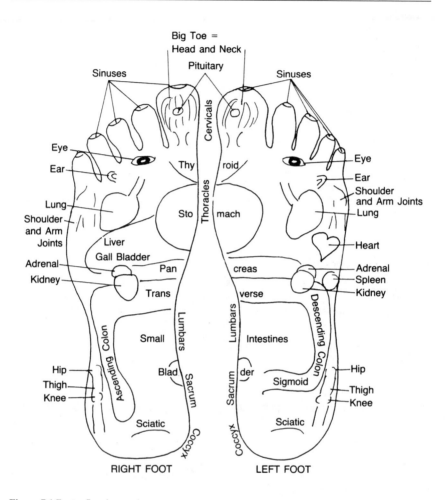

Figure 7.1 Foot reflexology points.

Sources: Extracted from *The Foot Book,* D. Berkson, New York: Harper & Row, 1977; *The Massage Book,* G. Downing, New York: Random House, 1972.

Reflexology Assessments

Figure 7.1 presents the foot reflexes used for assessment and treatment. Berkson (1977) suggests the following assessments be made:

- What does the skin color tell me?
- Are the heels of the shoes worn evenly?
- Are the eyes clear?
- Is the tongue coated?
- Are the nails strong and the hair shiny?
- What do the client's voice and posture tell me?
- Which joints rotate easily?
- Which reflex points are the most tender or the most difficult to relieve?
- How does bone feel under the skin?
- How do muscles feel?
- What temperature differences are there? (an even, warm temperature indicates balance)
- What differences in texture are there? (bunions and callouses can indicate imbalances)
- What areas on the foot indicate a hard resistance? (indicating tension, deposits, or degeneration, unless a bone, tendon, or ligament resides there)
- What areas feel hollow or recessed? (indicating lack of nutrition and energy imbalance)

SMOKING CESSATION: A SELF-CARE INTERVENTION

Table 7.8 provides suggestions for smoking cessation. A recent intervention for smoking cessation is the use of nicotine gum. Although originally thought to be a panacea, recent research shows it is most effective when used in combination with other approaches (Clavel & Benhamou, 1984). Additionally, nicotine chewing gum is suggested primarily for smokers who are heavily addicted to nicotine (Glantz, 1984).

Table 7.8 Smoking Cessation Suggestions

- Keep a notebook of current and past successes. Use the list as a reminder of your ability to succeed in new ventures.
- Identify a personal reason for quitting, not a "should" do because it's bad for me.
- Make a list of things that are personally pleasurable; choose one as a reward (instead of a cigarette) when feeling uncomfortable or bored.
- Make a list of reasons smoking began and compare with a list of current reasons for smoking.
- Write down all the missed opportunities that are regretted; choose one that is reachable and take action on it.
- Keep a log of each cigarette lit, including: purpose (to get up, to get to work, to relax, to appear calm, to celebrate, to quell hunger, after sex, after eating, etc.); focus on smoking the cigarette and sensations occurring during and after smoking.
- Write a list of stress enhancers; learn structured relaxation and stress reduction approaches to deal with each stressor; see pp.73–90.
- When using cigarettes as an energizer, substitute six small high-protein meals, sufficient sleep, a glass of milk, a piece of fresh fruit, fruit or vegetable juice, exercise or movement, or a relaxation exercise.
- End all meals with foods not associated with smoking, e.g., a glass of milk or half a grapefruit rather than a cup of coffee or a drink.

- Switch to noncaffeinated cofffee or tea, or bouillon.
- Eat a couple of sunflower seeds, or chew licorice, instead of having a cigarette.
- Have carrot sticks, celery, and other crudités ready to chew instead of smoking a cigarette.
- Eat more foods that leave the body alkaline and reduce the urge to smoke: vegetables, seeds, fruits.
- Use affirmations, such as "I no longer smoke," "I can quit," "It's getting esier and easier to quit smoking," or "It's getting easier and easier to think about quitting smoking."
- Use deep breathing or breath for unity when the urge for a cigarette appears.
- Work with a peer who can be called for positive feedback when the urge for a cigarette occurs. Be sure the peer is positive about ability to quit and does not nag or induce guilt.
- Stay away from friends who smoke and from places where people smoke.
- Buy different brands of cigarettes and avoid smoking two packs of the same brand in a row.
- Buy cigarettes only by the pack, not by the carton.
- Smoke with the opposite hand from the one usually used.
- Brush the teeth right after eating.
- Put cigarettes in an unfamiliar place.
- Every time a cigarette is reached for, ask: "Do I really want this cigarette?"; "Do I really need a cigarette?"; "What can I do instead of smoking this cigarette?"
- Develop and prepractice responses to peer pressure to smoke, including: "Come on, one won't hurt," "Smoking makes you independent, like an adult," "Here, have one," "Are you a sissy?" Take an assertiveness course if necessary to develop the skill of saying "NO."
- Tell six people, "I've quit smoking, and it was easy."
- Ask friends and co-workers not to leave cigarettes around or offer them.
- When the urge for a cigarette occurs, picture the word "STOP" in big red letters.
- Ask for a hug instead of having a cigarette.
- Choose a time to stop smoking when a peak mental or physical performance is not expected.
- Write and sign a contract with a trusted person so continuing to smoke will prove embarrassing or will result in great loss.
- Read articles and books by people who have successfully quit smoking or helped others to.
- To prevent weight gain: switch to low- or non-fat foods, fresh and dried fruit for snacks.
- When feeling depressed, talk with people who have successfully quit smoking and ask for information about why they are glad they quit.
- Chew gum to quell the urge to smoke.
- Go to the morgue and look at someone who died from lung cancer.
- Talk to someone in the hospital who has incurable lung cancer about the course of the disease; get to know what that individual is like as a person.

NOTE: Programs for children have been most successful when they are focused on showing smokers losing control and on teaching kids how to take control. For further information, contact: Clearinghouse on Drug Abuse, P. O. B. 416, Kensington, MD 20795, Tel.: (301) 443-6500.

Sources: Extracted from J. Rogers, *You Can Stop,* New York: Pocket Books, 1977. D. Van Deusen, "Kicking the Cigarette Habit: Some Reflections from an Old Pro," *The Wellness Newsletter* 5(2):3-4, 1984. National Institute on Drug Abuse, "Life Skills Program," Clearinghouse on Drug Abuse: Kensington, MD, 1984. M. Katahn, *How to Quit Smoking Without Gaining Weight.* New York: Norton, 1994.

TOUCH AND HEALING INTERVENTIONS

Behavioral Kinesiology Interventions

Diamond's research (1979, pp. 32–124) suggests the following activities may be helpful in balancing the cerebral hemispheres and activating the immune response, via thymus stimulation:

1. Center and balance the hemispheres by placing the tongue on the roof of the mouth. The intervention can be used to regain balance when threatened by an event.
2. Activate the thymus 3–4 times a day as a preventive measure; tap at the level of the sternomandiblular joint10–12 times in a rhythmic manner.
3. Read poetry in a rhythmical manner; this is a dual-brained activity: reading is a left-brained activity and rhythmical qualities require the right hemisphere.
4. Take an energy break to look at a landscape painting (beautiful scenes in nature strengthen thymus right-brained activity).
5. Tap the thymus and change ears frequently when listening on the telephone (listening with the left ear encourages left-brained activity and listening with the right ear encourages right-brained activity).
6. Practice contralateral walking and crawling to balance brain hemispheres.
7. Practice thymus thumping after homologous or homolateral movements such as jumping jacks, weight lifting, rowing, bicycling.
8. Concentrate on turning negative emotions (hate, envy, suspicion, and fear) which weaken the thymus into positive emotions (love, faith, trust, courage, and gratitude) which activate the thymus. Diamond does not suggest suppressing negative thoughts and emotions; people expressing negative emotions tested weak using the thymus test in Diamond's studies. (See Stress Management for suggestions regarding how to change negative thoughts and feelings into positive ones.)
9. Use facial expressions (smiles) and gestures (outstretched arms, nodding the head yes) to strengthen the thymus; avoid frowns and shaking the head no; they weaken the thymus. For those who cannot smile: tweak the cheek, and the smile muscle (zygomaticus major) linked to the thymus will activate the mechanism.
10. Avoid listening, reading about, or watching violence (hijackings, floods, fires, murders, and other disasters) that adversely affect the thymus.
11. Avoid being around people who use negative comments, e.g., "You're ugly," "I hate you," "You're stupid!" Such statements weaken the thymus response.
12. Avoid attempting to be "therapeutic" with a client if under stress; stress subtly distorts speech via the hyoid bone and this distortion is picked up by the listener. When under stress, use a centering technique or thump the thymus prior to working with a client.
13. Avoid the following or at least test individually, as Diamond has found them to produce weakness in the thymus for many individuals:

- tinted sunglasses
- electronic pulse and quartz-crystal watches (varying the position in which they are worn may not disturb thymus function; individualized testing is necessary to determine response)

- hats made of synthetics weaken the activity of the thymus gland
- synthetic wigs
- high-heeled shoes (the brain is confused by sensory messages from the ankle signalling that both feet are at the end of forward step)
- synthetic clothing and bedclothes
- disposable diapers
- toiletries
- ice cold drinks or showers
- fluorescent lighting
- fiberglass insulation
- household fuel and chemicals (e.g., cooking gas, cleaning agents)
- smoking, smoke filled rooms, watching someone smoke, or viewing a picture of someone smoking
- auto exhaust
- not breathing equally through both nostrils; if this cycle has been disturbed, breathing through the left nostril (increasing negative ions necessary for well-being)
- x-rays, electrical generators, and microwaves; Diamond's studies found the walk-through screening device did not weaken the thymus, but anyone within 10 ft of the carry-on baggage machine tested weak; even microwave ovens that operate safely weaken the thymus; CB radios affect thymus, but only for a short distance; microwave transmitters and electrical transmission lines weaken the thymus
- Viewing certain symbols weakens the thymus, including the pitchfork, crosses (only those that have vertical arms longer than horizontal arms), swastikas (depending on which cerebral hemisphere is dominant; clockwise or counterclockwise swastikas weaken the thymus). Diamond found that a circle with four intersections and a dot in the middle balanced the hemispheres and reduced stress
- Rock music with an anapestic beat that stops at the end of each bar or measure is correlated with cerebral imbalance and weakens the thymus. Listening to specific sounds strengthens the thymus: running water, bird sounds, cats purring, and classical music strengthen.
- Refined sugar and additives weaken the thymus. Over 90% of Diamond's clients tested weak with beef, wheat, and dairy products.

14. Good posture stimulates the thymus; metal folding chairs and soft, comfortable chairs weaken; firm chairs with straight backs do not. Crossing the legs while sitting weakens, and driving while sitting on a soft seat also weakens. Diamond recommends sitting on a firm board or sheet of hard plastic when driving or flying to counteract fatigue.

15. The Alexander Horizontal Position aligns the body and permits the free flow of energy, enabling the thymus to correct imbalances. (Lie supine on the floor, knees bent, with a book or two under the head so that the neck is at about a 45-degree angle to the body.

For further information see: Diamond, J., *Behavioral Kinesiology,* New York: Harper & Row, 1979.

Therapeutic Touch Interventions

The main therapeutic touch intervention is "unruffling the field." As the practitioner sweeps the hands down the client's body, any areas that feel like pressure or congestion are "unruffled."

Prior to any intervention, the practitioner centers and holds the intention to heal. This is accomplished by placing the hands "with palms facing away from the body at the area where you felt the pressure and then move the hands away from the body in a sweeping gesture . . ." (Krieger, 1979, p. 54). Energy can also be directed from a higher energy area to a low energy area by moving the hands in the appropriate direction in a brushing movement.

Another use of therapeutic touch is to act as a channel for energy to bring it to the client from a universal energy source. This is particularly helpful if the client is fatigued or needs concentrated energy to heal. In this case, the practitioner centers, protects herself or himself, and pictures an energy source such as the sun, God, or another light or energy source. With eyes closed, the universal source of energy can be pictured being channeled through the practitioner's hands to the area in need of healing or energizing. For further information, see Krieger, D., *The Therapeutic Touch*, Englewood Cliffs, NJ: Prentice-Hall, Inc., 1979, or *Accepting Your Power to Heal, the Personal Practice of Therapeutic Touch*, Santa Fe, NM, 1993.

Yoga Interventions

Yoga is a discipline devoted to balance; all forward bending postures are recommended to be balanced by a backward bending one. Forcing, straining, or stretching to the point of pain is the opposite of the needed approach. Postures are meant to be performed slowly, almost meditatively, while breathing consciously. Postures should be done on a cushioned floor, before eating, and while wearing loose clothing. Breathing should be in and out through the nostrils.

1. *The Bow.* Reported useful for gastrointestinal disorders, constipation, upset stomach, sluggish liver, abdominal fat. While lying flat on the stomach, grasp ankles, inhale, and lift legs, head, and chest, arching the back into a bow. Hold, then exhale and lie flat. Repeat 3–4 times, resting in between to note effects.

2. *Cobra.* Reported to tone ovaries, uterus, and liver, relieves constipation, limbers spine; excellent for slipped discs. WARNING: not recommended for those with peptic ulcer, hernia, or hyperthyroid. Lie on the stomach, arms at shoulder level; push the upper body up with the arms, arch the back and look up while inhaling; hold and exhale while lowering the upper body slowly to the floor.

3. *Corpse Pose.* Reported to stimulate blood circulation, alleviate fatigue, nervousness, neurasthenia, asthma, constipation (enhance by visualizing increased circulation and movement of material through the intestines), diabetes (enhance by visualizing circulation to and from the pancreas), indigestion, insomnia, lumbago (enhance by visualizing enhanced circulation to nourish back muscles), mental concentration, and generalized relaxation. Lie flat on the back, legs and arms a comfortable distance from the body; let the body sink into the floor. During the

second and third trimester of pregnancy, lie on the side using pillows as necessary.

4. *Knee to Chest.* Reported to relieve stiffness and soreness of back and extremities, constipation, diabetes, flatulence. Lie flat on back and bring knees to chest; rock back and forth gently, massaging the spine. Lower the legs one at a time slowly. Bring one leg to the chest, pulling it in in a controlled stretch with interlocked fingers. Hold the position and breathe. Slowly bring the head toward the knee, hold and exhale. Inhale and bring knee to nose and hold for a count of 10; exhale and repeat 5–10 times. Repeat with other leg. Draw up both legs so knee moves toward the nose; hold while breathing and exhale. Return legs to floor and rest, noting the effect.

5. *Kneeling Pose.* Reported to increase circulation to prostate gland and uterus. Sit on heels, keeping back straight. While breathing through nostrils, separate the feet and slowly sink in between, moving buttocks toward the floor. Move gently, avoiding straining knee ligaments. Keep feet facing straight back.

6. *The Lion.* Reported to relieve sore throat; stimulates circulation to throat and tongue (enhance by visualizing relaxation of throat and improved circulation to the area). Sit on the heels, palms on knees, fingers fanned out. Protrude the tongue as far as possible, open eyes and mouth as far as possible, roll eyeballs upward. Exhale saying "Ahhhh" and feeling the sensation in the back of the throat.

7. *Locust.* Reported to relieve problems of abdomen and lower back. WARNING: not recommended for those with hernia or acute back problems. Lie flat on stomach, head facing ahead, chin on the floor; relax and breathe. Keeping arms close to the body, palms up, slowly raise one leg toward the ceiling using the lower back muscles. Hold briefly and then exhale while lowering the leg to the floor. Rest. Repeat with the other leg. Repeat 2–3 times but not to point of fatigue.

8. *The Mountain.* Reported to strengthen lungs, purify blood, improve digestive system, tone nervous system. Sit cross-legged on the floor; stretch arms up toward the ceiling, fingertips together. Stretch up while breathing slowly and deeply 5–10 times; exhale and lower arms.

9. *Neck and Eye Exercises.* Reported to relieve headache and eyestrain, improve eyesight, relax neck and shoulder tension. Sit cross-legged on the floor, wrists at rest on knees. Nod head forward slowly 3–4 times; nod toward the left and right shoulder 3–4 times, allowing the mouth to fall open. Inhale and shut the eyes tightly; hold, then exhale, opening the eyes wide and blinking rapidly 8–10 times. Hold the eyes open wide while looking around the entire circumference of the eyeballs; reverse the circle. Look diagonally from left upper to right lower and vice versa. Look up and down 10 times. Remember to breathe throughout. Rub palms together, close the eyes, and cover them with the palms, while completing 5 slow breaths. Repeat until eyes relax. Visualize energy and brightness moving into the eyes.

10. *Uddiyana.* Reported to alleviate constipation, indigestion, gastrointestinal problems, diabetes, and obesity. WARNING: Avoid if pregnant or hypertensive. Stand with feet apart, knees slightly bent; lean forward and arch the back. Keep hands on thighs. While exhaling, suck abdomen toward the spine and hold for several seconds. Relax and repeat on exhalation. Work up to 20 repetitions with one exhalation.

11. *Cat Stretch.* Reported useful in relieving back pain of pregnancy and aids in generalized relaxation. While on all fours on the floors, arch the back and then concave it.

12. *Spinal Twist.* Reported to increase spinal flexibility, aids in the return of the uterus to its nonpregnant size, strengthens oblique abdominals (stretched during pregnancy), and stimulates elimination from the intestines and bladder. Sit on the floor, right knee bent at 90° angle to left leg. Bend left knee and place the left foot in front of the right knee. Place right hand directly behind right hip. Place left hand directly behind right hand. While exhaling, move the left hand in a circle (feeling spinal stretch) to rest on the floor behind left hip; hold, then rest. Return the left hand to the position behind the right hand by completing a slow semicircular movement in front of and to the side of the body. Switch legs and repeat, twisting first to the right and then to the left.

13. *Triangle Pose.* Reported to prevent degenerative arthritic changes, tone the sides of the body, and maintain joint health in the feet, ankles, knees, and hips. Stand with feet 3–5 feet apart, right foot at a 90° angle to left foot. Gradually reach down with right hand to grasp right ankle; hold left arm straight up in the air directly above right arm; eyes watch left hand while breathing and holding the pose. Repeat on left side of the body.

14. *Shoulder Stand.* Reported to regulate the thyroid, increase flow of venous blood from the lower extremities to the heart, prevent varicose veins, and reduce gravitation pressure on internal organs. WARNING: contraindicated in cases of hypertension, neck problems, ear, throat, or eye infection and obesity. Lie on the back, palms facing the floor; press palms down and lift legs up and over the head, supporting the back with the hands and resting so the chin is on the chest. Align the chin with navel and big toes. Relax, breathe, and enjoy.

15. *Sun Salutation.* Reported to invigorate, calm, exercise arms and spinal cord, prevent and relieve stomach ailments, reduce abdominal fat, improve digestion and circulation, limber spine, tone abdominal, thigh, and leg muscles, strengthen nerves and muscles of arms and legs, shoulders, arms, and chest. An all around preventive posture that should be done at least every day by everyone.

Figure 7.2 provides directions for the Sun Salutation (Berkson, 1977; Lasater, 1984; Lowe & Nechas, 1983).

For further information see: Lowe, C. and Nechas, J., *Whole Body Healing,* Emmaus, PA: Rodale Press, 1983, pp. 508–552; or, Weiss, K., (ed.) *Women's Health Care: A Guide to Alternatives,* Reston, VA: Reston Publishing Co., pp. 294–309; and *Easy Pregnancy with Yoga* by Stella Weller (1991), Thorsons.

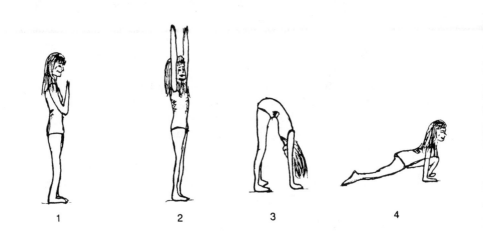
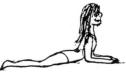
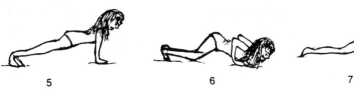
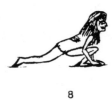
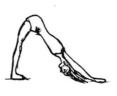
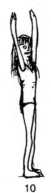
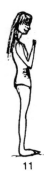

Figure 7.2 Sun salutation.

Massage Interventions

Mechanical pressure is used in massage to:

> . . . rid the muscles of toxic products by "milking" these acids into the lymphatic and venous flow toward the heart. As the muscles relax, fresh blood flows into them, bringing necessary nutrition to the area. It is obvious that massage should *not* be given if there is a possibility of spreading inflammation; or of dislodging a thrombus; thus causing embolism; or if there is such obstruction that the mechanical assistance of massage could not improve the blood flow. However, massage given *first* to the proximal aspects of an injured limb will ensure that these circulatory pathways are open enough to carry the venous flow along toward the heart. (Tappan, 1984, p. 260)

There are five basic massage strokes.

1. *Effleurage* is the stroke that glides over the skin on the surface. It is the most common stroke. Effleurage is often used to begin a massage to explore for areas of tenderness or tightness. The hand is molded to the skin, stroking with firm and even pressure, usually upward,

2. *Petrissage* strokes lift the muscle mass and wring or squeeze it gently. Kneading manipulations are completed with the hands or fingers pressing and rolling the muscles. It stimulates muscular and nervous tissue, frees adhesions, and stretches adipose tissue to release toxins, pesticides, and additives stored there.

3. *Friction* with the heel of the hands, thumb, or fingertips (according to the area to be covered) penetrates into deeper tissue. The tissue under the skin is moved, not the fingers on the skin. The stroke is used to massage deep into joint spaces or around bony prominences, and can break down adhesions; it cannot affect a deep abdominal fibrositis, however.

4. *Vibration* is a fine, tremulous movement, sometimes only fluttering above a body part. It is used for its soothing effect which can also be accomplished via an electrical vibrator.

5. *Tapotement* is the use of the fists, or cupped palms, or the loose flinging of the hands to percuss a body area. The movement is done parallel to the muscle fibers to prevent trauma or spasm. This stroke is especially effective on tight shoulders or necks.

Experiment with a peer, friend, or family member with the various strokes and their effects prior to working with a client.

When practicing massage, it is wise to communicate with the client, asking where tense or tight spots are, experimenting with different strokes and asking for client input, and teaching the client self-massage measures. A massage is not a good time for general conversation, but practitioner and client should be focused on the massage experience. It is not unusual for clients to experience strong positive or negative feelings during massage; the body work releases unresolved feelings. If this should occur, stop the massage and use listening skills until the feelings and thoughts have been expressed. Resume when the client is ready.

There is little agreement about oil use; some practitioners recommend it for its reduction of friction; vegetable (not mineral) oil is suggested because it is easily absorbed by the skin, whereas mineral oil tends to clog the pores. Practitioners who do not recommend the use of any oil believe oil interferes with energy exchange and finger sensitivity.

The best surfaces for giving a massage are: a massage table, a water bed, the floor. Most beds are too soft to offer the support needed to apply the appropriate amount of pressure. When giving a massage on the floor, it will of necessity be shorter in duration to prevent damage to the practitioner. To counter some of the fatigue and stress, use foam knee padding or several sleeping bags to kneel on. A single mattress taken from a bed and placed directly on the floor will work, but its height is inconvenient. Working outside on the grass is a beautiful, serene experience for practitioner and client. A massage is best received in the nude, but if the client is uncomfortable, negotiate this item.

The practitioner's hands should be clean and fingernails trimmed down so the fingerpads are available for massage. Warm them if cold; either use warm water or rub them together vigorously. Be sure the client removes all jewelry, contact lenses, glasses, etc. The practitioner removes wristwatch, rings, and anything that will detract from the massage for the client.

Approach the client's body slowly, gradually working up to stronger strokes. Always keep at least one hand on the client; stopping and starting touch is disruptive to the flow of massage. Use body weight rather than hand and arm muscle to apply pressure. Use good body mechanics, bending the knees and relaxing into massage movements; breathe regularly, avoid holding the breath. Massage is intense, hard work. Remember to keep yourself well by altering the procedure with gentler approaches such as therapeutic touch, Jin Shin Jyutsu or reflexology.

Begin a massage by holding the palms lightly against the client's forehead for a few moments, applying no pressure. Center and then begin massage. Table 7.9 gives information concerning massage.

Table 7.9 Massage

1. Ask the client to lie down on his or her back. Stand, sit, or kneel in back of the client's head. Massage the forehead with the balls of the thumbs ending at the temples.

2. Use the tips of the forefingers to press against the bony rims of the eye sockets.

3. Massage the chin between the thumb and forefinger.

4. Use the palms to massage both sides of the face.

5. Bring both hands under the neck (be careful of the ears); hold the head firmly and straight out from the neck. Knead the neck with one hand with the other hand moving from the bottom of the neck to the nape. Cradle the head firmly in your hands and pull out with a moderate pressure, hold the head, and begin making a cloverleaf (see Figure 7.3).

 This is an integrating brain movement that also releases tension. As you work, watch the client's chest for breathing changes; note skin color and sighs indicating relaxation. After completing the butterfly pattern, hold the head cradled in the hands for several practitioner and client breaths. Slowly place the client's head on the work surface and slowly move hands to the shoulders.

6. Push down on both shoulders with moderate to heavy pressure using body weight; hold the shoulders down through several slow breaths and then release the push, but keep the hands on the shoulders. Press in on the trapezius shoulder muscles looking for tight, hard, sore spots and lumps (muscle knots). When any is found, very gradually apply pressure with the ball of the thumb until reaching a point where it is sore; ask the client to tell you "when it's sore." Stop increasing the pressure at that point and hold the pressure you have. Wait for the client to relax; this can be enhanced by asking him or her to "breathe into my finger." Observe for signs of relaxation (muscle loosens, breath deepens and moves lower in the body) and then increase pressure with the ball of the thumb until another sore layer is reached. Repeat above. Move to locate and relax other sore areas in the shoulders.

7. Place the fingertips under the shoulders and move down to the shoulder blades, moving slowly if resistance is encountered, allowing the client to breathe in and out prior to moving the hands down. Watch for change in breathing and an opening up of the chest. When noted, go to number 8.

8 Place one hand on each side of the neck; turn the head to the left and to the right until resistance is met. If the neck is extremely tight, ask the client to "breathe into my hands" and gradually work the neck to the right and then to the left.

9. Holding the upper, back part of the head in both hands, lift the head as far forward as is comfortable. Stop when resistance is met, then gently nudge the head an inch farther forward. Slowly return the head to flat again.

10. Place the heel of the hands on the upper chest and push down and hold through several of the client's breaths, then release.

11. Place the hands under the client's armpits and gradually and firmly pull back and hold through several client breaths, then release.

12. Make fists of the hands and start at the middle of the chest below the collar bone and slide the knuckles out and down the torso following the ribs. Do successive movements until the entire rib cage has been covered. Avoid the abdominal area. Go lightly.

13. Move to the right side of the client and make a firm, circular motion several times, radiating out from the navel and down toward the bladder. Knead the abdominal area.

14. Grasp the client's right arm with both hands; pull the arm firmly and slowly toward the foot, keeping it in proper alignment with the shoulder; hold through several client breaths, then release.

15. Starting at the wrist, knead up the forearm and upper arm; glide the hands down to the wrist. Knead the hand and down each finger, pulling each finger out with firm, strong pressure (you will get some resistance and/or hear a crack as pressure is released.

Table 7.9 (*continued*)

16. Repeat no. 14 and no. 15 with the other arm and hand.
17. Move to the client's feet. Grasp the right ankle with both hands and exert firm, even pressure by leaning back; this will release tension in the hip joint. Knead up from the ankle to the hip. Glide the hands down to the ankle.
18. Make a fist with the right hand and make circles on the bottom of the foot. Knead the rest of the foot and pull out firmly on each toe.
19. Complete no. 17 and no.18 on the left leg and foot.
20. Ask the client to turn over on the stomach. Use pillows to support the abdomen, neck, etc. Knead up the back of the right leg. Grasp both ankles with the hands, lean back, and hold for one or two breaths, releasing any additional tension in the hip.
21. Knead up the back of the other leg.
22. Move to face the client's head. Using the weight of your body, push the client's shoulders down, hold through several client breaths, release.
23. Move to the right side of the client. Drum the outer edges of the hands lightly, but rapidly across the right shoulder and back several times. Drum down the spine and the leg and up the other leg to the top of the spine, down the spine and down the other leg, and back up to the top of the spine.
24. Place the heel of the right hand at the middle of the right shoulder and the heel of the left on the middle of the left buttock; alternately rock the body, pushing down first with the right heel (hand) and then with the left heel (hand). Complete this rocking motion 2–3 times. Then place the heel of the left hand in the middle of the left shoulder and the heel of the right hand in the middle of the right buttock; rock 2–3 times, remembering to breathe and bend (see Figure 7.4).
25. Place the right hand underneath the lower abdomen and the left hand directly above on the lower back; push up with three fingers with the right hand and work down all five meridians (see Figure 7.4).
26. Right (or lower hand) pushes on the coccyx (sitbone) towards head; upper hand works from the spine outward, working one vertebra at a time (see Figure 7.4).
27. Find coccyx, then go 2" out to the right from it; client will feel some pain/pressure; when area has been located, release the pressure and work on the left shoulder and neck area with the other hand (keep the hand in place on the coccyx). Repeat, reversing hands and moving 2" out to the left from the coccyx (see Figure 7.4).
28. Stand on the left side of the client, left hand to the left of the cervical spine, right hand just below it; work down the side of the spine with fingertips of both hands, making two clockwise circles into each spinal process; this soothes. Work around the coccyx and up the other side of the spine making two counterclockwise circles, up and into the spinal processes; this stimulates.
29. Place the hands on the client's head and quickly run both hands down the head, shoulders, arms, legs, and off the end of the feet. Return to the head and repeat until the entire back of the body has been covered with this quick, light movement.
30. Ask the client to slowly turn over when ready. Place the hands lightly on the client's cheeks and hold for a minute or two.
31. Move to the right side of the client, facing his or her head, and repeat the quick movement of the hands from the head down and off the body until every spot on the body has been covered.
32. Let the client rest for a few minutes while you meditate or close your eyes and relax.

Note: If, during massage, any muscle knots are found, use deep, hard pressure with the thumb; if that does not release the muscle, use acupressure, pushing straight in with the thumb for 8–10 seconds, release, and repeat until muscle relaxes. Additionally, ask the client to picture that muscle relaxing. For further information, see: Downing, G., *The Massage Book,* New York: Random House, 1972, or D. Baloti Lawrence, *Massage Techniques,* New York: Perigee, 1986.

Schneider (1979) advocates the use of *infant massage* as a relaxation and *bonding* procedure.

> The most important elements that form the bond between mother and child include skin-to-skin contact, prolonged and steady eye-to-eye contact, and the soothing high pitched sounds of mother's voice in response to her infant's cry. Infant massage which serves as communication between parent and infant helps cement that bond. Baby learns to enjoy the wonderful comfort and security of loving and being loved. She acquires knowledge about her own body, as mother shows her how to relax a tense arm or back, or helps her release some painful gas. (p. 17)

Fathers are encouraged to learn infant massage. It is an excellent tool, providing quality experience for father and infant. The infant learns father can touch gently and lovingly and can be counted on to satisfy physical and emotion needs. The father learns to satisfy his infant and enhance his self-esteem and self-confidence.

Schneider (1979, p. 25) suggests the first 9 months are the ideal time to start. Daily massages up to 6 or 7 months of age are recommended. As the child becomes more active, once or twice a week is sufficient, but "growing pains" can be reduced through a pre-bedtime massage. Children who are not introduced to massage until age 3 or 4 can be offered a brief, gentle back massage at bedtime; in time, children begin asking for a massage. Older children can be taught to give their brothers and sisters a massage; this will increase bonding between the children, enhance the older child's self-esteem, and help resolve being replaced when a new infant is born. Rolling, milking, and circular strokes can be used with the infant. The arms and legs can be kneaded just as in adult massage.

All babies will fuss and cry at some times during massage; this is expected. It may be that parts of their bodies they were not aware of are sore to the touch; a gentler massage in those areas will relax the infant. For the first 3 months of life, infants may resist having their arms massaged since moving the arms so far from the body may seem unnatural; gentle shaking and patting movements are suggested in this case. Back massage is usually enjoyed at this time.

From 4 to 7 months, soreness and tension often moves to the back (crawling and sitting begins) and face (sucking and teething). At the end of the first year, tension may move to the legs. Infants who have been massaged from infancy will help by massaging themselves and by one and a half years will massage their dolls and teddy bears, and often their mothers.

Schneider (1979, pp. 31, 76) suggests the following interventions when the infant fusses:

1. Breathe deeply and relax. Use affirmations including, "I now let go of tension. My body is relaxed. I now let go of thoughts. My mind is open and free. I am the gentle power of love, flowing through my hands to (baby's name)."

2. Stop in the middle of the massage to cuddle, hold, or walk the baby.

3. Give the baby a teether or small toy to play with or chew on.

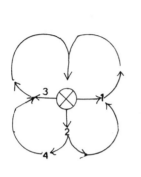

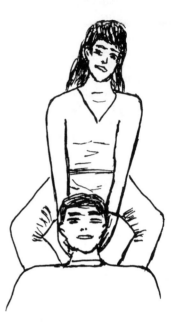

Figure 7.3 Integrating and relaxing the brain.
Sitting on the floor facing the back of the client's head, or standing behind the head of the massage table or bed, the practitioner exerts a slight, equal pull straight back with both hands from underneath the neck. Beginning and ending at midpoint **X**, the head is guided through two loops on the right side of midpoint and then two on the left side of midpoint. The head is gently placed on the floor, table, or bed, and hands are very slowly released from underneath the neck.

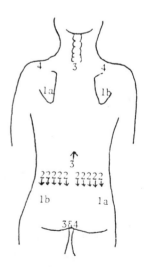

1a = rock
1b = rock
2 = work down meridians
3 = right or lower hand on coccyx/sitbone,
  other hand works up and outward from spine
4 = right or lower coccyx, left hand works
opposite shoulder and neck area

Figure 7.4 Back massage.

Acupressure Interventions

The palms of the hands, the thumbs, or the four fingers apply 3–5 kg of pressure to the client's body for 3–5 seconds in acupressure. Pressure is gradually increased until the maximum pressure is reached; then it is decreased. The direction of pressure is toward the center of the client's body. The weight of the whole body, not just the hands, is used (Serizawa, 1972, pp. 24–25).

Nickel (1984) suggests preventive acupressure for sports activities. (See Figures 7.5, 7.6). Areas of common injury are focused on prior to engaging in the activity, thus strengthening the body against injury during play. Nickel (1984) also suggests an overall balancing point using ear acupressure techniques; see Figure 7.6. The points suggested in the two illustrations can also be used once an injury is incurred; acupressure should not be used to avoid the pain associated with a strain, tear, or fracture in order to continue with vigorous exercise, but can be used in conjunction with other treatments.

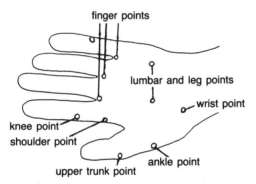

Apply firm pressure with ball of thumb; five seconds on and five seconds off for 30 seconds. Do both hands.

Figure 7.5 Prevention acupressure
(increases circulation to the most commonly injured areas)
(*Source:* Nickel, 1984, pp. 24–73.)

Lowe and Nechas suggest specific acupressure points of relief of pain. The Hegu point is the key to relieving pain in the head, neck, and arms. To locate the point:

> . . . lay your left hand on a flat surface. Position the thumb so that it forms a right angle with the index finger. Now feel along the bone that extends back from the knuckle of the index finger. Along the index finger bone is the Hegu point. The point actually lies a little down and under the index finger bone. If you press down right alongside the bone, you have to press sideways, after you reach a sufficient depth, to reach a point under the bone. . . . As you press harder you should feel the pressure radiating along the nerves in your hand. This sensation signals that you are on the Hegu point. (p. 15)

Early morning stiff necks, dental pain, and headaches respond well to hard pressure on the Hegu point.

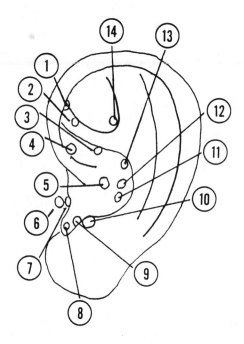

① **sympathetic point** (perspiration, stomach spasm, pain, coordination)

② **sciatic point** (sciatica)

③ **kidney point** (fractures, dizziness, ear ringing, edema, hearing loss, weariness, electrolyte imbalance, kidney injury)

④ **large intestine point** (constipation, diarrhea, hemorrhoids, respiration)

⑤ **stomach point** (indigestion, nausea, belching, heartburn, peptic ulcer, distension)

⑥ **hunger point** (under or overweight, anorexia, bulimia)

⑦ **adrenal point** (inflammation, swollen joints, muscles, tendons, allergies, cellulitis, common cold, fatigue, respiration, fever, frostbite, sinuses)

⑧ **steroid point** (allergies, inflammation, shock)

⑨ **ovary point** (painful menstruation, amenorrhea, infertility)

⑩ **occiput point** (jet lag, car and sea sickness, convulsions, lock jaw, stiff neck)

⑪ **spleen point** (abnormal uterine bleeding, indigestion, prolapsed viscera)

⑫ **relax muscles point** (liver, pain)

⑬ **liver point** (headaches, circulation, iron deficiency anemia, arthritis, muscle spasm, stomach gas, seizures)

⑭ **neurogate point** (body pain, allergies, anxiety, asthma, coughing, hypertension, insomnia, itching)

Figure 7.6 Overall balancing: ear acupressure.

Apply firm pressure with thumb ball and index finger for 1 minute, in 5-second on and 5-second-off intervals. Use right ear.

(*Source:* Nickel, 1984, pp. 83–103.)

Another location for headache is the Fengchi points on the back of the head, in the depressions on either side of the cervical vertebrae below the occipital bone. Pushing hard up and into the skull will relieve some headaches. One or the other points, or a combination of Hegu and/or Fengchi works for most people; experimentation is necessary. Tenderness of a meridian point is the best indicator the point has been located.

A point that brings neckache relief is Xuehai, located on the inside of the thigh, just back of the knee cap. The Liangqui point is located on the outside of the thigh behind the knee cap. The Tiantu point can help asthma; it is at the base of the throat right above the suprasternal notch; pressing this point on children may cause a slight choking sensation that may frighten the child.

The Yuyao point in the middle of the eyebrow eases fatigue, and Taichong, at the place where the big and second toes meet, energizes. Zusanli, about 3" below the knee, relieves abdominal pain and motion sickness as well as energizes. Yongquan, located just behind the ball of the foot, energizes and revives after a faint (Lowe & Nechas, 1983, pp. 1–29).

Patterson (1984) suggests the following acupressure points for specific problems: all points in Figure 7.7, Neck and Shoulder Release.

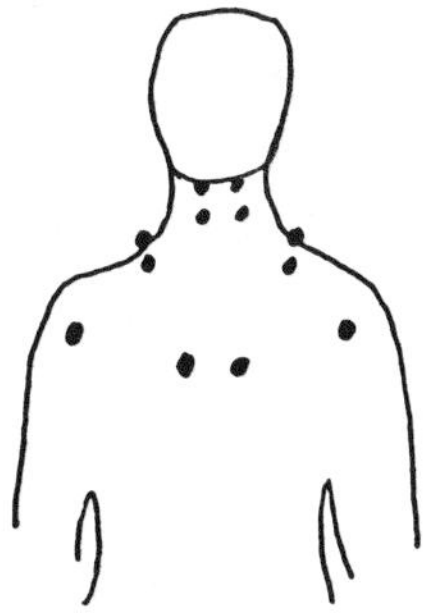

Figure 7.7 Acupressure for neck and shoulder release.

Jin Shin Jyutsu is a gentle form of acupressure which can be very effective. Three fingers of each hand—index, middle and ring—are used to assess pulses indicating the flow of bodily energy. There are 26 specific points on the body used to treat specific symptoms. The practitioner (or client) first learns to assess the pulses, then to keep the fingers on that area until all three pulses in both hands flow evenly. Points are usually used in a certain pattern to achieve release or balance. Figure 7.8 shows the energy release points.

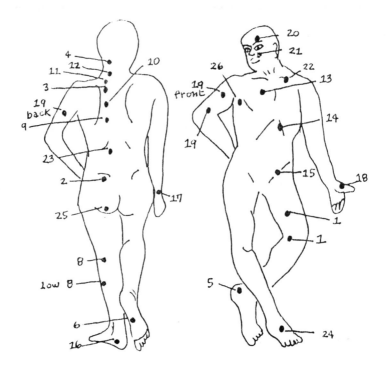

Figure 7.8 Jin Shin Jyutsu Pressure Points

S = same side O = opposite side

Abdominal bloat: Hold 2 and O-High 1
Abdominal congestion: Hold1 and O-26, then 1 and 8; then 13 and O-11
        then 23 and S-1 or high 1
Allergies: Hold 3 and S-15; then 10 and S-hi 19
Appetite: Hold 13 and O-11; 14 and S-19
Arms: Hold 3 and S-15; 11 and S-25; 12 and O-4
Arthritis: Hold 10 and S-3
Back, Low pain: Hold 2 and S-8; S-2 and O2; 4 and O-21
Balance (emotional/physiological): Hold 14 and S-19
Birth (pelvic opening): Hold hi 1s, 2s; 2s and O1s and O-8s
Bites (bug): 9s, left hand over right hand on bite
Bladder problems: Hold S-15s, S-2s, 2 and O-15; O1 and O-8
Bleeding: Left hand over right on top of bleeding
Bowels: S-15s; 2s; 2s and O8s; then O-1s
Brain: 4 and O-21; S-12 and 4; S-19,21 and O-23; 22 and S-3
Breasts (lumps): S-10s; S-19s
Burns: Palms on top of burn, then place palms (with fingers
        pointing toward the head) on calves and hold for
        20 minutes or more

Cancers: 15 and S-3; 16 and S-12; 17 and O-16;18 and S-4; 19 and S-14; 23
     and S-1; 25 and S-11
Circulation: 13 and O-1; both hi 19s; 3 and S-15
Colds: 10s; 11s; 12s; 1s; 17s
Constipation: L18 and R11, then R2
Diabetes: 23s, 9s
Diarrhea: R8 and L11, then L2
Digestion: Hold both hi 1s (on self, cross hands); hi 19 and O- hi 1
Dizziness: pinch under nose hard; 8 and S11
Ears: 13s; S-12 and 4; 21 and O-23; 22 and S-3
Emphysema: 10 and S-hi 19; 13 and O-11; 15 and S-3
Energy, Lack: hi 19s; 2 and O-9; 23 and S-1; 25 and S-11
Eyes: 4s; 10s; 3s
     Twitching: Hold opposite eye, hold 4 and opposite 20,21, 22
Face, tension: 21s
Fat: 1s; hi 1s; 23s; 25s; hi 19s
Flatulence: 11 and S-25
Flu/Fever: 3 and S-15; 4 and O-21; 15 and S-3
Gout: 16 and S-8
Groin: 2 and S-1; 3 and S-15
Headache: 8s; 11s; 16s; 24s; hold big toes or thumbs
     Migraine: 20s; 21s; 4s; 7s; 16s; 10s; 9s; 4s
Heart, attack: 3s; 9s; 14s
Hemorrhoids: O-8 and O-1
Hip: S-11 and S-15
Hormone, imbalance: 2s; ring fingers; on self, hold 12s
Hyperactivity: 13s
Hypertension: 19s; 16s; 15s and 3s together
Hypoglycemia: 12s; 19s; 13s and 9s
Insomnia: 18s and thumbs, 16s; l7s; l8s; 19s
Jet lag: 25s; lock fingers or hold each finger
Joint pain: 19 and 3
Kidney: 23s; 5s; 6s
     Stones: 3s; 23s; 2s; 25 and hi 11s same side
Knees: 24s
Labor: 2s; hi 1s
Legs: 25 and center back of leg; 25s
     Charley horse: 25 and 12; then S-15 and S-7
     cramps: S-15 and toes; S-25 and11
     fall asleep: 25s same side and O-1s
Leukemia 9s; 26s
Lungs: 9s; l0s; 22s
Mastectomy: 5s; 6s; 7s; 8s; 16s; 17s; 18s; 19s
Menopause: 22s
Menstruation: 2 with O-8 and 1o 8 to 16; lo 8s and 15s
     ovulation distress: 1 and O-8
Motion sickness: 14s; 25s
Muscles, tension: 8s; 16s; 25s
Nausea: 14s; 18s
Nervous system: 17s
     nervousness:11s
Newborn: 2 and O-9
Nightmares: 10 and S-hi 19
Nose: 3s; 4s; 11s

Overeating: Hold hi 1s (fingers pointing down)
Overweight: 21s; 23s; 25s
Pain: S-20s; right hand over left and cover pain area, 9 and 15 and hold 10 on opposite side
        of pain with same side 9, then 15
Paralysis: for left side, hand on right 8; for right side, hand on left 8
Parkinson's: 3 and S-15;10 and S-hi 19; 15 and S-3; 23 and S-1; 25 and S-11
PMS: 1 and O-26; 2 and O-9; 13 and O-11; 11 and S-19; 15 and S-3
Prostate: 23s
Sciatica: Hold left 11 as anchor, and L hand on L23, then L2 (for left pain use R pulse points)
Shingles: 9s
Shock: Thumbs on R temple, fingers on R 4; then Thumbs on L temple, fingers on L4
Shoulders: 3s; 19s (opposite side)
        To release: 8s; 1s; 16s
Sinuses: 4s and O-21
Snoring: 14 and S-19
Throat: 4s; 10s; 11s; 12s; 13s;
TMJ: 21s
Tonsils: 4 and O-16; then opposite lo 8
Varicose veins: 15 and S-13; 23 and S-1; 25 and S-11
Viruses: hold 3s and 11s together; then 9s; and 10s
Whiplash: 2s; 8s; 9s; 10s; 23s; 25s;
Yeast infection: 13s; 23s

Source: Extracted from *High Touch, Hands on Energy Workbook II,* Betsy Dayton, Edgewater, Colorado: Betsy Dayton, 1984.

Reflexology Interventions

Prior to attempting reflexology, sensitivity of the fingers must be developed. Placing a thread under the page of a book is a good exercise. When that can be sensed, try two pages, three, and so on. Using different materials, dental floss, rubber bands, and seeds of different sizes also works. As with other body therapies, it is not wise to practice them when feeling depleted or ill oneself since it is possible to drain energy from the client. Protecting oneself, using energizing affirmations, and attending to other dimensions of wellness (nutrition, stress management, relationships, environment) will tend to make depletion an uncommon happening.

Pressure in reflexology should evoke a "good hurt" or pressure that is comfortably tolerated. To estimate the pressure needed, practice pressing a bathroom scale to 20–25 lb. of pressure. Very sore spots may require a buildup to this amount of pressure. Once the appropriate amount of pressure is found, hold it until a rhythmic pulsation is felt or until the client experiences a release (observe for change to a deeper breathing pattern, change to a better skin tone, relaxation in facial expression, and/or the client's words). For very painful spots, return to them again and again rather than trying to relieve the pain all at once; too much work all at once may bruise the capillaries.

Practice strengthening and using the *thumb,* for it is the most sensitive of the fingers. Continued experimentation with reflexology will strengthen them. As with other body work, working with the fingertips in reflexology promotes the practitioner's physiological balance; every time the foot is pressed, spinal and brain energy are activated in both practitioner and client (Berkson, 1977, p.33).

Preparation for reflexology with a client:

1. Remove nail polish from fingernails and cut nails so nailpads are exposed. Shake, stretch, squeeze, and wash hands so they are relaxed and warm.

2. Find a quiet spot and ask the client to assume a comfortable sitting or lying position. Avoid music, disruptions, and any conversation except that related to the effects of the strokes.

3. Assume a relaxed position; a relaxation exercise can assist both practitioner and client to prepare for a reflexology session. Visualizing a protective covering of light and affirming that no negative energy will be transferred from client to practitioner is a safety measure.

4. Ask the client to relax and let go and avoid trying to assist.

5. Hold the client's feet in the hands for a few minutes while centering to orient both to the physical contact. Remember to breathe throughout the session.

6. Begin with the right foot. Avoid removing the hands from the foot until all steps have been completed. Each petrissage stroke (releases toxins) should be followed by an effleurage stroke (encourages removal of toxins to the bloodstream).

    A. Take the foot in both hands and stretch the sole gently, toes toward ankle and toes toward sole several times; note callouses, bunions, degree of flexibility, etc.

    B. Hold the front of the foot in the left hand (reverse if left-handed) and the heel in the right hand; rotate the heel slowly and gently clockwise and then counterclockwise; note reistances and range of motion.

    C. Grab hold of the foot and wring it like a sponge, one hand above the other, twisting in opposite directions; continue up and down the foot from ankle to toes, using steady, firm pressure. In this movement as in many others, the tendency for novices is to be too gentle; a firm pressure is needed to counteract tickling and to obtain results.

    D. Stimulate the lymphatic drainage by pressing the lymphatic drainage point between the big and second toe (Figure 7.1). Use the thumb to stretch the skin from the heel along the outside of the foot to the toes using 20–25 lb. of pressure. Remember to breathe.

    E. Sandwich the foot in between the two hands; use the knuckles to rub over all points on the foot. Breathe.

    F. Start at the end of the big toe and use the thumbs to stretch the tendons toward the ankle up into the lymphatic area. Do all toes and the spaces in between. Breathe.

G. Anchor the heel with one hand and push on the ball of the foot with the other palm to the client's limit; hold for 15–30 seconds, then release. Breathe.

H. Anchor the heel with one hand and press the toes and foot toward the floor with the other to the client's limit and hold for 15–30 seconds, then release.

I. Rotate the foot laterally and hold and then medially and hold. Rotate the whole foot clockwise and counterclockwise.

J. Hold heel firmly in left hand and firmly press all inside and outside ankle reflexes for 3–5 seconds on each spot (see Figure 7.1). Rub ankle in an upward movement (effleurage).

K. Stabilize the foot with one hand, using the other to grasp the big toe firmly with thumb on top and forefinger on the back; make stretching movements from the base to the top of the toe; repeat on each toe. Work each toe medially, laterally, forward, and back. Breathe.

L. Hold the big toe close to its base, thumb on top where it meets the foot and forefinger beneath the joint connecting the toe to the foot. Support the foot well with the other hand and pull the toe straight out to the toe's maximum stretch for 10 seconds, then use a firm jerk straight back, listening for a cracking sound; some toes will "crack," while others will not; avoid forcing it. Jerk once or twice on each toe and then move on to the next one; return later to release tension; this movement stimulates tendons and clears the head and neck of congestion since all meridians and nerve endings for the brain and neck are stimulated (Berkson, 1977, p. 47).

M. Begin with the big toe; hold each toe in succession firmly and work down its corresponding tendon toward the ankle.

N   Begin with the big toe and rotate each toe three times in a full circle clockwise and then counterclockwise; observe for resistance and gritty sounds (indicating crystal formation).

O. With the fingers on one hand on the top of the toes and the other hand anchoring the heel, push forward firmly, hold a stretch, go a bit further, then release (toe extension release).

P. Grasp the toes firmly with hand, thumb on top of toes downward while pushing up from underneath at the lung reflex; this movement will release tension in the shoulder girdle. Optional: flex and extend each toe individually.

Q. Hold the big toe firmly and pull it toward the other foot; smack the side of the thoracic reflex (bony ridge beneath the toes) with the top of the palm as if clapping the hands; repeat 8–10 times. Releases tight shoulder blades, clears the neck, throat, eye, and ear, and reduces bunions (Berkson, 1977, p. 49).

R. Press firmly on all points of the big toe, front, back, side, and top. Repeat with each toe using very firm thumb pressure. Stimulate the web of each toe with the thumb and forefinger, top and bottom; use a pinching movement. Effective for eyes, ears, and sinuses.

S. Inch along the top of all toes with fingernail and flick each toenail up and away from the toe. Nails store electromagnetic current; flicking and stimulating the periphery stimulates meridians and releases energy (Berkson, 1977, p. 52).

T. Stimulate the eye and ear points at the base of the toes and stretch the skin from the small toe to the inside of the big toe; this will drain the sinuses and soothe the eyes and ears (Berkson, 1977, p. 52).

U. Stimulate venous drainage by rubbing each toe from its tip to its base.

V. Start with the spinal points on the sole of the foot (Figure 7.1), working the sacral and lumbar area by the heel up to the cervical area by the big toe, then work down the other side to the heel; follow with friction and effleurage.

W. Press all points on the lateral, medial, and top of the foot and ankle using knuckles; follow with effleurage.

X. Use a wringing motion up the leg; push the middle three fingers under the tibia from the ankle to the knee. Observe for swelling, granular tissue, and deposits; work them out with rubbing and pressure.

Y. Support the leg and use the middle finger or knuckle to press up the center of the calf from the Achilles tendon to the knee, stimulating the endocrine glands; highly stressed clients are tender there (Berkson, 1977, p. 56).

Z. Push firmly all the way up the leg from the ankle to the thigh, increasing the lymphatic and blood flow. Close by clapping the foot from heel to toe, and then brushing the hands down the legs several times from the knee off the end of the toes and then several inches away from the body. Repeat A–Z with left foot.

Figure 7.1, p. 210, can be used to treat specific conditions, e.g., pancreas for diabetes; small intestines area for digestive or assimilation difficulties; stomach for heartburn, nausea, bad breath, vomiting, or tightness under breastbone. Working on the toes will assist with headache, tension, congestion, sinus trouble, weak eye muscles, fatigue, etc. Although reflexology can be used this way, it is recommended the steps from A–Z be completed daily as a preventive measure. For further information, see: Berkson, D., *The Foot Book: Healing through Reflexology,* New York: Harper & Row, 1977, Ingham, E., *Stories the Feet Tell through Reflexology*, St. Petersburg: Ingham Publishing, Inc., 1984.

OTHER SELF-CARE MEASURES

Herbal Remedies

Long before modern medical practices, wise women, medicine men and other healers used herbs to heal. Many have not had a rigorous history of scientific testing, but they have stood the test of time, some having been used safely for thousands of years.

Herbs can be steeped for a cup of tea (1 teaspoon, steep for 3-5 minutes). They can also be used in salves. Combine 3 ounces powdered herb with 7 ounces cocoa butter or any pure vegetable shortening, and 1 ounce of beeswax. Blend the ingredients and let heat over low heat in a covered pot for one to two hours. When cool, it firms up and is ready for use. Poultices are used to reduce swelling and encourage healing. They are applied directly to the skin. Add enough hot water to the herb to make a thick paste, then cover with a hot moist towel. Plaintain leaves will draw out toxins. To relieve pain and muscle spasms, Lobelia, Kava Kava, Catnip or Valerian can be used. Extracts are used by those who cannot swallow capsules; 12–15 drops of an extract are placed into a glass of water. Exact dosages are recommended on individual bottles. Capsules, plasters, and fomentations are methods of preparing and using herbs. Consult a herbalist for exact directions/uses. As with any new food, piece of clothing or household furniture, or essential oil, use a muscle test (see p. 207) to determine if the substance is right for you or a client at that moment in time.

Herbs are potent substances. Some have their main ingredients duplicated in the laboratory (e.g., aspirin from white willow) and are used as medical prescriptions or over-the-counter drugs. Herbs, however, have not had the therapeutic portion extracted and so are considered safer. Still, safe use of herbs is important.

After muscle testing, start with 1 capsule with an 8 ounce glass of water, or a teaspoon of herb steeped into 1 cup of tea twice a day. In a wellness approach, like foods, supplements, or exercise, herbs should be used in moderation. During times of acute illness, more may be needed. However, some herbs should not be taken for maintenance. For example, golden seal can depress the immune system if taken regularly; it is to be used during an acute phase of an illness. As with any new procedure, when using herbs, read extensively, talk to experts, keep careful records and be conservative in approach. Some herbs, such as peppermint and raspberry leaf are extremely safe and can be used daily and have no known side effects. When using drugs or medications, seek the counsel of a physician or wellness practitioner who is an expert in both modalities to insure the appropriate combinations are used. Table 7.10 presents some common herbal remedies.

Table 7.10 Herbal Remedies

Symptom/Function	Herbs
acne	aloe vera, bee pollen, echinacea, ginseng root, kelp, or basil oil
age spots	dandelion, gotu kola, licorice
AIDS	garlic, St. John's wort
allergy	chickweed, eyebright, fenugreek***, or parsley
anemia	dandelion (builds blood), yellow dock (high in iron)
appetite	camomile, dandelion, fennel***, horseradish, or peppermint
arteriosclerosis	cayenne, garlic, rose hips
arthritis pain	aloe vera, or capsicum (cayenne pepper ointment, taken externally) licorice root, parsley, yucca, or oat straw
asthma	cayenne, marshmallow, mullein, parsley or saw palmetto
bad breath	parsley, myrrh, cloves (+ eat lots of greens to clear up congestion in the colon)
bedwetting	oat straw, parsley, uva ursi, St. Johns' wort, cornsilk
bites/stings	blue cohosh, cinnamon, witch hazel (externally), clay (as a poultice)
blood pressure	high: cayenne pepper, garlic, hawthorne, or valerian
	low: dandelion, parsley, rosemary
bone loss	horsetail, yellow dock
burns	aloe vera, cayenne, chickweed, plantain, apply vitamin E
cholesterol	garlic, lecithin, fenugreek***, cayenne
poor circulation	cayenne, ginkgo leaf, licorice root, ginger, kelp, or witch hazel leaf
colds/flu	peppermint, ginger, echinacea root, golden seal root, or raspberry
colic	catnip, fennel***, or peppermint
colitis	fenugreek***, kelp, peppermint, or slippery elm
colon irritation	aloe vera, camomile, fenugreek***, peppermint, or slippery elm bark
constipation	slippery elm bark, psyllium seed, or aloe vera (internally)
coughs	licorice root, horehound, fenugreek*** seed, or golden seal root
cramps	peppermint, cayenne, kelp, or ginger
diabetes	parsley, raspberry leaves, buchu leaves, saw palmetto berries, dandelion root or bladderwrack
diarrhea	slippery elm bark, raspberry, peppermint or nutmeg
poor digestion	aloe vera, papaya leaf, fenugreek*** or peppermint leaf
diverticulitis	camomille, papaya, peppermint, psyllium seed, or slippery elm
dizziness	peppermint, camomile
ear infection	mullein drops in ear, tincture of Lobellia, ice bags, or an onion poultice
energy (lack of)	garlic, ginkgo leaf, ginseng root, licorice root or green barley
eyes	eyebright, bilberry, fennel seed***, or ginkgo leaf, cayenne, hyssop packs for black eyes
fatigue	gota kola, cayenne, ginseng, kelp, peppermint, or ginger root
fever	echinacea root, myrrh gum, goldenseal root, licorice root garlic or kelp

Table 7.10 (*continued*)

Symptom/Function	Herbs
gas	fennel seed ***, spearmint leaf, dill, or star anise
gout (pain)	fennel seed***, nettle, cherries, or safflower
gum disease	myrrh
hay fever	wild cherry bark, mullein leaves, horehound
headache	peppermint leaf, fenugreek seed***, or ladies slipper root
hearing	ginkgo
heart	peppermint leaf, gota kola, licorice root, rosemary, gingko, kelp, cayenne, or garlic
hemorrhoids	witch hazel (externally), slippery elm bark or aloe vera (internally), mullein, goldenseal root
herpes	comfrey, licorice, mint oils, uva ursi (externally), echinacea and ginseng (internally),
immune system	garlic, echinacea root, astragalus, or Pau d'Arco
infection	echinacea, garlic, peppermint, rosemary, or myrrh
infertility	damiana leaves, ginseng, sarsaparilla root, kelp, licorice
inflammation	camomile, marigold, white willow, witch hazel, or St. John's wort
kidneys/bladder	uva ursi, marshmallow, parsley, cinnamon, garlic, or buchu leaf
lead poisoning	apple, garlic
leg pain	ginkgo
liver	dandelion root, licorice root*, milk thistle, cayenne, wild yam root, or yellow dock root
lungs	red raspberry leaf or mullein
menopause	black cohosh**,***(digestion, hot flashes, pain) damiana leaf, kelp, red raspberry leaf, oatstraw (depression, sleep), nettle (sleep, hot flashes), grape juice (palpitations) fennel***, fenugreek***, red clover***, or yarrow flower, dong quai (hot flashes, dry vagina, palpitations, insomnia), licorice (calms heart), ginseng (alternate every two weeks with dong quai for hotflashes and anxiety, but not at bedtime), motherwort (anxiety, sleep, palpitations, vaginal wall), fenugreek (libido, nourish glands, restore blood sugar balance, improve digestion), red clover*** (sore joints, anxiety and energy loss), raspberry (strengthen bones, moderate mood swings)
menstrual discomtfort	camomile flower, papaya leaves, dong quai, fennel***, anise, red clover***, or red raspberry leaf
morning sickness	ginger, mints, raspberry (consult with health care provider)
motion sickness	ginger
mouth sores	blackberry
nausea	ginger root, licorice root, or cayenne
nervousness	wild yam root, spearmint leaf, skullcap, passion flower, ginger root, black cohosh root***, or dong quai
overweight	fennel seed***, kelp, plantain, or nettle leaf
pain	raspberry leaves, rosemary, kelp, marjoram, white willow, red pepper, witch hazel, or valerian
parasites	garlic, black walnut, or butternut bark
PMS	buchu, celery, dandelion, horsetail, nettle, parsley, uva ursi
poison ivy	aloe vera
postpartum hemorrhage	goldenseal, shepherd's purse
prostate	saw palmetto berry, echinacea root, parsley, cayenne, pumpkin seeds, anise, fennel***, or buchu leaves
senility	peppermint, gotu kola, kelp

Table 7.10 (*continued*)

Symptom/Function	Herbs
sexual passion	damiana leaf, ginseng root, dong quai root
sinus	blue violet flower, echinacea, golden seal root, mullein leaf, or myrrh gum
skin	aloe vera (internally and externally), kelp, comfrey poultice, red clover*** tea, echinacea, cayenne, licorice root, or yellow dock root
sore throat	fenugreek***, licorice, marshmallow, mullein, sage, or slippery elm teas
stroke prevention	ginkgo
thyroid	kelp, saw palmetto berries, cayenne
tinnitus (ringing in the ears)	ginko
toothache	allspice oil or clove oil (externally)
tooth-decay	mints, tea
toxicity (after exposure to x-rays, surgery etc.)	camomile, dandelion, echinacea, licorice, red clover***, kelp, apple pectin or algin
ulcer	peppermint leaf, slippery elm bark, or ginseng root
ulcer prevention	camomile, licorice
urethritis	uva ursi
urinary incontinence	cranberry
varicose veins	bayberry bark, golden seal root, gota kola or white oak bark
water retention	buchu leaf or uva ursi leaf, cornsilk, kelp, parsley or cayenne
wound healing	aloe, comfrey, garlic, marshmallow, mints, turmeric, witch hazel (externally)
yeast infections	goldenseal root, buchu leaves, witch hazel leaves, myrrh, camomile, cinnamon, dandelion, garlic, echinacea gum, juniper berries, or squaw vine

*Long-term use may lead to water retention, elevated blood pressure, headache. Avoid if taking digoxin-based drugs.

**Can depress heart rate.

***Has estrogenic action.

Sources: Extracted from *The Scientific Validation of Herbal Medicine* by Daniel B. Mowrey, New Canaan, CT: Keats Publishing, 1986; *The Complete Medicinal Herbal*, by Penelope Ody, New York: Dorling Kindersley, 1993; *The Healing Herbs*, by Michael Castlemen, Emmaus, Pennsylvania: Rodale Press, 1991; *Menopausal Years, the Wise Woman Way*, by Susan S. Weed, Woodstock, New York: Ash Tree Publishing, 1992.

Aromatherapy

Aromatherapy is not new. *Aromatherapy* is the practice of using naturally distilled essences of plants to promote well-being. Essential oils, or essences, promote balance and harmony. Nearly all ancient cultures recognized the value of botanicals and aromatic plants and used them to maintain health. Essential oils are essences that are extracted from the bark, leaves, petals, resins, rinds, roots, seeds, stalks and stems of certain aromatic plants. They are extremely concentrated. Essential oils circulate in plants and send messages that help them function efficiently, much as hormones do in humans.

Essential oils work on several levels. The first is through the sense of smell. Receptors in the nose identify an odor and nerve cells relay this information directly to the limbic system of the brain. Here, odors trigger memories and influence emotions and behavior. The limbic system works in coordination with the pituitary gland and the hypothalamus to regulate the hormonal activities of the endocrine system. Odors can trigger the production of hormones that govern appetite, insulin production, body temperature, metabolism, stress levels, sex drive and thoughts. Through their action on the limbic system, essential oils can impact all these functions,

The limbic system also affects the nervous system. Because smells act on this system, they have the potential for affecting desires, motivation, intuition, moods, and creativity. Odors affect psychological well-being by stimulating the release of neurotransmitters and endorphins in the brain. Odors can also trigger long-forgotten memories and alter attitude. Inhaling essential oils can calm and relax or stimulate and energize. When essential oils are inhaled, their minute molecules attach to oxygen molecules in the lungs. They are then circulated throughout the body, having the potential to activate the body's ability to heal itself. Essential oils work through the skin to stimulate circulation and encourage the formation of new skin cells. They can calm inflamed or irritated skin, release muscle spasms, soothe sore muscles, and relieve muscular tension. European physicians use essential oils as part of their treatment program (Wilson, 1995).

Essential oils are very strong and should never be used near the eyes or taken internally. Do not buy or use essential oils that you don't like the smell of. They are just not for you and caution clients to follow the same advice.

A few drops of essential oil can be placed in a carrier oil and massaged into the skin. Some possible carrier oils are apricot, canola, olive and peanut. Apricot kernel oil soothes and smooths dry or inflamed skin and is high in vitamin A. Canola oil promotes skin health and resists rancidity. Olive oil is beneficial to skin and hair but because of its strong odor, works better with stronger smelling oils such as basil, rosemary, and tea tree. Peanut oil can be used on any skin type and is absorbed readily. Wheat germ oil nourishes dry or cracked skin and soothes eczema and psoriasis, may prevent stretch marks, and helps reduce scarring (Wilson, 1995).

Essential oils can be inhaled directly to achieve the desired result, or a few drops can also be dropped into a warm bath. Table 7.11 gives some essential oils and their uses.

Table 7.11 Some Essential Oils and Their Uses in Aromatherapy

Essential Oil	Uses
Basil	relieves sinus congestion, averts asthma attack, soothes stomach, clears head, soothes mouth ulcers, fights gum infection, reduces pain of menstrual cramps, relieves pain of arthritis/muscular aches/pains, insect repellent, soothes mosquito bites and wasp stings, relieves some symptoms of chronic fatigue syndrome
Camomile	eases symptoms of PMS, menopausal symptoms, vaginitis, scanty/irregular periods, reduces inflammation, calms irritated skin, fights infection, relieves sprains/swollen muscles, soothes inflamed joints, reduces fluid retention, antidepressant action, minimizes pain of headaches and migraine, treats fatigue symptoms, calms crying and hyperactive children, eases earaches, soothes stomach aches and colic, relieves toothache and teething pain
Cedarwood	eases coughs and decreases cold discomfort, expectorant, promotes urination and is useful against urinary tract infections and prostate problems, combats infection, controls the pain and swelling of arthritis, heals skin rashes, fights fungal infection
Coriander	relieves pain and muscle spasms, stimulates the appetite and digestion, fights bacteria and fungi, boosts circulation and stimulates the heart and nervous system, encourages menstrual flow, arouses sexual desire
Cypress	detoxifying effect, relieves congestion and eases coughing, stops cuts and wounds from bleeding, soothes bleeding gums and periodontal disease, relief from hemorrhoids, eases foot odor/swelling, relieves sore muscles, can avert an attack of asthma when used in an inhaler, decreases excess flow of fluids (runny nose, diarrhea, excessive menstrual flow, perspiration), balances female hormones, reduces hot flashes, speeds recovery from cystitis when used in a sitz bath, may inhibit the growth of ovarian cysts when massaged over the area
Rosemary	tightens and tones tissues, promotes new cell growth, regulates oil secretion, fights infection, relieves joint pain, eases muscles spasms and digestive disorders, improves functioning of many internal organs and systems (heart, nervous system, adrenal glands, liver, gall bladder). CAUTION: elevates blood pressure, may irritate sensitive skin, can trigger epileptic seizures in susceptible individuals.
Rosewood	diminishes depression, stimulates sexual feelings, relieves pain, fights infection, stimulates the brain and clears thinking, improves immunity, soothes skin disorders, maintains healthy skin
Sandalwood	releases negative emotions, promotes understanding, increases sociability, clears thought processes, strengthens resolve, stabilizes, helps fight infection (especially of the urinary tract), relieves muscle spasms, releases mucus and clears congestion

Table 7.11 (*continued*)

Essential Oil	Uses
Tea Tree	restores energy, calms during times of emotional stress, kills insects, fights infections and fungi, heals wounds, relieves respiratory congestion, increases immunity. CAUTION: may be irritating to sensitive skin
Vetiver	stimulates the production of red blood cells, improves circulation and immunity, relieves muscular aches, stiff joints, sprains, strains, calms nervousness, may help with anorexia nervosa, helps induce restful sleep, balances female hormones, tones the reproductive organs, may help overcome sexual dysfunction caused by nerves or stress
Ylang Ylang	lowers blood pressure, regulates respiration, calms heart palpitations, relaxes tense muscles, PMS and menstrual disorders, calms menopausal women, soothes dermatitis, fights bacterial infection, controls acne and blemishes, relaxes facial muscles to ward off wrinkles, lifts depression, arouses sensuality.

Source: Extracted from *Aromatherapy for Vibrant Health and Beauty* by Roberta Wilson, Garden City Park, New York, 1995.

NOTE: Prior to using essential oils with clients, consult an aromatherapy text for further instructions.

Natural Treatments for Common Ailments

In addition to the treatments already discussed, there are other self-care measures to use. Table 7.12 presents self-care suggestions for various conditions, but there are also suggestions and ideas in the Stress Management, Nutritional Wellness, and Fitness Chapters, as well as this chapter.

Giller (1994, p. xxiv), a physician, strongly recommends that everyone take a basic vitamin/mineral antioxidant supplement daily that includes at least the following (in addition to amounts suggested below): 50 mg of B_1, B_6, and B_{12}, 1,000 mg vitamin C; 400 to 600 IU vitamin E; 10,000 to 25,000 IU beta-carotene, and 100 to 200 mcg of selenium.

Additionally, fresh vegetable juices are an especially useful way of getting nutrients (especially enzymes) into the bloodstream quickly without stressing the digestive system. Buy a juicer from a health food store or buy juices at their juice bar. When making your own, use organically grown produce or soak them in a sink filled with water, four tablespoons of salt and the juice of one fresh lemon or use a soap specifically for washing vegetables (to remove pesticide sprays). Use the tops and roots of beets, dandelion, radish and turnips. Cut the tops one-half inch below the ring where green stems start on carrots as well as snipping the tail.

When using self-care measures it is wise to use common sense: (1) start with a small dose of the substance or procedure, then assess results before building to a higher dose or continuing on; (2) rashes, stomach upsets, reactions the opposite of those intended, are examples of reasons to at least consult with a(nother) health care practitioner; (3) use muscle testing to determine if a substance is positive for the body at the moment or not.

It may take three months for a supplement, herb or practice to show results, so don't give up too quickly. On the other hand, as with any new behavior, go easy. Consult more detailed references and health care practitioners, and evaluate the results. NOTE: (Do not double supplement amounts if bothered by two conditions.)

Additionally, herbs and oils may or may not combine well with traditional medicines. Be aware there are few, if any, studies of the interactions of medications, let alone herbs, oils and medications. Since each person is unique each client is a one-person case study in areas where research has not yet provided the answers. Although many herbs and oils have few unwanted effects, read the cautions for each one and abide by them. Also, do additional study if you are unfamiliar with the procedure. Above all, pay attention to client reactions and adjust doses or discontinue the approach when deleterious signs appear.

Table 7.12 Self-Care Measures for Various Conditions

Condition	Measures
AIDS	• Take additional selenium, chromium, coenzyme Q_{10} combined with vitamin B_6, vitamin C (700 mg up to 200 grams), copper, vitamins B_6, B_{12}, and A (9,000–20,000 IU), and licorice extract according to directions on label. Also follow directions under "Cancer"
Alzheimer's	• Avoid all potential sources of aluminum, including cookware, antacids, buffered aspirin, douches, or diarrhea medicines • Investigate the following as a possible source of memory loss: interactions of drugs/medicines taken, high blood pressure, depression, infection, poor thyroid function, food allergies (use muscle testing to determine this) • In addition to daily supplements take the following daily to improve memory: 1,000 mg Vitamin D; 44 IU vitamin E; 10,000 IU beta-carotene; 50 mcg selenium; 1,000 mcg vitamin B_{12}, 50 mg zinc; 6 grams evening primrose oil; 2.5 g L-carnitine and 1,000 mcg vitamin B_{12} dissolved under the tongue; 40 mg ginkgo 3–4 times a day; and 650 mg choline three times a day
Arthritis	• Maintain optimum body weight and focus meals around whole grains, fresh vegetables and fresh fruits, reducing sugar, refined carbohydrates (doughnuts, cakes, pies, candy, etc.

Table 7.12 (*continued*)

Condition	Measures
Arthritis (cont'd)	and saturated fats (meat,hard cheeses, and other dairy products unless nonfat) • Eat more fish, especially herring, salmon, and tuna to add fish oils to your diet • Avoid foods from the nightshade family: tomatoes, potatoes, eggplant, peppers, paprika, cayenne, and tobacco for one month. If no relief, reintroduce slowly to see if they affect your symptoms • Test for other food allergies (see p.207) (people with rheumatoid arthritis are often sensitive to wheat, corn, milk/dairy products and beef) • For very bad symptoms, try a vegetable juice fast for three or four days, using no nightshades and checking with your health care practitioner first • Drink two cups fresh grapefruit juice daily in the morning • Drink 10 ounces fresh carrot juice mixed with 6 ounces fresh spinach juice and 10 ounces of carrot juice mixed with 6 ounces of celery juice, after noon, spaced at least two hours apart • Avoid Aspartame (artificial sweetener) • Exercise 20 minutes daily: yoga and/or swimming, walking • Do daily exercises to rotate joints • Castor oil packs on noninflamed joints • Rub grated onion, garlic and potato into inflamed joints • Massage body daily with castor or olive oil • Soak in a warm tub or use moist heat for relief • Brush skin all over with body brush before taking alternate cold and hot showers • Take an afternoon nap to relax the body • Take the following daily in addition to your regular supplements: 3 g pantothenic acid, 2 mg Boron, and 400 IU vitamin E • For rheumatoid arthritis, in addition to the above and daily supplements, take: 100 mcg selenium, 2,000 mg vitamin C, and 22.5 mg zinc daily; 2 mg copper salicylate once a day with a meal (try for 6 weeks, then discontinue if no improvement), 500 mg ginger powder three times daily, 500 mg sea cucumber capsule twice a day • Try acupuncture, acupressure, therapeutic touch or massage • Learn stress reduction measures and practice them, see Stress Management Chapter • Picture your joints being soothed by a cool, healing salve or liquid • Say affirmations aloud, for example, "My joints are healing, my body is well." "I release all negative thoughts and feelings." • Use therapeutic touch, yoga and reflexology, see pp. 215

Table 7.12 (*continued*)

Condition	Measures
Asthma	• Learn your triggers for attacks and avoid them • Drink at least one-half cup of warm fluid every hour • Deep breathe for five minutes at least twice a day • Morning and night complete the following: Sit on your heels and clasp hands behind you; pull shoulders back to open chest; and take a deep breath; exhale as you lean forward, stretching straight arms above head and in front of body (forehead resting on floor) • Avoid pollen, and pets with fur or feathers • Buy a HEPA-type air cleaner • Check food labels and avoid all food additives (especially MSG, sulfites, tartrazine yellow food dye, and foods with salicylate in them (almonds, apples, apricots, blackberries, boysenberries, cherries, cucumbers, currants, gooseberries, grapes, nectarines, oranges, peaches, plums, prunes, pickles, raisins, strawberries, tomatoes, beer, birch beer, cider, cider vinegars, diet drinks, distilled liquors, Kool-Aid and artifically flavored beverages, tea, wine, wine vinegars) • Drink 10 ounces fresh carrot juice mixed with 6 ounces of fresh spinach juice and/or 13 ounces of fresh carrot juice mixed with 3 ounces of radish juice daily after noon • Mix the juice of one fresh lemon with 4 ounces ground horseradish and take once a day • Use muscle testing to identify food allergies/sensitivities) Milk and cheese are common ones • Avoid aspirin and nonsteroidal anti-inflammatory drugs: ibuprofen, indomethacin, fenoprofen, mefenamic acid, naproxen, phenyl- butazone • Avoid eating after 6 p.m. and raise the head of your bed or elevate your head with pillows to prevent nighttime attacks • In collaboration with your health care practitioner, exercise daily. Take 1,000 mg of vitamin C before each session • Learn relaxation and imagery techniques to avoid attacks, see pp. 35–38 • Say affirmations, for example, "My breath is easy, my body is well" • Supplements: In addition to usual supplements, take additional B-complex, 1,000 mg vitamin C and 1,000 mg before exercise; 400 mg magnesium daily; 50 mg zinc daily; 100 mcg selenium daily • Eat at least one onion every day. They have anti-asthmatic and anti-inflammatory effects. • Use therapeutic touch, reflexology and yoga, see pp. 215
Athlete's Foot	• Take one teaspoon of acidophilus mixed in water on an empty stomach every morning and evening to restore healthy bacterial balance • Drink 10 ounces fresh carrot juice with 6 ounces fresh spinach juice after noon daily; at least two hours later, take 10

Table 7.12 (*continued*)

Condition	Measures
Athlete's Foot (*cont'd*)	ounces fresh carrot juice with 3 ounces each fresh beet and cucumber juice • Puncture a capsule of vitamin E and squeeze it directly on any irritated skin • Use a brush to remove dead skin from your feet (only after irritation clears) and shower daily • Put on clean socks (washed in hot water) at least once a day and use a hair dryer to dry feet before putting on socks • Avoid wearing the same pair of shoes two days in a row • Wear shower shoes or sandals at the beach, pool or gym • Use imagery to picture your body attaining a bacterial balance
Back Problems	• Follow directions on p.218 • Complete Feldenkrais movement, p.170 • Lie on back, knees to chest and gently rock back and forth • Drink 10 ounces fresh carrot juice mixed with 6 ounces fresh spinach juice daily after noon or carrot with a little fresh beet and apple juice • Eat at least 1 large green salad every day • Practice stress reduction measures, p. 70 • Do reflexology to back points, therapeutic touch and gentle yoga • Use imagery to picture your back relaxed and healthy • Affirm many times daily: "My back is strong and flexible. I am healthy and well."
Burns	• Splash apple cider vinegar on sunburn or other burn every few hours • Topically apply tea-tree oil, aloe vera, or vitamin E • In addition to usual supplements, take: 1,000 mg vitamin C 400 IU vitamin E, 50 mg zinc, and 10,000 IU beta-carotene daily • Use imagery to picture your burns healing and scars melting away
Cancer	• See *Nutritional Wellness*, (Chapter 5) • Avoid taking extra iron • Drink 1 pint of fresh juice combining 3 ounces fresh beet, 10 ounces of fresh carrot juice, asparagus, or cabbage juice daily after noon • Drink 1–2 cups of fresh grape, black cherry, or apple juice in the morning every day • Eat onions and garlic (Kyolic is an odorless form) • Include whole grains, nuts (especially almonds), seeds, brown rice, millet cereal, oatmeal, broccoli, brussel sprouts, cabbage, cauliflower, cantaloupe, carrots, pumpkin, squash, yams, apples, berries, chickpeas, lentils, red beans and plums • Avoid processed foods (white bread, pies, cakes, candy,

Table 7.12 (*continued*)

Condition	Measures
Cancer (*cont'd*)	canned foods), luncheon meat, hot dogs, smoked or cured meats, meats, salt, sugar, alcohol, coffee, tea (except herbal) • Avoid oral contraceptives and menopausal estrogens: both are associated with increased risk of breast cancer • Look into a macrobiotic diet • Start an exercise program (see p.170) • Avoid chemicals, see pp. 275 plus (they weaken the immune system) • Practice stress management procedures, p.70. (Severe stress has harmful effects on the body's defense system and disease progression.) • Use imagery (and imagery tapes) to picture the body healthy releasing resentments • Say affirmations many times daily, for example, "My immune system is getting stronger and I am getting well." "I forgive all the people in my life, including myself." • Use herbs, including: dandelion, echinacea, pau d'arco, and red clover • In addition to daily supplements take: 10,000 IU beta-carotene, 100 mg coenzyme Q_{10}, 200 mcg selenium, 5,00–10,000 mg vitamin C with bioflavonoids
Cold Sores	• Apply topical Lysine cream and take 3,000 mg L-lysine daily, 1,000 mg with each meal until symptoms subside, then take 500–1,000 mg a day depending on what works; 50 mg zinc daily; 500 mg vitamin C with bioflavonoids; zinc lozenges— let them dissolve on the lesion • Avoid arginine-rich foods, including chocolate, peanuts and other nuts, seeds and cereal grains during outbreak and as a preventive • Use imagery to picture sores leaving
Cystitis (bladder infection)	For Prevention: • Wipe from front to back after having a bowel movement • Avoid feminine hygiene sprays, douches, and bubble bath • Avoid tight clothing and wear cotton underpants • Urinate as soon as you feel the urge and stop and start the stream as often as you can; these Kegel exercises strengthen the urinary muscles and keep bacteria out of the bladder • Drink lots of fluids, including at least six eight-ounce glasses of water each day • Drink 10 ounces fresh carrot juice combined with 3 ounces each beet and cucumber juice after noon and then 10 ounces carrot juice combined with 6 ounces fresh spinach juice at least two hours later • Drink fluids and void before and after intercourse For Treatment during an infection: • Take one capsule of cranberry concentrate three times a day with an eight-ounce glass of water • Include the natural diuretics, celery, parsley and watermelon in your diet

Table 7.12 (*continued*)

Condition	Measures
	• Avoid taking iron supplements until healed (bacteria require iron for growth) • In addition to daily supplements, take: 500 mg buffered vitamin C every 4 hours for duration of infection, then cut down to 1,000 to 1,500 mg daily for maintenance, 1 g bioflavonoids daily, 25,000 IU vitamin A during the infection and 50 mg zinc every day • Picture your bladder healthy and functioning well • Say affirmations, for example, "My bladder is healing, my body is well."
Digestion/Indigestion	• Have a green drink at least three times a week: spinach, celery, beet greens, endive, parsley with unsweetened pineapple juice; chew each mouthful • Focus on greens, fresh fruits, garlic, onions, potatoes, papaya, pineapple, and nonfat yogurt with active cultures • Reflexology: hook in under the ball of the foot and press under the bone with each finger • To calm stomach/intestines, lie down in a comfortable position and hold hand over abdomen; breathe into your hand, releasing tension and negative feelings • Drink 2-6 ounces aloe vera juice daily and two cups of fenugreek tea
Diverticulosis (constipation alternating with diarrhea, gas and pain the left side of the abdomen)	• Adopt a high-fiber diet centered around fresh fruits and vegetables, whole grains and cereal. Substitute whole grain bread for white, a whole apple for apple juice • Put a teaspoon of psyllium seed in a glass of warm water, let it thicken a bit, then drink it down. If that doesn't bring on a bowel movement, add a teaspoon of coarse miller's bran to cereal, muffins or juice. Expect minor cramping or bloating until the colon adjusts (1 month) • Drink 6-7 glasses of water every day • Avoid seeds, nuts and foods with hard particles (strawberries, figs, tomatoes, zucchini, cucumbers, baked goods that have cracked wheat, poppy, sesame, or caraway seeds • Picture your digestive system clear and healthy • Say affirmations, e.g., "My colon is healthy and pink."
Earwax/Dizziness	• Use a few drops of hydrogen peroxide, glycerin or mineral oil; rinse the ears using a bulb syringe and warm water; dry ears thoroughly after showering/swimming with a hair dryer and use a drop or two of rubbing alcohol and vinegar
Eyestrain/Irritation	• Eat a diet high in vegetables and fruits, especially radishes, carrot juice, berries, kale and yellow squash • Sit with spine erect and hold motionless while completing each of the following ten repetitions: inhale slowly and look up to ceiling, exhale while looking down to the floor; do ten circles clockwise and then ten counterclockwise; focus on a far away object, then one close up; squeeze eyes shut as fast as possible; squeeze eyes shut and hold for the count

Table 7.12 (*continued*)

Condition	Measures
	of ten, rub the palms of your hands together then cover your eyes with the fleshy part of your palms for several minutes until you see only black • Make a healing affirmation for your eyes
Gallbladder distress, bloating, gas, nausea, after fatty meal, or sharp pain in upper right corner abdomen, due to gallstones	• Lose weight gradually if overweight, focusing meals around whole grains, fresh fruits and vegetables • Avoid fatty and fried foods and increase fiber with whole grains, fresh fruits and vegetables • Eliminate any possible food allergies (Use muscle testing to see which foods test weak; avoid those) • Drink six to eight glasses of water daily • Eat a complete breakfast daily, for example, cereal, fresh fruit and yogurt • Have the juice of 1 fresh lemon in a glass of hot water in the morning and 10 ounces of fresh carrot juice combined with 3 ounces each of fresh beet and cucumber juice after noon, and then 10 ounces of fresh carrot juice and 6 ounces of fresh spinach juice at least 2 hours later • Avoid caffeine • In addition to regular supplements, take 500 mg lecithin three times a day to promote the ability of bile to keep cholesterol in solution and prevent stones. • Picture your gallbladder healthy and well. • Say affirmations, for example, "My gallbladder is healthy and well."
Gout	• Eliminate foods that promote uric acid (meat, gravies, rich foods such as cakes and pies, white flour and sugar products, dried beans, cauliflower, fish, lentils, oatmeal, peas, poultry, spinach, and yeast products) • Avoid purine-rich foods (anchovies, asparagus, consomme, herring, meat gravies and broths, mushrooms, mussels, all organ meats, sardines, and sweetbreads). • Lose weight gradually if overweight • Increase fruit and vegetable consumption • Drink 7 ounces of fresh carrot juice combined with 4 ounces fresh celery, 2 ounces fresh parsley and 3 ounces fresh spinach juice, daily after noon and/or drink 10 ounces fresh carrot juice combined with 6 ounces spinach juice (at least 2 hours apart) • Drink 3 quarts of liquid daily • Eliminate alcohol drinks • Eat one-half pound of cherries or strawberries daily to neutralize uric acid • Eliminate or reduce niacin; avoid more than 100 mg daily • Eliminate vitamin A intake if attacks continue • Use stress-reducing techniques • Picture your body healthy and well • Use reflexology and therapeutic touch

Table **7.12** (*continued*)

Condition	Measures
Hay Fever	• Avoid aspirin and ibuprofen as well as foods containing salicylates (see "Asthma") • Stick to low-fat foods • Avoid wheat, sugars, salt, flours, and coffee • Combine the juice of 1 whole lemon mixed with 4 ounces of horseradish, daily in the morning • Drink10 ounces of fresh carrot juice combined with 3 ounces each fresh beet and cucumber juice, daily after noon • In addition to daily supplements, take: 2,000 mg vitamin C daily during hay fever season, and 1,000 mg citrus bioflavonoids, and 200–300 mg pantothenic acid every day. Take 500 mg evening primrose oil three times a day • Morning and evening do sinus exercise: lie on abdomen, arms crossed, chin rested on hands, knees bent, legs up; stretch legs out to side, then cross them, then out to side again; repeat 50–100 times • Avoid drinking alcohol (it swells bronchial tissue) • Use a dehumidifier and get rid of damp articles • Limit houseplants and terrariums • Vent clothes dryers and bathroom fans to the outside • When symptoms are worse in the morning (probably due to dust and dust mites): —vacuum mattress, then use a plastic cover over it —avoid storing anything under your bed (to discourage mites) —avoid rugs and carpets, and vacuuming (or use an accessory filter or central vacuum system) —install an HEPA filter on your furnace • Use reflexology to stimulate all toes, spinal reflexes, and sciatica. • Use imagery to picture nose and bronchial tubes unplugging and breathing becoming easier • Say affirmations many times a day, for example, "I breathe easily, I am well."
Heartburn/Hiatal Hernia	• Eat smaller, more frequent meals and never within three hours of sleep • Eat low-fat foods (fatty foods increase stomach acid) • Avoid antacids: both aluminum and magnesium in them can be problematic • Drink 7 ounces of fresh carrot juice combined with 4 ounces fresh celery, 2 ounces fresh parsley and 3 ounces fresh spinach juice after noon, daily • Elevate the head of the bed • Avoid bending, stooping, leaning forward or lying down for two hours after eating • Lie on your left side (right side allows stomach acid to irritate esophagus) • Stop smoking and drinking alcohol • Avoid coffee, tea, chocolate, liquers, citrus fruits and juices, onions, tomatoes and any food or drug that is irritating • Take l-2 acidophillus capsules to relieve heartburn

Table 7.12 (*continued*)

Condition	Measures
	• Strengthen stomach muscles by doing safe situps. • Picture your diaphragm and stomach muscles strong and healthy • Practice stress management procedures, see Chapter 4 • Say affirmations, for example, "My hernia is healing. I am well.
Hemorrhoids	• Apply witch hazel (for itching) and vitamin E (for burning) • Sit in a warm bath with your knees raised for 5-15 minutes 2-3 times/day • Sit on a "doughnut" to relieve the pressure of sitting • Shift to a diet centered around fresh fruits and vegetables, whole grains, and beans • Take 1–2 tablespoons of linseed oil daily to soften stools • Drink 2–6 ounces of aloe vera juice daily to heal digestive track • A peeled whole clove of garlic or a raw slice of potato serves as a beneficial suppository when taken 3 times a week • Drink 8 ounces fresh carrot juice mixed with 4 ounces fresh spinach juice, 2 ounces fresh turnip and 2 ounces watercress, daily after noon • Vitamin K is good for bleeding hemorrhoids; eat more kale and all dark green leafy vegetables to obtain it • Drink psyllium powder (1 teaspoon in water) 1–2 times/day • Only move your bowels when you feel the urge and use premoistened towelettes or cotton balls to wipe • Avoid lifting heavy objects (puts stress on circulatory system) • Use reflexology, imagery, massage, and therapeutic touch to open up blocked channels and release constricting feelings • Picture your digestive system healthy and well • Say affirmations many times daily, for example, "My digestive system functions perfectly. I am well. I release all anger."
Herpes	• Keep affected area clean and dry • Avoid touching the lesion and then touching your face • Avoid arginine-rich foods, including chocolate, peanuts, nuts, seeds, cereal grains such as oatmeal, gelatin, carob, and raisins • Use ice packs to the affected areas (ten minutes on, five minutes off, 2–3 times) • Practice stress reduction measures (stress stimulates outbreaks) see Chapter 4 on Stress Management • In addition to daily supplements, take: L-lysine, 1000 mg at each meal at the sign of cold sore outbreak; reduce to 500 mg a day when symptoms lessen or increase to 1000 mg daily if you break out on the lower dose; 22.5 mg zinc, 1,000–2,000 mg, vitamin C with bioflavonoids, 400 mg vitamin E and 500 mg L-lysine daily

Table 7.12 (*continued*)

Condition	Measures
Herpes (*cont'd*)	• Apply lysine cream or alternate vitamin E and vitamin A topically to lesions • Warm Epsom salts or baking soda baths will help itching and pain • Take three lactobacillus acidophilus capsules a day; one per meal • Refrain from sexual intercourse until gential sores have been completely healed for two weeks • Picture yourself well • Say affirmations, for example, "I am well and healthy."
Kidney Stones (due to calcium oxalate or uric acid crystals in the urine)	• Increase your fluid intake to at least 8 glasses of water /day • Avoid the amino acid L-cystine (crystallizes stones) • Avoid oxalic acid-containing or, -producing foods (asparagus, beets, parsley, rhubarb, sorrel, spinach, Swiss chard, vegeables of the cabbage family), as well as alcohol, caffeine (tea, coffee, sodas) chocolate, dried figs, lamb, nuts, pepper, and poppy seeds • Drink 9 ounces fresh carrot juice combined with 5 ounces fresh celery and 2 ounces fresh parsley juice after noon • Reduce intake of animal proteins (meat, milk, yogurt, ice cream, cream, chicken, fish) to no more than 3 ounces at lunch and dinner; animal protein results in excess calcium in the urine • Reduce salt intake • Eat watermelon often (by itself) as a diuretic and cleanser • Drink cranberry juice to acidify the urine • Avoid naturally carbonated and mineral waters (high calcium content) • Eat foods rich in magnesium (barley, bran, corn, buckwheat, rye, oats, brown rice, potatoes and bananas) • In addition to daily supplements, take: 400-500 mg magnesium oxide or chloride daily, 100 mg vitamin B_6 (pyridoxine) twice daily and 100 mg potassium every day • Picture the kidney stones dissolving and leaving your body • Use affirmations, e.g., "My kidneys are well. I am well."
Liver Health	• Avoid all meats except fish and chicken • Avoid sugar, alcohol, coffee or caffeinated tea, fried foods, processed foods or flours, salt, strong spices preservatives, additives and synthetic vitamins • For breakfast, every other day for two months, drink liver flush drink: blend two oranges or apples with 1 clove of fresh garlic,1 tablespoon olive oil, and juice of 2 fresh lemons; follow drink with two glasses of dandelion/parsley tea; no solid foods until lunch • Eat fruit salad or vegetable salad/steamed vegetables and 2 tablespoons of sesame butter for lunch

Table 7.12 (*continued*)

Condition	Measures
Liver (*cont'd*)	• At both lunch and dinner, have 2 tablespoons of raw grated beets combined with 1 tablespoon olive oil and 1/2 teaspoon fresh lemon juice • Morning and night (or more often), complete the following exercises: stand with arms hanging freely, then twist vigorously from side to side, inhaling and exhaling fifty times; inhale and stretch arms up, clasping hands above head, then bend all the way to one side, hold for five slow counts before inhaling up and repeating on opposite side (3 times each side); kneel on floor, extend right leg to the side and stretch right arm down that leg as far as is comfortable, keeping other arm over opposite side ear and elbows and outstretched knee straight (3 times each side) • Do reflexology for liver, gall bladder, colon, spinal and glandular reflexes five times each twice a day
Memory loss	• Test for allergies/food sensitivities • Avoid eating junk foods and fried foods • Increase intake of whole grains, tofu, farm fresh eggs, legumes, wheat germ, soybeans, fish, brewer's yeast, nuts, millet, and brown rice • Avoid dairy and wheat products for one month; if no improvement, gradually add these foods back to your diet • Avoid candy, cake, pies, doughnuts and all refined sugars which "turn off" the brain • Start a daily exercise program, especially walking • Practice breathing deeply • Read aloud, do crossword puzzles, balance your checkbook, and devise games and phrases to remember items • Keep active, doing things that satisfy you • Picture yourself with a good memory and a well mind • Use affirmations, for example. "My memory is getting better and better." • In addition to daily supplements, take: 40 mg ginkgo biloba 3-4 times a day, 650 mg choline three times a day, 1,000 mg vitamin C/400 IU vitamin E /10,000 IU beta-caroten/50 mcg selenium/1,000 mcg vitamin B_{12} sublingually/ and 50 mg zinc daily • Use reflexology: using thumbnail, stimulate tip of big toes, both feet

Table 7.12 (*continued*)

Condition	Measures
Ménière's Syndrome	• Eat regular meals primarily of whole grains, fresh vegetables, and fresh fruits • Eliminate sugar including candy, ice cream, cakes, cookies, frozen yogurt, sodas, diet sodas, honey, chocolate and dried fruit • If overweight, lose weight • Eliminate alcohol, smoking and caffeine • Check for hidden food allergies • Exercise daily (walk, swim, yoga) since impaired blood flow to the brain from clogged arteries and poor circulation may be the cause • In addition to daily supplements, take: 5 mg manganese daily (a deficiency may be the cause), 100 mcg chromium, fish oil capsules (1,000 mg three times/day), 40 mg ginkgo biloba three times daily, coenzyme Q_{10} (improves circulation), 1 capsule or tbsp lecithin before meals (for cellular protection and brain function) • Picture yourself well and healthy • Say affirmations, for example, "I am well. I am healthy."
Menopause	• Eliminate simple sugars (cakes, pies, candy, ice cream, frozen yogurt, etc.), meat, and dairy products, except nonfat plain yogurt, to control hot flashes • Increase intake of soy-containing foods (tofu, soy flour, soy burgers, tempeh) • Eat more whitefish, blackstrap molasses, broccoli, dandelion greens, kelp, salmon with bones, sardines and nonfat plain yogurt • Exercise at least 30 minutes five times a week • Stop smoking (increases risk of earlier menopause, osteoporosis, heart disease, cancer) • Choose herbs from Table 7.10 depending on symptoms • Drink 7 ounces fresh carrot juice combined with 3 ounces fresh beet, 4 ounces fresh lettuce and 2 ounces fresh turnip juice daily, after noon and/or 10 ounces fresh carrot juice with 6 ounces fresh spinach juice • In addition to daily supplements take: 2 mg boron daily, 1500-2,000 mg calcium citrate,* 1,000 mg magnesium (to ward off osteoporosis and irritability), 400 mg to 1,600 mg vitamin E daily (increase slowly until hot flashes cease), 100 mcg chromium three times daily • Take primrose oil or black currant oil capsules as directed on label to reduce hot flashes, fluid retention and insomnia • Prick a vitamin E capsule and apply the oil to vaginal area for itching or dryness • Avoid stress and practice stress management procedures • Picture your body healthy and well • Say affirmations, for example, "I love my body. I am well"

* No more than 1000 mg/day if prone to kidney stones and follow other recommendations for kidney stones.

Table 7.12 (*continued*)

Condition	Measures
Migraines	• Avoid fried foods, yellow cheese and other cheeses that contain tyramine, hot chocolate mixes (and other foods) containing phenylalanine and tyramine, nitrites (preservatives found in hot dogs and luncheon meats), aspirin, MSG, chocolate, and citrus fruits • Test for food sensitivities • Keep a headache diary for at least three weeks to find a pattern between food, drinks, medications and headache (birth control pills can affect migraines) • Eat regular small meals and snacks (low blood sugar can trigger a headache) • Drink 10 ounces fresh carrot juice combined with 6 ounces fresh spinach juice after noon every day • Take chromium to stabilize blood sugar (100 mcg 3 times daily) • Eat more fish (their oils have anti-inflammatory properties effective for migraines • Eat more high magnesium foods (apples, apricots, bananas, brown rice, figs, garlic, kelp, lima beans, millet, nuts, peaches, black-eyed peas, salmon, sesame seeds, tofu, green leafy vegetables, and whole grains • Avoid staring at movie, TV, or computer screens • Listen to soft music (helps relieve migraines) • Use full-spectrum or natural soft light bulbs (avoid fluorescents and harsh sun known to trigger migraines in some people) • Avoid changing daily routine even on weekends and holidays • Eat sufficient high fiber foods (fresh fruits and vegetables, whole grains) to ward off constipation • Exercise daily • Reduce stress and practice stress management procedures • Use feverfew (has the same anti-inflammatory effects as aspirin without the side effects) following directions on bottle • For headaches due to muscle cramping, take four, 500 mg evening primrose capsules in the morning and evening, and 1,200-1,500 mg calcium at bedtime • Use imagery to picture pain becoming a color, then a liquid, then draining out of the body and flowing far away; release negative feelings
Mitral Valve Prolapse	• If on antibiotics, take acidophillus capsules to promote friendly bacteria killed by medication • Exercise daily to control stress • Drink 10 ounces fresh carrot juice daily combined with 6 ounces fresh spinach juice, after noon • Practice stress management procedures • In addition to regular supplements, take: 30 mg coenzyme Q_{10} three times a day and 400 mg magnesium daily • Picture the heart healthy and well

Table 7.12 (*continued*)

Condition	Measures
Morning sickness	• Avoid greasy foods • Have frequent protein snacks and keep your stomach full • Apply pressure to the acupressure points on the wrist (three finger-widths up the inside of the wrist from the crease), pressing for several minutes • In addition to daily supplements, take: 50 mg vitamin B_6 (no longer than first three months of pregnancy) and 250 mg ginger capsules three times daily
Motion sickness	• Eat a small, low-fat starchy meal before traveling • Avoid fatty, greasy foods before and during travel • Take whole grain crackers with you to eat on the trip • Avoid smoke and food odors • Lie down and close your eyes at first sign of motion sickness • Keep busy but don't read • Stay as still as possible • Take two or three ground ginger root capsules before your journey and additional capsules every 3-4 hours, or drink ginger tea • Use stress reduction procedures
Multiple Sclerosis	• Reduce the amount of saturated fat by limiting whole milk, eggs, cheese, and meat • Increase intake of polyunsaturated oil (safflower oil, sunflower seeds, pumpkin seeds, wheat germ, wheat germ oil) • Drink up to 3 quarts of fresh raw juices daily after noon, including 10 ounces carrot combined with 6 ounces spinach, 9 ounces carrot/5 ounces celery/2 ounces parsley, 12 ounces carrot and 4 ounces parsley, 7 ounces carrot/ 4 ounces celery/ 2 ounces parsley/ 3 ounces spinach, and/or 16 ounces carrot • Take omega 3 fish oils or eat fish to reduce inflammation • Use muscle testing (p.207) for allergens and avoid those items • Eat low-pectin fruits: strawberries, blueberries, raspberries, peaches, apricots and cherries, avoiding apples, plums, red currants, gooseberries and cranberries (myelin may be damaged when pectin is incompletely broken down) • In addition to daily supplements, take: 1,000 mg vitamin C, 400 IU vitamin E, 1,000 mg vitamin B_{12} (dissolved under tongue), 10,000 IU beta-carotene,100 mcg selenium, 22.5 mg zinc,1,200 mg calcium, 400 mg magnesium, and one teaspoon of cod liver oil daily. Also take black currant seed oil or borage oil capsules (1,000 mg three times daily) • Exercise daily (especially swimming, yoga and movements which do not overheat the body) • Massage and therapeutic touch may be beneficial • Use imagery to picture the body healthy and strong

Table 7.12 (*continued*)

Condition	Measures
Osteoporosis	• Increase foods containing calcium (nonfat dairy products, buckwheat, dandelion greens, flounder, molasses, nuts and seeds, oats, tofu, seaweed, broccoli, kale and turnip greens) and add powdered milk to puddings, muffins, etc.
	• Eat sulphur foods; sulfur is necessary for calcium uptake: eggs, onions, garlic and asparagus
	• Reduce protein intake from meat, fish, poultry or cheese to 6 ounces daily
	• Avoid adding salt to cooking or meals
	• Eliminate sugar, caffeine and alcohol
	• Stop smoking
	• Exercise daily; walking, bicycling and movement that works weight-bearing joints is best
	• In addition to daily supplements take: 1,2000–2,000 mg calcium citrate at bedtime; 400 mg magnesium and 2 mg boron daily
	—To aid in calcium absorption, consider L-lysine (follow directions on label), digestive enzymes (with meals as directed on label), horsetail, oatstraw tea, and kelp (up to 10 tablets daily)
	• Use imagery to picture the bones strong and well
Parkinson's disease	• Eat a diet high in fiber to ward off constipation: including fresh fruits and vegetables; put a teaspoon of psyllium seed in half a glass of water and drink just when it starts to gel if food alone isn't enough
	• Eat foods high in vitamin C and E (which seem to delay progress of the disease) (See Table 5.3). If on levodopa, avoid foods or supplements containing vitamin B_6 (especially bananas, beef, fish, liver, oatmeal, peanuts, potatoes and whole grains)
	• Use the following exercises to gain better physical control: (for stooping) line up the spine against a doorjamb or wall several times a day (for shuffling) raise the feet over books placed at regular intervals along the floor, (for difficulty arising) lean forward 45 degrees and push with hands, (for speaking difficulties) read aloud
	• Limit intake of protein to 4 ounces of chicken or fish daily if on drugs because these foods may interfere with absorption—check with health care practitioner
	• Limit intake of manganese as it can aggravate symptoms (see p.115)
	• In addition to daily supplements, *gradually* increase vitamin E to 2,000 IU daily and 3 grams (3,000 mg) vitamin C daily
	• Picture the body healthy and well

Table 7.12 (*continued*)

Condition	Measures
PMS	• Increase fiber (fresh fruits and vegetables, whole grains clear estrogen and cut down symptoms) • Eliminate caffeine drinks, chocolate, alcohol, salt, and sweets—they all stress the body and increase symptoms • Eliminate animal fats (meat, dairy products) and increase intake of olive, safflower and linseed oil • Exercise daily, especially walking • In addition to regular supplements, take:10,000 IU vitamin A daily, 100 mg vitamin B_6 three times a day for two weeks prior to period, 400 to 600 IU vitamin E daily, 1,200 mg calcium at bedtime, 400 mg magnesium daily, 100 mcg chromium three times a day, 50 mg zinc daily, four 500 mg capsules of evening primrose oil in the morning and four in the evening • Picture the body healthy and functioning at optimal wellness
Prostate problems	• Follow a low-fat diet, avoiding margarine, hydrogenated vegetable oils and fried foods that interfere with prostaglandin metabolism • Avoid alcohol • Use a food diary and test for food allergies that could affect urination • Always void when feeling the urge and fully empty the bladder by relaxing the muscles in the pelvic floor • Drink 10 ounces fresh carrot juice combined with 3 ounces each beet and 3 ounces cucumber and/or 10 ounces carrot and 6 ounces spinach, and/or 8 ounces carrot, 4 ounces asparagus and 4 ounces lettuce • Exercise daily, walking is good, but avoid biking • Eat one ounce of pumpkin seeds or take pumpkin seed oil capsules as directed daily (zinc tends to shrink the prostate) • Hydrotherapy can increase circulation to the prostate • In addition to daily supplements, take daily: 1-2 flaxseed oil, 400 mg vitamin E, 60 mg zinc, and saw palmetto (160 mg) twice a day • Bleeding and frequent nighttime urination may be helped by horsetail (can be combined with hydrangea for an enlarged gland) • Ginseng as a general tonic and a decoction of equal parts of gravel root, sea holly and hydrangea root, taken 3-4 tablespoons three times daily may ease inflammation and reduce the discomfort of urination (add marshmallow to reduce burning and heat) • Picture the body healthy and well

Table 7.12 (*continued*)

Condition	Measures
Shingles	• Increase intake of fresh fruits and vegetables, brown rice and whole grains • Avoid arginine-rich foods: chocolate, peanuts, nuts, seeds and cereals • Squeeze vitamin E capsule directly on lesions and apply lysine cream twice daily • Use cayenne capsules (capsicium) as directed on label for postherpetic pain • Calamine lotion may help, too • Acupuncture, therapeutic touch and injections of vitamin B_{12} may help relieve symptoms • In addition to daily supplements, take: 500 to 1,000 mg lysine three times a day during an outbreak, 2-3 grams (2,000 to 3,000 mg) vitamin C every six hours at first sign of pain until lesions clear, and 600 IU vitamin E daily • Picture the body healthy and well
Sinusitis	• Drink 6-8 glasses of fluid daily, such as water, herb teas, low salt broth or soup • Reduce salt intake • Increase intake of raw fruits and vegetables to 75% • Avoid mucus-producing foods like cheese, milk, frozen yogurt, and ice cream • Take the juice of 1 whole lemon mixed with 4 ounces ground horseradish • Drink 10 ounces fresh carrot juice mixed with 6 ounces spinach juice daily after noon • Use a cool-mist humidifier • Take hot showers and baths, tenting a towel over the head and inhaling several times a day • Use warm compresses to relieve nose and eye pain • Use acupressure (see pp.194) several times a day • Test for food or inhallant allergies • In addition to daily supplements, take: 1,000 to 10,000 mg vitamin C plus bioflavonoids in divided doses, 10,000 IU vitamin A daily, and a vitamin B complex with at least 100 mg pantothenic acid three times daily • Avoid blowing nose forcefully and instead, draw the secretions to the back of the throat, then expel • Picture the sinuses draining like a stopped up sink • Affirm your ability to breathe easily daily many times, for example, "I breathe easily."

Table 7.12 (*continued*)

Condition	Measures
Stiff neck/ Shoulders	• Avoid pasteurized dairy products, refined foods, too many proteins at one meal, excessive eating • Drink water with the juice of one fresh lemon squeezed in it, and fresh fruit and vegetable juices and eat fresh green salads, at least once a day • Use reflexology, rotating all toes, especially the big toe vigorously; shoulder, arm, sciatic and hip • Picture tension, worry, responsibility flowing down your neck across your shoulders, down your arms and out your fingertips • Try to clasp hands behind back (bend right arm down over back of right shoulder, left arm bent up so left hand can try to clasp right hand); repeat, left arm over back of left shoulder • Use Feldenkrais to loosen tight shoulders, p. 170
Tinnitus (noises in the ear)	• Protect ears with plugs when exposed to noise • Remove excess earwax (see earwax/dizziness, p. 246) • Rule out any problem with the nerves in your ear with a health care practitioner • Test for food allergies, and eliminate any food that contains salicylates; see asthma p. 235 • Stop smoking • Avoid caffeine • Eat low-fat, low-cholesterol foods • Have hearing checked • If taking any of the following, consult your health care practitioner to see if they affect your tinnitus: aspirin, atropine, chloroquine, Flexeril, ergotamine derivatives, nicotine, Talwin, quinidine, and quinine • Eliminate sugar and keep a food diary to see what other foods may be affecting your tinnitus • Use stress management procedures, pp. 70–76 • Use imagery to picture your ears healthy and well • In addition to your daily supplements, take 10,000 IU vitamin A, 50 mg zinc, and 1,200 mg calcium at bedtime daily; 100 mcg chromium and 40 mg ginkgo biloba three times/ day • Affirm your ability to hear
TMJ (due to clenching) jaw, and grinding teeth)	• Get teeth aligned by your dentist • Eliminate caffeine, sugar, all white flour products, candy, colas, potato chips, pies and fast foods • Focus on steamed vegetables, fresh fruits, whole grain products, clear water fish, skinless chicken and turkey, brown rice and homemade soups and breads • When talking on the phone, use a headpiece so you do not cradle the phone against your shoulder or stress your arm holding the phone • Avoid chewing very large pieces of food or hard brittle foods

Table 7.12 (*continued*)

Condition	Measures
TMJ (cont'd)	• Sleep on your back • Drink a cup of hops, passionflower, skullcap or valerian root tea before bed • Practice stress management techniques, pp. 70–76 • Use imagery to picture your jaw relaxed and healthy and to release negative feelings (anger, resentment, etc.) • In addition to daily supplements, take: 1,200-2,000 mg calcium (chelate or citrate) and 600–1,000 mg magnesium in divided doses after meals and at bedtime, 100 mg vitamin B complex with extra pantothenic acid (B_5) 3 times daily (depending on symptoms)
Ulcers (stomach)	• Avoid all of the following which irritate the stomach's protective lining: fried or spicy and acidic foods, aspirin and non-steroidal anti-inflammatory drugs, smoking, alcohol, sugar, food allergies (use muscle testing), Tums, Alka-2 and other antacids (have a rebound effect and create even more stomach acid) • Gradually increase fiber intake of fruits, vegetables, and whole grains • Drink 2-6 ounces aloe vera juice alone or in water or juice daily • Rule out the source of ulcers as a bacteria by having a physician or nurse practitioner order a blood test • Drink 10 ounces fresh carrot juice mixed with 6 ounces fresh spinach juice after noon and, at least two hours later, drink 10 ounce fresh carrot juice mixed with 3 ounces each fresh beet and cucumber juice • Eat small, frequent meals • Avoid milk • Exercise daily, swimming and walking are good • Practice relaxation, see p. 69 • Use imagery to picture your stomach healthy and well • Affirm your wellness by saying many times daily, "My stomach is well, I am well." • Drink 1 quart of raw cabbage juice, divided into 3-4 doses daily • In addition to regular supplements, take: 1,000-1,500 DGL (a licorice extract) twenty minutes before eating to protect the stomach, 500 mg evening primrose oil three times a day, 10,000 IU vitamin A daily, 500 mg buffered vitamin C twice a day, and 400 IU vitamin E daily
Varicose veins	• Lose weight if overweight • Adopt a high-fiber diet including plenty of fresh fruits and vegetables and whole grains • Daily, after noon, drink 7 ounces fresh carrot juice mixed with 4 ounces celery, 2 ounces celery and 3 ounces spinach; at least 2 hours later, drink 10 ounces fresh carrot juice mixed with 3 ounces each beet and cucumber juice

Table 7.12 (*continued*)

Condition	Measures
Varicose veins (*cont'd*)	• Eat raw foods, whole grains, seeds and avoid refined foods • Practice deep breathing, see p.73 • Get up every fifteen minutes, walk, stretch, deep breathe • Use reflexology to stimulate heart, glands, spine, toes, and hips • Exercise daily by walking, running or cycling for 20-30 minutes as well as stretching the legs or elevating them for 3-15 minutes throughout the day • Wear support stockings • Use a slant board twice a day, elevating legs for 5-15 minutes to encourage blood flow • Lie on back, knees to chest, gently rock back and forth • Butcher's broom, parsley or uva ursi herbs may help (see Table 7.10) • In addition to your daily supplements, take: 400-1,000 mg vitamin E, 1,000 mg bioflavonoids or Psynogenol daily • Use imagery to picture your legs healthy and release negative feelings many times every day • Affirm healthy veins, for example, "My blood circulates easily and completely," many times a day
Wound healing (pre- and post-surgery)	In addition to daily supplements, take: • Acidophilus (in high potency, powdered form), 3 times a day (to stabilize the intestinal bacterial flora) • 60 mg coenzyme Q_{10} daily (to improve tissue oxygenation) • 100 mg geranium (oxygenation and pain relief) • protein supplement of free form amino acids to aid healing • 2 garlic capsules three times a day to enhance immune function • 500 mg L-cystine twice daily to speed healing • 5,000-10,000 mg vitamin C to aid tissue repair • 400 mg vitamin E daily and apply to wound after stitches have been removed • 80 mg zinc plus 1,500 mg calcium plus 1,000 mg magnesium vitamin B_3 daily • In addition to daily supplements, take lactobacillus acidophilus, 1 capsule three times daily; garlic capsules or in its natural form • Eat garlic and fresh fruits and vegetables • Drink water with the juice of a lemon in it throughout the day • Use reflexology to stimulate genital reflexes and lymphatics 25 times • Use imagery to picture your body returning to a healthy state

Table 7.12 (*continued*)

Condition	Measures
Yeast Infections (white coating on tongue, allergic rashes, gas and bloating)	• Eliminate antibiotics, birth control pills, corticosteroids, and ulcer drugs • Begin a yeast- and sugar-free diet including no bread or baked goods with yeast, cheese, mushrooms, vinegar, soy sauce, fermented foods, alcohol, cookies, candy, ice cream or sweetened yogurt, soda, diet soda, dried fruit, chocolate, and sweeteners including fructose, malt, barley, and juices

Adapted from: *Natural Prescriptions* by Robert M. Giller, M.D. and Kathy Matthews, New York: Carol Southern Books, 1994; *Prescription for Nutritional Healing* by James F. Balch, M.D. and Phyllis A. Balch, C.N.C., Garden City Park, NY: Avery Publishing Group Inc., 1990; *Raw Vegetable Juices* by N.W. Walker, D. Sci.,New York: Jove, 1970; *The Foot Book*, by D. Berkson., New York: Harper &Row, 1977; *Your Health and the Indoor Environment* by Randall Earl Dunford and Kevin G. May, Dallas TX: NuDawn, 1991.

INTEGRATIVE LEARNING EXPERIENCES

Beginning Level

1. Assess yourself using the following measures:
   A. Breast/vaginal self-exam or testicular exam
   B. Sexual communication (Table 7.4)
   C. Diamond's behavioral kinesiology
   D. Krieger's Therapeutic Touch

2. Develop and try out appropriate interventions based on the above assessments with a peer; also ask your peer if she/he has any symptoms that you have not assessed via the above assessments, and develop and try out interventions for those. Use Table 4.7 to organize the data.

3. Work with a peer to complete a therapeutic touch assessment of each other.

4. Work with a peer to complete a reflexology assessment and appropriate interventions.

5. Complete a massage with two peers (See p. 219); compare your results.

6. Role play responses to the following client responses with a peer using assertiveness criteria to evaluate your efforts:
   A. "Doesn't yoga have something to do with winding yourself up like a pretzel? How can that be healthy? Sounds harmful to me!"
   B. "Thump my thymus! What good can that possibly do?"

     C. "How can my feet affect my heart? Hogwash!"

     D. "I let my doctor examine me; I don't want to know what's happening with my body unless there is something really wrong."

7. Role play a discussion with a client (using a peer to play the client) regarding which detection tests she should have so she will not miss an illness process. Use assertiveness criteria to evaluate the outcome.

Advanced Level

1. Complete assessments of one child, one young adult, and one senior client using assessments based on the frameworks of:

     A. Diamond
     B. Krieger
     C. Berkson (reflexology)
     D. Yoga
     E. Acupressure

2. Develop appropriate intervention for the three clients assessed. Organize your results using Table 4.7.

REFERENCES

Abrams, H. (1979). The "overutilization" of x-rays. *NE J Med* 300:1213–1216.
Balch, J.F., and Balch, P.A. (1990). *Prescription for Nutritional Healing.* Garden City Park, NY: Avery Publishing Group.
Berger, B.G., and Owen, D.R. (1992). Mood Alteration With Yoga and Swimming: aerobic exercises may not be necessary. *Percept Motor Skills* 75(3, part 2): 1331–1343.
Bergman, A. (1977). The menace of mass screening. *Am J Pub Health* 67(7):601-602.
Berkson, D. (1977). *The Foot Book: Healing The Body Through Reflexology.* New York: Harper and Row.
Berry, C. (1980). Doing your own vaginal self-exam. In *Medical Self-Care,* T. Ferguson, Ed. New York: Summit Books, pp. 281–284.
Borysenko, J. (1985). Healing motives: An interview with David C. McClelland. *Advances* 2(2):29–41.
Diamond, J. (1979). *Behavioral Kinesiology.* New York: Harper and Row.
Diamond, J. (1985). *Life Energy. Using the Meridians to Unlock the Hidden Power of Your Emotions.* New York; Paragon House.
Downing, G. (1972). *The Massage Book.* New York: Random House.
Galen, R. (1974). False-Positives. *Lancet* (Nov. 2): 1081.
Giller, R.M., and Mathews, K. (1994). *Natural Prescriptions.* New York: Carol Southern Books.
Hale, E.H. (1986). A Study of the relationship between therapeutic touch and the anxiety of hospitalized patients. Unpublished doctoral dissertation, Texas Women's University.
Harrold, F. (1992). *The Complete Body Massage: A Hands-On Manual.* New York: Sterling Publishing Co., Inc.
Heidt, P. (1979). An investigation of the effects of Therapeutic Touch on anxiety in hospitalized patients. Unpublished doctoral dissertation, New York University.
Institute of Noetic Sciences. (1984). The new field of psychoneuroimmunology. *Investigations* 1(1):n.p.
Iyengar, B. (1966). *Light on Yoga.* New York: Schocken Books.
Kawaski, I., Colditz, G.A., Ascherio, A., et al. (1994). Prospective study of phobic anxiety and subsequent risk of coronary heart disease. *Circulation* 89(5): 1992-1997.
Knaster, M. (1984). Massage: The roots of women's healing. In *Women's Health Care: A Guide to Altneratives,* K. Weiss, Ed. Reston, VA: Reston Publishing Co.
Koenig, S. (1981). Touch for health. In *The Holistic Health Lifebook.* E. Bauman et al., Eds. Berkeley, CA: And/Or Press, pp. 44–51.
Kramer, N.A. (1990). Comparison of Therapeutic Touch and Casual Touch in stress reduction of hospitalized children. *Ped Nsg* 16(5):483–485.
Krieger, D. (1993). *Accepting Your Power to Heal. The Personal Practice of Therapeutic Touch.* Santa Fe, NM: Bear & Company, Inc.
Lasater, J. (1984). Hatha yoga for women's health. In *Women's Health Care: A Guide to Alterntives,* K. Weiss, Ed. Reston, VA: Reston Publishing Co.
Lowe, C., and Nechas, J. (1983). *Whole Body Healing.* Emmaus, PA: Rodale Press, pp. 508–552.
McClelland, D., et al. (1985). Stressed power motivation, sympathetic activation, immune function and illness. *Advances* 2(2):43–52.
Meehan, J.C. (1985). the effect of therapeutic touch on the experience of acute pain in postoperative patients. Doctoral Dissertation, New York University.
Napodano, R. (1977). The functional heart murmur: a wastebasket diagnosis. *J Fam Prac* 4(4): 637–639.
Nickel, D. (1984). *Acupressure for Athletes.* Santa Monica, CA: Health AcuPress.

Patterson, A. (1984). Acupressure for women's health. In *Women's Health Care: A Guide to Alternatives,* K. Weiss, Ed. Reston, VA: Reston Publishing Co., pp. 270-283.

Quinn, J. (1982). An investigation of the effects of therapeutic touch done without physical contact on state anxiety of hospitalized patients. Unpublished doctoral dissertation, New York University.

Rice, R. (1975). Premature infants respond to sensory stimulation. *APA Monitor* 6(11):8–9.

Robinson, N., and Dirnfeld, F. (1967). The ionized state of the atmosphere as a function of meterorological elements and the various sources of ions. *Int. J Biometerol* 11(11):279–288.

Schneider, V. (1979). *Infant Massage,* 2nd ed. Aurora, CO; Vimala Schneider.

Serizawa, K. (1972). *Massage the Oriental Method.* Elmsford, NY:Japan Publications, Inc.

Tappan, F. (1984). Massage, reflexology, and women. In *Women's Health Care: A Guide to Alternatives,* K. Weiss, Ed. Reston, VA:Reston Publishing Co., pp. 258–269.

Udupa, K., Singh, R., and Settiwar, R. (1971). Studies on physiological, endocrine, and metabolic response to the practice of yoga in young normal volunteers. *J Res. Indian Med* 6(3):345–353.

Wirth, D.P. (1990). The effect of non-contact therapeutic touch on the healing of full dermal thickness wounds. *Subtle Energies* 1(1): 1-20.

Wilson, R. (1995). *Aroma therapy.* Garden City Park, NY: Avery Publishing Group.

8

ENVIRONMENTAL WELLNESS

This chapter discusses the following topics:

* Environmental factors influencing wellness
* Accessing environmental wellness
* Environmental interventions

The most difficult challenges for environmental wellness today come from the uncertainties about toxic and ecologic effects of fossil fuels and synthetic chemicals. An estimated 82 percent of major industrial chemicals have not been tested for their toxic properties and links to specific diseases, and only a small proportion have been adequately tested for their ability to cause or promote cancer. Still, enough is known to target improvement in exposure to lead, air pollution, radon, drinking water, air and soil quality, solid waste contamination, hazardous waste sites and recycling of materials and toxic waste (*Healthy People 2000*, 1990, p. 66).

ENVIRONMENTAL FACTORS INFLUENCING WELLNESS

Researchers have found many environmental factors influencing wellness, including: waste disposal and transport, air quality, smoking, drinking water, crowding, radiation, consumer products, occupation, noise, acid rain, ions, light, and color. Many of these factors interact to enhance or detract from wellness.

The Environment and Cancer

Of current interest is the relationship between the environment and cancer. "It has been estimated that 50–90 percent of human cancer is due to known or unknown environmental factors. It is necessary to regard all agents demonstrated to be carcinogenic in animals as potentially carcinogenic in humans since present information precludes any reliable distinctions" (NIH, 1980, p. 33). Specific environmental risk factors include: cigarette smoking, personal habits, occupation, drugs, food, water pollutants, atmospheric contaminants, and some consumer products.

Solid Wastes

Billions of gallons of municipal waste are produced daily, industry dumps millions of tons of waste materials annually into the environment, and 2 billion tons of solid waste are produced by farm animals in the United States. In the recycling of municipal waste, it can be contaminated by industrial, hospital, research, wastes, and pesticides; all these can enter plants grown on the soil using recycled sludge or waste water and be consumed on the dinner table (NIH, 1980, p. 28).

Dioxin is an unintended byproduct of several industrial processes, including municipal incineration, chlorine bleaching of paper, and manufacture of chlorinated chemicals, such as wood preservatives, pesticides, and herbicides. Low-level exposure to dioxin and related chemicals may already be causing immune suppression, reproductive difficulties, and endocrine-related disorders. Dioxins persist for decades in the environment. They build up in fat cells of animals that eat animals. People get exposed primarily from eating animal fats from meat, fish, and dairy products (Dioxin risks sound greater than had been thought, 1994).

Women, Health and the Environment project is a grassroots cancer movement redefining cancer as an environmental issue. Studies by Falck et al. (1992), Wolff et al. (1993) and others have linked blood levels of pesticides to breast cancer.

Air Quality

A major factor influencing environmental wellness is the quality of indoor and outdoor air. Some variables lowering the quality of outdoor air are: industries that vent dangerous chemicals into the air (both the areas nearby are affected and those far away due to high smokestacks and acid rain that falls many miles away), vehicle exhaust (especially from diesel engines), emissions from toxic waste dumps, nuclear plants, and nuclear testing areas. A major factor in air quality is the presence of smokers. Smoking not only affects those who smoke in terms of increasing risk for lung cancer and heart conditions; it also affects the passive smoker (EPA, 1993).

> Known harmful effects of maternal smoking on the fetus include retarded fetal growth in utero, premature labor, mental retardation, hyperkinesis in childhood, higher perinatal mortality, spontaneous abortion, congenital neural tube defects, other birth defects, cardiac effects, higher breathing frequency, and elevated hemoglobin and hematocrit. Pathophysiologically, it is reported that smoking causes (1) lowered

arterial pressure of the mother; (2) permanent damage to the uterine arteries; (3) lowered uteroplacental perfusion; (4) lowered caloric intake of the mother; (5) uterine artery vasospasm; and (6) fetal carboxhemoglobinemia. In normotensive mothers, smoking one cigarette raises arterial blood pressure (both systolic and diastolic), producing decreased placental blood flow; normal flow is restored only after 15 minutes. (Voldman, 1983)

Additionally, children of smoking parents are apt to have more upper respiratory ailments (Bryce & Enkin, 1984), lower scores on spelling and reading tests, shorter attention spans, more hyperactivity (Naeye & Peters, 1984), and infantile colic and ear inflammation twice as frequently as children of non-smokers (Forskningsroen, 1984). Cancer risk in adulthood may also be increased (Sandler et al., 1985).

Indoor air pollution is a relatively new problem. Older homes, offices, hotels, and hospitals were not hermetically sealed. Prior to the interest in energy conservation, buildings were not composed of double-glazed windows, sealed windows, and synthetic materials, and there were sufficient cracks and leaks in walls and windows to let stale air out and fresh air in. Synthetic building materials and equipment and gas and kerosene stoves give off irritating gases and fumes. When combined with cigarette smoke and the fungus growth and spread of organic matter through air conditioning and humidifying equipment, air to breathe is severely compromised (Ager & Tickner, 1983; Epstein, 1978, pp. 450–453; George, 1985; Indoor air pollution and S. 1198 fact sheet, 1985). The problem is compounded in hospitals where bacteria, viruses, particles of fecal material, etc., are circulated to distant parts of the building via the air conditioning, plumbing, and laundry chute systems. The problem of hospital-acquired infection is growing and requires control (Mendelsohn, 1979, pp. 72–73; NIH, 1980, p. 26).

Smoking

Compared to nonsmokers, an average young male smoker (30–40 years of age) who smokes more than 40 cigarettes per day loses an estimated 8 years of life. Cigarette smoking acts synergistically with alcohol and toxic substances in the air to increase the risk of cancer (Office of Disease Prevention and Health Promotion, 1988).

There is a 62.5% mortality rate in hospital fires due to cigarette ignition. Measures to limit rather than eliminate smoking by clients have proven unsatisfactory, since most burn-related deaths occur while the clients are unattended (Bongard et al., 1984).

Smoking affects the quality of life in other ways; for example, it is correlated with higher absenteeism and health costs, excess office maintenance, increased ventilation needs, and lowered employee morale (Weis, 1984).

Drinking Water

Water quality is another factor affecting environmental wellness. Drinking water contains contaminants of varying harm: perhaps the most insidious are the organic compounds from sewage treatment plants and industrial discharge. Keough (1980, p. 10) states that an estimated 500–1,000 new chemicals are introduced into industry yearly, leading to increased drinking water contamination. Preliminary studies suggest a link between cancer and some organic and inorganic contaminants in drinking water. The higher incidence of heart disease in soft water areas may be due to the cadmium leached from plumbing by the corrosive action of the water. Soft water may leach lead from the plumbing and contribute to mental retardation in children (NIH, 1980, p. 23).

Drinking water has also been contaminated by parasites and microbes (Water-drinking disorder, 1995).

Measures to destroy organisms found in drinking water also present potential hazards. Drinking chlorinated water is associated with cancer, high blood pressure, and anemia. Chloroform is formed in the chlorination process; this chemical is rapidly absorbed in body fat and tissues. Other potentially dangerous offshoots of the chlorination process are tribromomethane and chlorobenzene, a CNS depressant.

Several authors have noted the potential dangers of water fluoridation, including the possibility of surpassing the acceptable level of fluoride by using substances containing natural fluoride (e.g., tea) and drinking fluoridated water (Keough, 1980, pp. 22–23). Diesendorf (1980) has reviewed the scientific studies on fluoridation and found that: (1) The use of fluoridated water in kidney dialysis may lead to severe bone disease. (2) There is evidence of low tolerance to fluoride. In one study 1% of the study group of 1,100 suffered dermatological, gastrointestinal, and neurological symptoms from receiving a daily tablet of approximately 1 mg/day of fluoride. (3) There is no guarantee that adding a fixed concentration of fluoride to the water supply delivers a controlled dose to individuals. Measurements in Canada found that workers received 2 to 5 mg daily with a 1 mg fixed concentration; skeletal fluorosis has been observed in concentrations of 0.8 to 4.0 mg/liter. A major study in an American hospital found 3.6 to 5.4 mg with a mean of 4.4 mg. Additionally, a review of the studies used to support fluoridation reveals statistical and methodological problems.

In addition to the dangers of consuming drinking water, a study (Brown, Bishop, & Rown, 1984) showed that the skin route of exposure to chemicals in drinking water accounted for 29–91% (64% on the average) of the total dose of chemicals received by the individual. The following compounds found in drinking water samples were studied: toluene, ethylbenzene, and styrene. Although not studied by the researchers, Regna (1984) points out toxins like benzene, carbon tetrachloride, vinyl chloride, and trichloroethylene are commonly found in surveys of drinking water supplies completed by the Environmental Protection Agency (EPA).

Personal Space

Amount and type of personal space is an environmental wellness factor. Crowding increases stress and contributes to the "spread of acute and contribution to the chronic disease morbidity and mortality" (U.S. Dept. of Health, Education and Welfare, 1977, p. 29). There is a variation in personal space required and individual and ethnic parameters must be assessed.

Radiation

Radiation can decrease personal wellness. The U.S. Academy of Sciences has confirmed that radiation exposure changes the electrical charge of atoms and molecules in cells and that there is no level considered safe since even very low levels affect the body and its processes and its effects are cumulative (Dickson, 1979). Toxic agent and radiation control is one of the 15 health priority areas addressed by the Public Health Service's Objectives for the Nation. Cancer is the chief concern of the overuse of diagnostic x-rays in medicine and dentistry. Diagnostic x-rays account for more that 90% of the total human-controllable ionizing radiation exposure for the U.S. population. Because of this problem, the Public Health Service has developed the following objective: By 1990, the number of medically unnecessary diagnostic x-ray examinations should be reduced by some 50 million examinations annually (Rall, 1984). Additionally, radiation is produced by microwave ovens, long-distance telephone microwave relay towers, police, weather, and airport radar systems, nuclear-generating stations, atom bomb tests, fluoroscopes, diathermy, radioactive isotopes, electron microscopes, some types of computers and office machines, high voltage electrostatic air filters, and AM-FM radio and TV broadcasting stations.

Radon comes from rock and soil, enters buildings through cracks in foundations or basements, and when inhaled releases ionizing radiation that can damage lung tissue and lead to lung cancer. As many as 8 million homes may have radon at a level requiring correction. Low-cost test kits are available to identify exposure (*Healthy People 2000*, 1990, p. 66).

Consumer Products

Many consumer products can affect wellness negatively, including: foods in cans with leaded seams (increase lead toxicity); drugs (interact with pollutants to increase their toxic effects; estrogens and chemotherapeutic agents increase the risk of additional cancer); cosmetics (many contain carcinogenic substances); clothes (in a study of 4700 women who wore bras more than 12 hours a day, they were 21 times more likely to develop breast cancer, apparently due to restrictions on the lymph system, an important filter of body toxins) (Singer & Grismaijer, 1995); pesticides (many have been linked with cancer and contaminate soil, surface water, animals, and fish); toys (accidents result most commonly from choosing toys that are not age appropriate); cleaners (can cause burns and eye and lung irritation); aerosols (can irritate lungs and affect ecological balance); waxes (irritation of lungs and nasal passages): cleaning fluid (irritation and cancer); deodorizers (allergic reactions); insect repellents (skin irritation); formaldehyde fumes released from new products including pressed wood materials, urea-formaldehyde foam insulation, permanent press fabrics, and wet strength paper (eye, nose, and throat irritation, difficulties in breathing, headaches, fatigue, memory loss, nausea, and cancer in laboratory animals); decorated glassware (lead decals are toxic); ice cube trays if cadmium-coated (this heavy metal can leach into sherbet if the trays are used to produce it); silver polish if not adequately rinsed from kitchen utensils contains the heavy metal cadmium; pesticide treated shelf liners (toxic and volatile); plastic food wraps containing PVC (a carcinogen); food toxins; and possibly even dental fillings (Isaacson & Jensen, 1992; Casdorph & Walker, 1995).

Occupation

A number of workers are at high risk. Hospital workers are at high risk for cancer due to occupational hazards related to handling laundry (liver cancer) and exposure to ionizing radiation (leukemia) (Mancinon, 1983). Other substances in hospitals linked with cancer include: anesthetic gases, benzene, formaldehyde, ethylene oxide, sex hormones, and alkylating agents used to treat cancer. Hospital workers are at risk for exposure to ethylene oxide, a sterilant linked with dermatitis, burns, eye irritation, pulmonary edema, leukemia, lymphoma, and possible stomach cancer, miscarriage, birth defects, and reproductive conditions.

The manufacture of consumer products increases the negative effects for those employed in certain work. Workers in high risk industries (asbestos, rubber, chemical, plastic PVC/VC, steel, smelting, and some mining operations) have increased rates of cancer, respiratory, and gastrointestinal disorders (Epstein, 1978, pp. 435–458).

Those who work with pesticides and grain workers (who must unload incoming cargoes of fumigated grain) are at high risk for short-term effects: nervousness, tremors, difficulty breathing, nausea, vomiting, skin irritation, collapse, coma, and death; and long-term effects: liver, kidney, CNS, and eye damage; allergic skin reactions, sterility, birth defects, stillbirths, and cancer (Fumigants used in the food industry, 1983).

Asbestos poses a major threat to 2.5 million workers in diverse occupations. Those at especially high risk are construction workers, brake mechanics, maintenance employees, and shipyard workers. Mt. Sinai Environmental Sciences Laboratory projects that there will be 200,000 excess cancer deaths from asbestosis by the year 2000.

Benzene is a major cancer hazard for 3 million workers in the chemical industry. A risk assessment by scientists from OSHA and the National Toxicology Program estimate that between 44 and 152 of 1,000 workers will contract leukemia if they are exposed to the current legal limit of asbestos for 45 years.

Roofers and waterproofers are exposed to asphalt and coal tar pitch fumes laden with hydrocarbons known to cause cancer in laboratory animals including lung, skin, bladder, and gastrointestinal cancers. More than half a million workers employed in cotton agriculture and yarn and fabric manufacture are at risk for brown lung, a chronic, irreversible respiratory condition worsening with exposure. It is estimated that 30,000 workers in the South Atlantic region are already totally disabled by the condition and that 83,000 will be afflicted in the future.

Industrial workers and gas station attendants are at risk from exposure to EDB, which is known to cause cancer in animals and is suspected of causing reproductive problems.

Up to 2.6 million workers may be exposed in the manufacture, installation, and use of formaldehyde products. Inhalation or skin contact has been linked with cancer since the mid-1970s. It is estimated that 6 million workers have work-related hearing loss and 15 million are currently exposed to hazardous noise levels.

Approximately 835,000 workers in diverse occupations are exposed to lead; exposure to the metal is known to cause intoxication, loss of appetite, constipation, nausea, tremors, weakness, numbness, colic, and kidney disease; long-term exposure has been linked with CNS and brain damage, reproductive conditions, and possible heart disease (OSHA Standards: 1981–1984, 1984).

Noise

According to the American Speech-Language-Hearing Association, noise is the most pervasive pollution in America (Ciccone, 1989). Continued exposure to sound at high decibels (noise) is correlated with hearing loss, elevated blood pressure, tension, nervousness, and imbalance in the fluid, electrolyte, and hormonal systems. The Environmental Protection Agency's rule of thumb is that if an individual has to raise his or her voice to be heard, the noise is too loud and should be avoided. Although it is believed hearing is lost during the aging process, a remote Sudanese tribe living in a noise-free culture has near perfect hearing past 80 years of age. Being exposed to daily rapid-transit trains, V-8 engines, or aircraft can result in psychological, psychosomatic, and cardiovascular symptoms. Some sound levels that create risk to hearing loss include live rock bands, jackhammers, heavy duty trucks, and living next to a freeway; a jet takeoff (100 meters away) or a jet engine (25 meters distance) can be harmful to hearing (Raloff, 1982).

Acid Rain

A by-product of high smokestack emissions is acid rain. Deaths of fish and entire ecological systems have been traced to industrial emissions hundreds of miles away. Weathering is accelerated and there are possible effects to human skin and hair (Rosenfield, 1978).

Ions

The air is filled with ions; "pos-ions" or positive ions are produced by various kinds of friction which tends to "knock off the negative electrons and produce an overdose of positive ions. On a dusty or humid day this overdose may be massive because the neg-ions promptly attach themselves to particles of dust, pollution, or moisture and lose their charge" (Soyka, 1977, p. 21). An overdose of "neg-ions" or negative ions seems to be beneficial to well-being while an overdose of pos-ions leads to fatigue, tension, and hyperactivity. Probably due in part to the overproduction of serotonin as well as interfering with the normal clotting mechanism, ". . . Pos-ions stimulate the metabolism and that alone could be responsible for an increased flow of blood from an open surgical wound. Whether the problem is thrombosis or hemorrhage depends on the patient" (Soyka, 1977, p. 63).

Neg-ions are associated with the calm after a storm (the pos-ions have been washed away), mountain areas (sun, clean air, and rock strata interactions), seashore (waves bounce on beaches and rocks), waterfalls, and showers. Pos-ions are associated with tall buildings, air conditioning systems, enclosed areas (e.g., riding in a car with the windows closed and vents open or spending hours in hermetically sealed buildings where windows cannot be opened), storms, certain desert winds, full moons (number of pos-ions close to the earth's surface increases as the negative outer face of the ionosphere is repelled), synthetic fibers (static electricity potential is high compared to natural fabrics), pollution, smoking, and any other situation setting up friction resulting in the loss of neg-ions.

Light

Full spectrum light is associated with well-being, whereas less than full-spectrum light, e.g., fluorescent lighting, is associated with decreased wellness (Liberman, 1991). Full spectrum light enters the eye and stimulates the pituitary. Studies of bird and animal migration and hen egg production "has led to strong evidence that mammals respond to particular wavelengths of *visible light* as well as other areas of the *total spectrum*, including the longer wavelengths of ultraviolet that penetrate the atmosphere" (Ott, 1973, p. 13).

One of Ott's experiments provides evidence for the effect of different types of light on well-being. Thirty pairs of mice were kept in a room lighted by white fluorescent bulbs; 30 other pairs were kept in another room lighted with pink fluorescent bulbs; a control group (of eight pairs) was kept in a room receiving daylight filtered through window glass. All mice were of C3H strain, which is highly susceptible to spontaneous tumor development. The mice in the control group developed cancer 2 months later than the mice in the white fluorescent light and 3 months later than those under the pink fluorescent lighting.

In later experiments with larger numbers of mice (over 2,000 in all) not only tumor development, but necrosis of the tail, calcium deposits in heart tissues, smaller litters, and behavioral problems were associated with pink fluorescent lighting. The effect of tinted pink glass on behavior was also noted by Ott. Mink placed behind deep pink glass became increasingly aggressive, as did students who wore "hot pink" sunglasses (Ott, 1977, pp. 155–157).

Ott (1977, pp. 192–202) reports studies of the effect of light on well-being. In one study, four first-grade classrooms in a windowless school in Sarasota, Florida, showed dramatic reactions in hyperactive children when new, full-spectrum fluorescent tubes (that duplicate natural light) were used in two of the classrooms. Under the standard cool white fluorescent lighting, some first-graders demonstrated nervous fatigue, irritability, lapses of attention, and hyperactive behavior. When the new full-spectrum fluorescent tubes were installed, a marked improvement occurred in the children's behavior. Films of classroom behavior for 4 months showed the children in full-spectrum light remained calm and more interested in their work while those in rooms with the standard cool white fluorescent light were observed fidgeting to an extreme degree, leaping from their seats, flailing their arms, and paying little attention to their teachers. Similar results were reported in studies in two schools in California. Additionally, the number of cavities and the extent of tooth decay in new teeth showed significant differences; the children in the improved lighting had one third fewer cavities.

Ott (1977, pp. 195–196) contended that since several conditions are treated with specific wavelengths of light (jaundice with blue light and psoriasis with black light), living under artificial light lacking these wavelengths might logically contribute to causing the condition originally. Contrarily, too much direct exposure to the sun (full-spectrum light) is correlated with skin cancer; however, it is not necessary to be in the sunlight to obtain full-spectrum light. Being outdoors during daylight hours (preferably not in direct sunlight), sitting in a room flooded with natural light, or using full-spectrum fluorescent lighting will all produce wellness enhancement without increasing the risk of skin cancer.

Dr. Richard J. Wurtman, Director of the Neuroendocrine laboratory at M.I.T., sheds further light on the benefits of full-spectrum light. "Light striking the retina stimulates the optic nerve, which . . . in turn sends out impulses to the hypothalamus, a part of the brain with a great influence on emotions. From there, stimulation travels through neuro-chemical channels to the pituitary and pineal glands, which release the hormones that control body chemistry" (Houck, 1979).

In Russia, daily exposure to low dosages of ultraviolet is prescribed by law for coal miners as an aid in fighting black lung. Researchers believe that ultraviolet light stimulates enzyme reactions, increases the activity of the entire endocrine system and increases immunological responses. And the U.S. Navy has been irradiating its personnel on submarine duty. There has been less illness among irradiated crewmen, the navy reports, and full spectrum lighting has had definite beneficial effect on the sailors' emotional lives. (Houck, 1979, p. 34)

Color

Each color has its own wavelength in the spectrum of light. Although working in red light has been shown to increase productivity and reduce fatigue, people tire more easily and are more prone to accidents than if they work in a green light vibration (Don, 1977, p. 17). Color can be used to decorate the environment, chosen in color of dress, used in serving attractive meals, and has been used as a treatment for various conditions; thus color can enhance or detract from the quality of life.

ASSESSING ENVIRONMENTAL WELLNESS

Assessments of environmental wellness can be made for the following issues: indoor and outdoor air pollution, water quality, crowding, radiation, consumer products, noise, ions, and use of light/color.

The reactions of household plants to toxic radiation and harmful gasses is one way to assess whether the environment enhances wellness. Impatiens, petunia, clematis, nicotiana, and tradescantia have all proven useful as detectors. In the case of tradescantia, the petals change color from blue to pink (a sign of mutagenesis) when the flower has been exposed to radiation or a gas that is harmful to humans (Liberati, 1982).

The National Cancer Institute found that in certain locales the incidence of canine bladder cancer is an early identifier of human cancers: it takes 20 years for the development of cancer in humans, but only a decade for it to develop in dogs (Watchdog, 1981).

The questions below can be used to assess indoor air pollution problems:

- Does the room seem stuffy and humid?
- Do odors linger for a long time?
- Do eyes get irritated when spending time in the room?
- Are headaches a common complaint after spending time in the room?
- Is there a complaint of difficulty with breathing in the room?
- Is there a complaint of sleepiness while in the room?
- Are cardiovascular symptoms present (associated with cellophane, plastics, extreme temperature changes, hazardous art and hobby supplies)?
- Is asbestos or formaldehyde used in building or consumer products?
- Are aerosols used?
- Are any cleaning agents or solvents used containing carbon tetrachloride, trichlorethylene, perchloroethylene, or benzene?
- Does the individual work in a high risk industry?
- Does the individual handle contaminated clothing belonging to other family members?

- Does the individual (or family member) use chemicals in arts and crafts pursuits?
- Are ventilation and air circulation systems inadequate?
- Does anyone in the work area smoke?

Outdoor pollution can be assessed by asking the following questions:

- Does the individual live near a major expressway or high risk industry?
- Are pesticides sprayed on the lawns or in the air?
- Are toxic waste dumps, nuclear plants, or nuclear testing nearby?

Assessing Water Quality

Water quality can be assessed in a gross manner by eyeballing a glass of it. Some questions to ask are:

- Does the water foam as it splashes into the glass? (can indicate detergent residue)
- Is the water murky? (could indicate clay, silt, metal, synthetic or natural chemical compounds, plankton, microorganisms, sewage, industrial waste, asbestos, soil, or rusty pipes)
- Is the water colored? (indicates the water has not been properly treated or decaying plant matter is entering the water source)
- Does the water have a peculiar taste or odor? (could be due to anything from industrial solvents to a dead animal in the cistern; chlorine adds an unpleasant taste and smell to water)

Most people become accustomed to the taste of their drinking water and may find it difficult to discriminate between good and bad quality water. If drinking water *suddenly* tastes bad, it is an indication that a water test should be completed. Water can be tested by state departments of public health, county health departments, or regional departments of environmental resources.

When it comes to fluoride, more is not better. A new study of 708 children in a city with fluoridated water found that 3 out of 4 had fluorisis, the mottled discoloration of teeth caused by excess fluoride. Mottled teeth can occur even in children who don't drink fluoridated water because many use fluoride supplements, fluoride toothpaste and foods and drinks prepared with fluoridated water.

Because of these risks, children younger than age 6 should brush only with small amounts of fluoridated toothpaste because they tend to swallow too much of their paste when brushing (Lalumandier & Rozier, 1995). The American Dental Association and the American Academy of Pediatrics no longer recommends fluoride supplements for babies under 6 months of age, and recommended doses of fluoride supplements have been lowered for children 6 months to 16 years old.

Crowding

Adverse effects from crowding must be assessed on an individual basis. Individuals of different ethnic groups, ages, or socialization processes may have different needs for personal space; these need to be assessed with each client.

Radiation

Exposure to radiation can be assessed by keeping a record of dental and medication x-rays and frequency of contact with microwave ovens, long distance telephone microwave relay towers, airport radar, nuclear-generating stations, atom bomb tests, fluoroscopes, diathermy, radioactive isotopes, electron microscopes, computers, office machines, high voltage air filters, and radio broadcasting stations.

Consumer Products

Many consumer products can create symptoms. Again, individual differences must be assessed. The listing on page 268, "Consumer Products," provides a starting point. Symptoms which appear to have no organic basis may be due to a hazardous substance. The Health Systems Agency of New York City (111 Broadway, New York, NY 10006) prepared a quick reference guide to the health effects of hazardous substances. The following information may assist in assessing whether symptoms are due to hazardous substances.

Skin Problems. Rashes, irritation, redness, or itching may be due to having touched a metal-cleaner, wood, or food, preserving chemical, a household soap or chemical, or could be a reaction to a food or cosmetic.

Respiratory Problems. Difficulty breathing or lung conditions may be due to exposure to construction or insulation materials, meat wrappings, paint, materials used in textile manufacture or arc-welding, radiological (x-ray) materials, improper ventilation and heating, traffic exhausts, animals, dust, industrial air pollution, or inflight airline services.

Heart and Circulatory Problems. May be due to exposure to traffic exhaust, diesel engine operation, sewage treatment, cellophane, the manufacture of plastic, repairing a motor vehicle, extreme temperature changes, pesticides, or hazardous art and hobby supplies.

Digestive Problems. The most common ones are pain in the abdomen, vomiting, diarrhea, blood stools, or liver disease. May be due to exposure to jewelry making materials, dry cleaning fluid, refrigeration manufacturing, food or printing processing, contact with lead based paints, batteries and electrical equipment, or improperly handled food.

Nervous System Disorders. May be due to exposure to woodworking materials, paints, traffic exhausts, fireproofing, plumbing materials, soldering, manufacture of textiles and petrochemicals, pesticides, or improperly prepared food.

Eye Irritation or Cataracts. Could be due to exposure to petroleum refining, chemical handling, paper production, laundering materials, photographic films, or glass blowing.

Reproductive Problems. May be due to exposure to operating room procedures, such as inhalation or exposure to chemicals, anesthetics, etc., pesticides, or battery components.

Blood Disorders or Cancer (especially leukemia). May be due to exposure to dye manufacturing, dry cleaning, chemical handling, hazardous art or hobby materials, or rodent bites or excretions.

Nose or Sinus Problems (especially inflammation and tumors). May be due to exposure to welding, photoengraving, glass, pottery, linoleum or textile manufacturing, wood or leather products, or battery components.

The relatively new field of clinical ecology examines the effect of the environment on well-being. According to Randolph and Moss (1980), the physical environment can be responsible for conditions ranging from fatigue to headaches, arthritis, colitis, hyperactivity, and depression. Randolph and Moss suggest that clients maintain a 4-day period between eating foods of the same family. Taking the pulse before and after eating offensive foods is used as a measure of allergic response to it. (Pulse either increases or decreases after eating an allergen.) Diamond's (1979) behavioral kinesiology assessments can also be used to determine negative reactions to consumer products.

Assessing Occupational Risks

The list of high risk occupations appears in the section entitled "Occupation." Individuals can be assessed based on this list.

Assessing Noise Risks

Living, working, and playing noise risks can be assessed using the EPA's rule of thumb.

Acid Rain Assessments

A walk around the nearest pond and statue can provide information about the effects of acid rain. There are no measures to date to assess the effects of acid rain on human skin and hair.

Assessment of Air Ions

Assessing the typical weather, proximity of bodies of water, waterfalls, mountains, frequency of showers (all neg-ion producers); use of synthetic fibers, smoking (active or passive), and time spent in hermetically sealed buildings or vehicles (all pos-ion producers) will give a gross ratio of pos-ions to neg-ions.

Light

The ratio of number of hours spent in full-spectrum light to fluorescent light will give a gross measure of well-being due to light source.

Color

Color can be used to stimulate or calm. An assessment of the client's needs in this regard will assist in choosing appropriate colors. Refer to the color intervention section for specific information.

ENVIRONMENTAL INTERVENTIONS

When discussing the environment, it is not unusual to hear a sigh followed by, "But everything causes cancer, so why worry?" The National Cancer Institute has developed a brochure entitled, "Everything Doesn't Cause Cancer" (1980), which may be helpful in these cases.

Points of interest in the brochure include:

- Many cancers can be prevented by reducing exposure to the carcinogens.
- Everything does not cause cancer if the dose is high enough. High doses of many chemicals are toxic, but they will not cause tumors. Other symptoms of toxicity, such as loss of hair or weight, various organic malfunctions and even death, should not be confused with carcinogenesis.
- The risk of cancer may be increased when people are exposed to several carcinogens at the same time, e.g., smoking and working in an asbestos factory.

Environmental interventions include conservation of natural resources, protection from pollutants, and active plans to mold a lifestyle and shape the environment to enhance wellness. The environmental dimension is only part of the whole wellness approach. Thus, interventions are planned to optimize nutritional, stress management, interpersonal, fitness, and self-care approaches.

Plants are a particularly pleasant way to enhance air quality. Some plants which protect against indoor toxins are: Boston fern, chrysanthemum, areca palm, ficus, peace lily, corn plant, dwarf date palm, English ivy, gerbera daisy, *Dracena Marginata* and warneckei (Sick building syndrome? March in plants, 1994).

Unity with the environment is difficult given the stresses and strains of modern life. Table 8.1, Breathe for Unity, provides an opportunity for reestablishing environmental unity.

Table 8.2 provides information regarding protection from some environmental influences.

Table 8.1 Breathe for Unity

Many of us never allow ourselves the luxury and potential well-being we could obtain from getting in touch with Mother Earth. In celebration of your unity with the earth:

- Go outside and find a bit of earth to stand on—your lawn or some grass in a park, sand, a forest, or seashore—somewhere where you feel contact with nature.
- Take off your shoes and socks.
- Undo tight, restrictive clothing.
- Look at the earth beneath your feet and imagine the tremendous energy source available to you.
- Inhale through your nose and visualize breathing in the earth's energy through your feet; imagine it rising up your legs and into your hip socket.
- Think of your feet as spreading and opening to the energy of the earth.
- Exhale through your nose, sending your breath from your coccyx down, down to the very center of the earth.
- Feel yourself beginning to exchange energies with the earth. Draw the earth's energy into your body and send back any darkness or negativity or problems you wish to be rid of.
- Repeat this breath until you feel one with the earth.

Use of Color to Enhance Wellness

Table 8.3 shows use of color to heal. Colors can be worn or colored gel filters can be taped over the bulb of a lamp and placed 4′–8′ away and used in natural, indirect light. Colored paper or fabric swatches can also be used.

The Effect of a Natural Setting on Wellness

One study examined the effect of environment on healing (Ulrich, 1984). The records of 46 post-cholescystectomy clients in a suburban Pennsylvania hospital were examined to determine whether assignment to a room with a window view of a natural setting might have restorative influence. Twenty-three clients assigned to rooms with windows looking out on a natural setting had shorter postoperative stays, received fewer negative evaluative comments in nurses' notes, and took fewer potent analgesics than 23 matched clients with windows facing a brick building wall.

Table 8.2 Protection from Environmental Influences

Harmful substance/ occurrence	Protective measures
1. Hazardous Solid Wastes	Become involved in the assessment and legal processes to monitor solid wastes more carefully; ask to be on local EPA mailing lists for meetings and hearings; talk to state officials to find out state laws and how they will be enforced; subscribe to *Exposure* (The Environmental Action Foundation, 724 Dupont Circle Bldg., Suite 724, Washington, D.C. 20036); obtain a copy of the House of Representatives report on hazardous waste disposal sites and Hunt the Dump instruction packet from A. Blakeman Early, Sierra Club, 330 Penn. Ave., S.E., Washington, D.C. 20003. Vote for politicians with a record of protecting the environment. Recycle and buy recycled products.
2. Air Quality Ventilation	Install a heat exchanger (pulls in fresh air and blows stagnant air out); many air conditioners recirculate the same air; clean reservoirs and change filters in air conditioners; biocidal water treatment can minimize growth of microorganisms in cooling towers (Ager & Tickner, 1983). Have name placed on mailing list to receive *Indoor Air News* (Consumer Federation of America, 1424 16th St., N.W., Washington, D.C. 20036). Vote for politicians with a record of protecting the environment.
Gas stoves	Use electric stoves; gas equipped homes are linked with allergies and respiratory conditions (Randoff & Moss, 1980).
Smoking	Ask visitors who smoke to use the front porch for smoking; stay away from areas where others smoke; increase intake of vitamins C and A.
Formaldehyde	Avoid urea-formaldehyde foam; cover particle board with vinyl wallpaper and paint plywood furniture with low density paint; avoid permanent press clothing, plastic, adhesives, and other items if they seem linked with eye irritation, headache, cough, or skin rashes.
Cars	Walk more often or bike; it's better for air quality and your fitness. Consider car pooling.
Other pollutants and toxic substances	Use recommended houseplants (see p. 278) to detect toxic substances; avoid using disinfectants, air "fresheners," insecticides, aerosols, floor waxes and moth balls (Indoor air pollution and S. 1198 fact sheet, 1985)

Table 8.2 (*continued*)

Harmful substance/ occurrence	Protective measures
3. Water Quality	Install activated carbon filter on drinking water tap or a line bypass system; change filters as product supplier suggests.
Soft water	Disconnect or never install water softener; check drinking water for sodium content; consider breast feeding infants; those at high risk for soft water include those with congestive disease, hypertension, renal disease, cirrhosis of the liver, and infants (Keough, 1980).
Fluoridated water	Those at risk include people who eat large amounts of protein, calcium, vitamin D, take alcohol, and are over 50; increase magnesium intake; use natural fluoride foods including fish, tea, milk, and eggs (Garrison,1985) and/or fluoride toothpastes to protect against dental caries instead of drinking fluoridated water.
4. Crowding	Redesign environment or use stress reduction techniques to decrease crowding effects.
5. Radiation	Use food substances that bind radioactive materials and help excrete them: sea kelp, apples, slightly unripe fruit, sunflower seeds, miso, calcium tablets or calcium-rich foods, B-vitamins, buck wheat, sprouted seeds, peanut or olive oil, raw leafy green vegetables, vitamin C tablets or vitamin C-rich foods.
x-rays	Avoid unnecessary x-rays; dental x-rays only every 3–5 years (American Dental Association) or every 6–10 years (other authorities); ask for thermography instead of x-rays; inquire about the reliability of the x-ray procedure; ask for specific dose that will be received; insist on hearing the benefits in detail; only have x-rays done by a specialist or in a radiology department by a certified technician using up-to-date equipment, small doses, and adequate body shields. Especially at risk are young women who suspect breast cancer, pregnant women, children, and unborn fetuses (Abrams, 1979; Epstein, 1978.)
Smoke detectors	Avoid standing under a smoke detector; discard when cracked (Clark, 1982; George,1985).

Table 8.2 (*continued*)

Harmful substance/ occurrence	Protective measures
Luminous dials	Avoid wearing a watch with a luminous dial or sleeping next to a clock with a luminous dial.
Microwave relay high relay towers for telephone and television	Look for neighborhood towers; avoid buying a home or living near one.
Microwave ovens	Check yearly for leakage; avoid opening and closing unnecessarily or banging its sides.
Checkpoints at airports or department stores	Move speedily through checkpoints; stay far away from x-ray of luggage and pick up belongings only at end of ramp.
Radon	Have house tested for radon emissions.
6. Consumer Products	Read labels and purchase only those products that enhance well-being; contact CPSC for guidelines (1111 18th St., N.W., Washington, D.C. 20207).
Alcohol	Avoid alcoholic drinks and increase intake of recommended vitamins and minerals when drinking.
Additives	Processed, junk foods contain high amounts of additives and are low in nutrient quality. Avoid saccharin, foods with red dye #40 and synthetic coal tar dyes, certified colors, cosmetic food additives, and nitrites found in sandwich meats, salami, bologna, hot dogs, smoked meats and fish, and bacon (Epstein, 1978). Vote for politicians who have a record of protecting consumers.
Aluminum cookware	Use iron, glass, or stainless steel cookware.
Cans with leaded seams	Choose food packaged in other types of containers; never leave opened cans in the refrigerator; place unused contents in a glass container and seal; increase intake of vitamins A, C, E, and selenium.
Benzene	Artists and hobbyists using products containing benzene can consider substitute products and increase their intake of vitamin C.
Cadmium in artist and hobbyist materials	Increase selenium and zinc intake; correct any iron deficiencies; use substitute materials.

Table 8.2 (*continued*)

Harmful substance/ occurrence	Protective measures
Cigarettes	Stop smoking to reduce risks of cancer of the larynx, lungs, esophagus, mouth, bladder, and heart disease.
Cleaners, aerosols waxes	Be aware that many cleaners contain unlisted toxic ingredients. Use organic cleaners (*Octagon* brown soap and cold water will remove most stains); *Twenty Mule Team Borax* softens water, disinfects and controls molds and odors and is made from a naturally occurring mineral; *Bon Ami Polishing Cleanser* (unlike other scouring powders) contains no chlorine; use *Murphy's Oil Soap and Arm & Hammer Baking Soda* to remove stains and odors; avoid aerosols, and use paste rather than spray waxes and only in well-ventilated areas; wear gloves when touching strong chemicals; contact Women's Occupational Health Research Center, School of Public Health, Columbia University, 60 Haven Ave, B-1, New York, NY 10032.
Constrictive clothes, especially bras	Avoid wearing tight clothing which impedes lymphatic flow and thereby the removal of toxins from tissue. Consider eliminating tight collars, ties, girdles, knee-high hose, belts, tight jeans, push-ups/restricting bras. If you suffer red marks or irritation after wearing, your lymph system has been restricted.
Cosmetics	Avoid purchasing any products carrying a warning label, 2, 4-toluene-diamine or 4 methoxy-in-phenylene-diamine, yellow #1, blue #6, and reds #10–13 (used in lipsticks and soaps primarily).
Estrogens	Use other forms of birth control; take additional magnesium if on "the pill"; refuse "morning after" pills (DES) offered in some clinics to disrupt pregnancy; use vitamin E for debilitating symptoms of menopause; take estrogens only at low doses for short periods of time.

Table 8.2 (*continued*)

Harmful substance/ occurrence	Protective measures
Hair dyes	Read labels carefully; write to manufacturers for information; medium and dark-haired people can use henna; streaking, tipping, or frosting are safer and should be used instead of dyes; use natural hair tints such as lemon juice, camomile tea, cloves and alka-net.
Prescribed drugs	Be apprised of *all* risks before deciding to submit to treatment; read all inserts and relevant portions of the *PDR*; choose less toxic alternatives when possible, e.g., brown soap assists in healing many skin conditions; application of vitamin E (oil capsules) assists in healing burns, cuts, sores, etc.; use preventive methods (stress reduction, nutrition, color, reflexology, etc.) so drugs are not needed.
Seat belts	Wear seat belts and ensure that all those riding in the car do.
Toys	Choose age-appropriate toys; supervise play and maintain ground rules.
Pesticides	Use natural repellents; use dormant oil sprays; plant native trees, vines, hedges and flowers instead of grass to deter insects conserve water and energy; energy; buy more organically grown fruits and vegetables and ask your store manager to carry them; plant marigolds and nasturtiums in the garden to deter insects; plant garlic or use as a spray on plant leaves; buy or feed ladybugs, praying mantises, wasps, birds, and toads; hang a bouquet of dried tomato leaves in rooms to repel mosquitos, flies, and spiders; place dried lavender, cedar chips, or rosemary in bags to deter moths; sprinkle crushed catnip or ant rails; use citronella and lavender oil to repel biting insects.
7. Occupation	Contact OSHA (Labor Dept., 200 Constitution Ave., N.W., Washington, D.C. 20210) regarding policies, laws, and programs. Demand informed consent regarding dangers and a surveillance program to follow up worker symptoms and treatment. Include occupational health in contract or collective bargaining agreements; serve on hospital planning

Table 8.3 (*continued*)

Harmful substance/ occurrence	Protective measures
7. Occupation (*cont'd*)	committees to ensure future additions; meet wellness and safety standards; report any hazards to appropriate superior or union representative in writing; keep a copy and send one to the appropriate agency if no action is taken; the law protects against firing for a workplace complaint. Workers (including nurses, dental assistants, x-ray technicians, and monitors at airport checkpoints) should wear a film badge; stand at least 6′ away from x-ray source; wear lead shields; limit time with clients with radioactive implants; and use gloves/forceps and appropriate disposal procedures for contaminated items. Parents should inspect schools for asbestos and unsafe laboratory or physical education practices (Mancino, 1983).
8. Noise	Wear earplugs if exposed to loud engines; plan some time daily in a quiet, restful environment; ensure employers monitor noise levels; union representatives have the right to observe monitoring and obtain records; by law, hearing protectors must be available to workers exposed to 85 DB or more (OSHA Standards, 1981).
9. Acid Rain	Wear protective covering on hair and skin when out in the rain; work with environmentalists to control the effects of acid rain. Vote for politicians who have a record of protecting the environment.10.10.
10. Pos-ions	Spend time out of hermetically sealed buildings, preferably at the seashore or mountains; take a shower daily; walk amongst plants and trees daily.
11. Light	
Sunlight	Wear a sunscreen (PABA) and protective clothing when in direct sunlight; avoid long hours in the sun.
Fluorescent light	Choose full-spectrum fluorescent light if full spectrum natural light is not available; if in a tightly sealed building during daylight hours, walk to work or park 20 minutes from work; go outside during lunch and breaks; avoid sunglasses; use Vitalites for desk or kitchen lighting.

Table 8.3 Use of Color to Heal

Red	Invigorates, stimulates, energizes. Good for anemia, poor blood circulation, liver and heart conditions. Not suggested for use in highly emotional states.
Pink	Use for pelvic probems, hip and buttock tenderness. Stimulates caring and love.
Orange	Invigorates and stimulates feeling and endocrine action; stimulates confidence, respiratory action, relieves gas and sluggish digestion, drains infections, decreases menstrual discomfort. Wearing an orange scarf around the neck is useful for thyroid conditions.
Yellow	Stimulates the nervous system and brain activity. Increases receptivity for knowledge, self-confidence, appetite, enhances liver and gall bladder functions. Assists in dissolving arthritic deposits.
Lemon (yellow with some green)	Cleans mucus, activates the thymus gland, builds bone, speeds up the healing process of a cold. Relieves the body of muscular tension.
Green	Stabilizes and calms. Used for high blood pressure, hot flashes, menopause, infections, and resistance to healing. Stimulates the pituitary.
Turquoise	Reduces aches and pains, skin conditions.
Blue	Stimulates the pineal gland and deep sleep. Assists with fever process.
Indigo	Sedative. Reduces swelling and pain. Firms skin.
Violet	Muscle relaxant. Builds white blood cells and depresses the appetite.
Purple	Slows heart rate and reduces heart pain. Increases venous drainage during systemic congestion and excessive menstruation.
Scarlet	Stimulates heart rate and arterial action. Revives kidney and adrenal function.
All colors	Sunlight. The great healer for all conditions.

Adapted from: D. Berkson., *The Foot Book.* New York: Harper and Row, 1977, pp. 204–206.

INTEGRATIVE LEARNING EXPERIENCES

Beginning Level

1. Assess the environmental factors influencing your level of wellness. Discuss these with a peer and devise an action plan (in writing with realistic dates for evaluating and rewarding progress). Refer to Table 8.2 for ideas.
2. Write one or more of the wellness-oriented organizations in the Resources Section, pp. 334–338 for further information.

3. Identify the specific environmental contributions for clients with the following conditions.

    A. Birth defects
    B. Spontaneous abortion
    C. Upper respiratory ailments/difficulty breathing
    D. Cancer risk
    E. High absenteeism
    F. High blood pressure
    G. Bone disease in clients receiving dialysis
    H. Neurological symptoms
    I. Skin irritation/rashes
    J. Asbestosis
    K. Loss of appetite, constipation, nausea, tremors, weakness, numbness, colic, and kidney disease
    L. Hearing loss, elevated blood pressure, tension, nervousness, fluid imbalances
    M. Fatigue, tension, hyperactivity
    N. Circulatory difficulties
    O. Cataracts

4. Investigate the use of color in your lifestyle and its effects. Devise a plan to use color as an environmental intervention.

Advanced Level

1. Collaborate with three clients to devise a plan to enhance their environmental wellness.

REFERENCES

Abrams, H. (1979). The "overutilization" of x-rays. *NEJ Med* 300(21):1213:1216.

Ager, B., and Tickner, J. (1983). The control of microbiological hazards associated with air-conditioning and ventilating systems. *Annals Occupt Hyg* 27(4):346–358.

Bongard, F. et al. (1981). Fatal hospital-acquired burns. *JAMA* 252(20):2813.

Brown, H., Bishop, D., and Rowan, C. (1984). Drinking water safety. *Am J PH* 74:479.

Bryce, R., and Enkin, M. (1984). Lifestyle in pregnancy. *Can Phys* 30:2127-2130.

Casdorph, H., and Walker, M. (1995), *Toxic Mental Syndrome*. Garden City Park, NY: Avery Publishing Group.

Ciccone, J.C. (1989). Noise: The most pervasive pollution in America. *Media Update Am Speech-Language-Hearing Assoc* (Fall):1.

Clark, C.C. (1981). Reader queries: safe ways to control insects. *The Wellness Newsletter* 2(5):3.

Clark, C.C. (1983). From the editor. *The Wellness Newsletter* 4(5):1-2.

Diamond, J. (1979). *Behavioral Kinesiology*. New York: Harper & Row.

Dickson, D. (1979). US academy denies threshold for radiation. *Nature* 279:90–91.

Diesendorf, M. (1980). Is there a scientific basis for fluoridation? A review of the report by the Royal College of Physicians. *Com IIIth Studies* 4(3):224–230.

Dioxin risks found greater than had been thought (1994). *EDF Letter* 25(6): 1,3.

Don, F. (1977). *Color Your World.* New York: Warner Destiny Books.

Environmental Protection Agency. (1993). *Respiratory health effects of passive smoking.* Washington, D.C.: United States Environmental Protection Agency. 4 pps.

Epstein, S. (1978). *The Politics of Cancer.* San Francisco: Sierra Club.

Fagerstrom, K. (1984). Effects of nicotine chewing gum and follow up appointments in physician-based smoking cessation. *Prev Med* 13(5):517-527.

Falck, F., Ricci, A., Wolff, M.S. et al. (1992). Pesticides and polychlorinated biphenyl residues in human breast lipids and their relation to breast cancer. *Arch Environ. Hlth.* (March/April): 143-146.

Forskningsroen, N. (1984). Passive smoking and the infant. *Tobaken Och Vi* 29(3):7–9.

Fumigants used in the food industry. (1983). *Staying Alive Safety and Health News of the Food and Beverage Trades* 22:1-2.

Garrison, R.H. (1985). *Nutrition Desk Reference.* New Canaan, CT: Keats Publishing Co., p. 65.

George, A. (1985). Measurement of sources and air concentrations of radon and radon daughters in residential buildings. Paper presented at the ASHRAE Semi-Annual Meeting, June 23-27, Atlanta, GA.

Health People 2000. (1990). Washington, D.C.: U.S. Department of Health and Human Services, Public Health Service.

Houck, C. (1979). Caution: artificial light may be hazardous to your health. *Review* March:27–34.

Indoor air pollution and S. 1198 fact sheet. (1985). Washington D.C.: Consumer Federation of America, p. 1.

Isaacson, R.L., and Jensen, K.F. (1992). *The Vulnerable Brain and Environmental Risks.* NY: Plenum Press.

Keough, C. (1980). *Water Fit to Drink.* Emmaus, PA: Rodale Press, Inc.

Lalumandier, J.A. and Rozier, R.G. (1995). Prevalence and risk factors of fluorosis among patients and pediatric dental practice. *Pediatric Dentistry* 17:19.

Liberati, L. (1982). *Lawrence Rev Natural Prods.* 3(1):1.

Liberman, J. (1991). *Light Medicine of the Future.* Santa Fe: Bear & Co.

Mancino, D. (1983). Creating a safe hospital environment. *The Wellness Newsletter,* 4(5):3–5.

Mendelsohn, R. (1979). *Confessions of a Medical Heretic.* Chicago, IL: Contemporary Books, Inc.

Naeye, R., and Peter, E. (1984). Mental development of children whose mothers smoked during pregnancy. *Obstetrics and Gyn* 64(5):601–607.

NIH. (1980). *Basic Concepts of Environmental Health.* Research Triangle Park, NC: NIH Publication #80-1254.

Office of Disease Prevention and Health Promotion. (1988). *Disease Prevention/Health Promotion: The Facts.* Palo Alto, CA: Bull Publishing Co., pp. 4–7.

OSHA standards: 1981 to 1984. (1984). *Exposure* 41:8–11.

Ott, J. (1973). *Health and Light.* New York: Simon and Schuster.

Rall, D. (1984). Toxic agent and radiation control: meeting the 1990 objectives for the nation. *Public Health Reports* 99(6):532–538.

Raloff, J. (1982). Noise can be hazardous to our health. *Sci News* 121: 377–381.

Randolf, T., and Moss, R. (1980). *An Alternative Approach to Allergies.* New York: Harper & Row.

Regne, J. (1984). More than what you drink. *Exposure* 41:2.

Rosenfield, A. (1978). Forecast: poisonous rain. *Saturday Rev* Sept:16–17.

Sandler, D., et al. (1985). Cancer risk in adulthood from early exposure to parents' smoking. *Am J PH* 75(5):487–492.

Sick building syndrome? March in the plants. (1994) n.a. *The Western Way* 20(2):17.

Singer, S.R. and Grismaijer, S. (1995). *Dressed to Kill: the Link Between Breast Cancer and Bras.* Garden City, NY: Avery Publishing Group.

Soyka, F. (1977). *The Ion Effect.* New York: Bantam.

Tedesco, P. (1982). ANA delegates take two strong environmental stands. *Health watch.* 3(2):1, 9.

Ulrich, R. (1984). View through a window may influence recovery from surgery. *Science* 224:420–421.

U.S. Dept. HEW. (1977). Statistics needed for determining the effects of the environment on health. Hyattsville, MD: Office of Health Research, Statistics, and Technology.

Voldman, E. (1983). Socially accepted drugs and pregnancy. I. Cigarettes and pregnancy. *Revista de Obstet y Gyn de Venezuela* 43(2):59–61.

Water-drinking disorder. (1995). *The Amicus J* 17(1):7.

Watchdog. (1981). *Exposure* 9 (July):1.

Wolff, M., Toniolo, P.G., Lea, E.W. et al. (1993). Blood levels of organochlorine residues and risk of breast cancer. *J. Nat'l. Cancer Inst.* 85(8):648–652.

9

COMMUNITY WELLNESS PROGRAMS

This chapter discusses the following information:

- Justification for community wellness programs
- Assessing wellness program needs
- A community assessment tool
- Suggestions for planning and implementing wellness programs
- Methods of evaluating wellness programs

JUSTIFICATION FOR COMMUNITY WELLNESS PROGRAMS

Healthy People 2000 (1990) provides specific objectives for enhancing community health. Table 9.1 (p. 292) provides selected health promotion objectives. Other priority areas include: alcohol and other drugs, family planning, mental health, violent and abusive behavior, and educational and community-based programs. *Healthy People 2000* also addresses areas of health protection and preventive services and can be obtained from the U.S. Government Printing Office, Superintendent of Documents, Mail Stop: SSOP Washington, D.C. 20402–9328.

Common sense dictates that preventing illness saves money, yet the majority of the health care dollar is spent treating illness, not preventing it. Even if the money were available, the question would be: Which individual habits affect the cost the most? A number of recent studies have provided information regarding how wellness programs reduce illness care costs or affect behavior positively.

One study combined the resources of Milliman & Robertson, Inc., a healthcare consulting firm, Staywell Health Management Systems, Inc., Chrysler Corporation, and the International Union, UAW (Anderson, Brink, &

Courtney, 1995). Health status information was provided by StayWell for Chrysler employees enrolled in a voluntary wellness program.

The researchers studied 10 different health behaviors: smoking, weight control, exercise, alcohol use, driving habits, eating habits, stress, mental health, cholesterol, and blood pressure. Medical utilization and cost data were analyzed for low and elevated levels of risk for each category.

They found a significant difference in the costs of medical care by health risk status. A person with an elevated level of risk generally uses more medical care. The extent of the effect varied by the behavior being analyzed. For example, persons who smoked experienced 31% higher claim costs than those who did not smoke. Employees outside the healthy weight range had a 143% higher hospital inpatient utilization than those in the healthy weight range. Those with poor eating habits generate 41% higher claim costs than employees with good eating habits. Overall claim costs for the elevated risk group were 24% higher than the low risk group. Employees at elevated risk for stress experience 13% higher hospital inpatient utilization and a 26% higher utilization of physician services than the persons at low risk. Costs experienced by employees classified as at an elevated risk for mental health (feels depressed some or most of the time) were 13% higher than the lower risk group (feels depressed only rarely).

Costs for employees with elevated (total cholesterol level of 200 or more) versus low risk cholesterol levels (total cholesterol level less than 200) were nearly the same. There remains a controversy over whether cholesterol levels are related to longevity. Also, given the long-term nature of cardiovascular conditions, a longitudinal study effect of high cholesterol level on costs may be more pertinent.

Claim costs for employees with a systolic reading of 140 or more and/or a diastolic reading of 90 or more were only 7% higher than those with a systolic reading of less than 140 and a diastolic reading of less than 90. However, hospital inpatient utilization was 24% higher and utilization of physician services was 11% higher for the high risk group.

Such information can be useful to companies and wellness programs who wish to enhance wellness in employees as well as save money. For example, a program to encourage employees to quit smoking would likely generate more near-term cost savings than an effort to encourage employees to lower their cholesterol level.

Interestingly, those at high risk for exercise-related claims (exercised aerobically for at least 20 minutes less than once a week), showed only 8% higher claim costs than those with low risk (exercised aerobically one or more times a week). However, the low risk requirement may not be sufficient to discriminate between groups very well. (Many fitness experts recommend exercising 3–4 times/week. See the fitness chapter for more information.)

Although the Anderson et al. study (1995) did not show a significant impact of exercise on cardiovascular fitness, another study did. Heirich et al. (1993) compared the impact of different program designs on cardiovascular risks. Four automotive manufacturing plants participated over a 3-year span, with one

PHYSICAL ACTIVITY AND FITNESS

1. Reduce overweight to a prevalence of no more than 20% among people age 20 and older and no more than 15% among adolescents age 12 through 19. (Baseline: 26% aged 20 and older, 15% aged 12 through 19 in 1976–1980)

2. Increase to at least 30% the proportion of people age 6 years and older who regularly (preferably daily) engage in light to moderate physical activity for at least 30 minutes per day.

3. Reduce to no more than 15% the proportion of people age 6 years and older who engage in no leisure time physical activity. (Baseline: 24% aged 18 and older in 1985)

4. Increase the proportion of worksites offering employer-sponsored physical activity and fitness programs as follows:

50–99 employees	20%	(1985 Baseline: 14%
100–249 employees	35%	23%
250–749 employees	50%	32%
≥ 750 employees	80%	54%)

5. Increase to at least 50% the proportion of primary care providers who routinely assess and counsel their patients regarding the frequency, duration, type, and intensiity of each patient's physical activity practices. (Baseline: 30% of sedentary patients counseled in 1988)

NUTRITION

1. Reduce growth retardation among low-income children age 5 years and younger to less than 10%. (Baseline: Up to 16% in 1988)

2. Reduce dietary fat intake to an average of 30% of calories or less and saturated fat intake to an average or less than 10% of calories among people age 2 years and older.

3. Decrease salt and sodium intake so that at least 65% of home meal preparers cook without adding salt, at least 80% of people avoid using salt at the table, and at least 40% of adults regularly purchase foods modified or lower in sodium. (Baseline: 54%, 68%, and 20%, respectively)

4. Reduce iron deficiency to less than 3% among children age 1 through 4 and among women of childbearing age.

5. Increase to at least 75% the proportion of mothers who breast-feed their infants in the early postpartum period and to at least 50% the proportion who continue breast-feeding until their infants are 5 to 6 months old. (Baseline: 54% and 21%, respectively)

6. Increase to at least 90% the proportion of restaurants and institutional food service operations that offer identifiable low-fat, low-calorie food choices, consistent with the Dietary Guidelines for Americans.

7. Increase to at least 90% the proportion of school lunch and breakfast services and child care food services with menus that are consistent with the nutrition principles in the Dietary Guidelines for Americans.

8. Increase to at least 75% the proportion of primary care providers who provide nutrition assessment and counseling or referral to qualified nutritionists or dietitians. (Baseline: Physicians provide diet counseling to 40 to 50% of patients in 1988)

Table 9.1 (*continued*)

TOBACCO

1. Reduce cigarette smoking to a prevalence of no more than 15% among people age 20 years and older. (Baseline: 29% in 1987)
2. Reduce the initiation of cigarette smoking by children and youths so that no more than 15% become regular cigarette smokers by age 20 years. (Baseline: 30% in 1987)
3. Reduce to no more than 20% the proportion of children age 6 years and younger who are regularly exposed to tobacco smoke at home. (Baseline: 39% in 1986)
4. Establish tobacco-free environments and include tobacco use prevention in the curricula of all elementary, middle, and secondary schools, preferably as part of quality school health education. (Baseline: 17% of schools banned smoking in 1988; 75% had curricula)
5. Increase to at least 75% the proportion of worksites with a formal smoking policy that prohibits or severely restricts smoking at the workplace. (Baseline: 54% of medium and large companies in 1987)
6. Enact in all 50 states comprehensive laws on clean indoor air that prohibit or strictly limit smoking in the workplace and in enclosed public places. (Baseline: 12 states in 1990)
7. Increase to at least 75% the proportion of primary care and oral health care providers who routinely advise cessation and provide assistance and follow-up for all of their tobacco-using patients. (Baseline: 52% of internists counseled 75% of their smoking patients in 1986)

PRIMARY CARE

1. Provide quality K–12 school health education in at least 75% of schools.
2. Provide employee health promotion activities in at least 85% of workplaces with 50 or more employees.

(Also see last objective under each section above.)

* Adapted from United States Department of Health and Human Services. (1990). *Healthy People 2000: National health promotion and disease prevention objectives. Summary report.* Washington, DC: U.S. Government Printing Office.

designated as the control site. Of the remaining three, the first site created a fitness facility complete with equipment and mandated every employee with a disability to use the facility. The second location employed two wellness counselors to provide one-to-one counseling for employees with cardiovascular risks, and encouraged them to create their own personal exercise program. The last plant used outreach and counseling for all employees in conjunction with organized fitness activities. The two programs using counseling and outreach were more effective in getting employees with cardiovascular risks to exercise three or more times a week. The plant with just a fitness facility showed a weight gain among employees who were 20% overweight before the study. The authors suggested employee fitness programs include health professionals who regularly inform the participants about the health risks of cardiovascular conditions, and combine counseling and outreach efforts.

Arbeit et al. (1992), found that a Heart Smart cardiovascular school health promotion—including a school lunch program reducing fat to 30% and sodium and sugar to 50%, a physical education program promoting personal fitness and aerobic conditioning, and cardiovascular risk screening— evoked decreased cholesterol levels and improvements in run/walk performance.

Kagan et al. (1995) conducted a 3-year field study of 373 employees in the emergency medical service of a municipal fire department. A framework for defining and categorizing psychoeducational stress reduction programs was developed. The overall effect of a single program as well as combinations of programs were determined. Findings supported the value of psychoeducational programs for preventive mental health in the workplace.

Ruffing-Rahal (1994) reported the evaluation of a group health promotion program with community-dwelling older women, a majority of whom were African American. The intervention group showed significant increases in well-being, health practices and life satisfaction, compared to controls.

Olds et al. (1993) completed a series of randomized trials showing that pre-natal and infancy nurse home visits improved a wide range of wellness out-comes (reduced smoking, improved diets, reduced pre-term deliveries, increased birthweights, reduced child abuse and neglect and emergency room visits, in-crease in mothers' participation in the workforce, decreased subsequent preg-nancies and government expenditures for poor unmarried teenaged women bearing their first child).

A randomized controlled trial of antismoking advice for 10 years (Rose et al., 1982) provided advice to 1,445 male smokers aged 40–59 at high risk of cardiorespiratory disease. After 1 year reported cigarette consumption in the intervention group (714 men) was one fourth that of the control group (731 men). At 10 years the reported reduction averaged 53%. Over 10 years death from coronary heart disease was 18% lower and mortality from lung cancer was 23% lower in the intervention group than in the control group. However, deaths from other types of cancers were significantly higher in the interven-tion group. The nonlung cancers seemed unrelated to changes in smoking hab-its.

Pillsbury Company's Be Your Best Program has offerings in three lifestyle areas: (1) fitness and exercise, (2) nutrition and weight control, and (3) mental well-being and stress management. Twice a year the complete program, featur-ing assessments to determine health risk factors and education workshops, is offered to 200 employees. The most signficant benefit is that employees who participate in the program submit fewer claims and that those claims submitted were less costly than claims made prior to involvement in the program. The program director estimates that for the years 1981–1982 there was a $3.63 return on every $1.00 invested in the program.

Some of the major difficulties in obtaining data to support wellness program efforts are: the time lag between starting the program and seeing an impact, difficulty in analyzing individual components of the program to distinguish cause and effect relationships, and self-selection of participants.

Although not focused on employees, a study completed by Vickery et al. (1983) provides support for the cost benefits of educating clients about their own care. A prospective randomized, controlled trial of self-care educational intervention conducted in an HMO showed statistically significant decreases in total medical visits and minor illness visits in three experimental groups as compared to the control group. The results were clearly linked to receiving books and a newsletter presenting self-care information. A telephone information service was available but was not used. Estimated savings in utilization were between $2.50 and $3.50 for each dollar spent on the educational interventions. The addition of a nurse counseling session to the written information was suggested as a way to further increase cost savings and appeared to be attractive to high utilizers of services.

Glanz (1994) reviewed and summarized evidence regarding the association of dietary factors including alcohol intake, with breast cancer risk and survival. Although the evidence is inconclusive, total fat intake, saturated fat intake, obesity, and moderate to heavy alcohol consumption have shown to be risk factors. Fiber, fruits and vegetables, vitamins A and C, and soy products may have protective effects. Clear evidence exists from clinical trials that intensive educational and behavioral interventions can be effective for promoting lower-fat diets. Clinical interventions and community-based studies using combinations of educational and environmental strategies have achieved significant, though smaller, changes across large populations. Research needs include investigating influences on the maintenance of dietary change, examining the role of readiness to adopt new eating patterns and continuous refinement of measures.

Angotti and Levine (1994) reported a 5-year clinical experience with combined dietary and exercise interventions to reduce cholesterol levels at NASA. They found that decreased cardiovascular risk could easily be accomplished at the worksite when dietary intervention, personal monitoring, and a reasonable exercise program were used.

ASSESSING WELLNESS PROGRAM NEEDS

All communities, schools, companies, and agencies can benefit from wellness programs. Many have already developed them; however, they may have been based on what the planners believed were important; a wellness view includes the client in the planning process. Some questions to ask and methods to use to begin to assess the wellness program needs have been suggested by Parkinson (1982, pp. 22–26):

- What are the sociodemographic characteristics of the population? (Determine age, sex, ethnic origin, occupation, employment status, education, and residence using a health history or risk-appraisal form.)
- What are the costs of health care, disability benefits, and insurance premiums for the population? (Determine number and cost, including any insurance claims, and average the rate by the number of people; determine the number, frequency, duration, and costs of incidental and disability absences.)
- What are the use patterns for health care by the population? (Determine what kinds of preventive and wellness issues are brought to health care providers; what chronic and acute conditions are being treated; talk with health care providers and obtain summaries of use patterns if possible.)

- What conditions or diseases are present or potential in the population? (Randomly sample the population or obtain a representative sample and use written questionnaires, phone interviews, or one-to-one interviews to obtain information); determine blood pressure, height, weight, lipids, blood sugar, and other information indicative of wellness state; survey current lifestyle habits (nutrition, exercise/movement, stress management skills, parenting skills, communication skills, knowledge of how to obtain wellness information, self-care skills, smoking, drinking, use of drugs and medications); if necessary, determine those at highest risk and plan programming accordingly.
- What wellness programs are currently available for the population? (Talk with providers of programs and participants or use questionnaires to obtain needed information; for certain populations, the media may publicize programs; in these cases, obtain information from the media or public relations department.)
- How effective are the current wellness programs in enhancing wellness? (Obtain evaluation information from program providers and interview or survey participants.)
- What wellness needs does the population identify? (Interview or survey the population or a representative sample.)
- What kinds of wellness programs does the population think should be included? (Interview or survey the population or a representative sample.)
- What are the levels of needs in the population—awareness, knowledge, change in attitudes, change in behavior, reduction in risk or reduction in disease or death? (If sufficient funds and time are available, all levels can be developed; if not, use interview, survey, and information collected from the results of answering the above questions to make a determination.)

Community Assessment

The Community Assessment (Table 9.2) gives information for assessing wellness in a community.

Table 9.2 Community Assessment

Who and What Is the Community?

1. How is space distributed and used? (Buildings, crowded areas, natural and physical barriers to social interaction, parks, playgrounds?)

2. How safe and healthful are work and school environments? (Are smokers and non-smokers segregated? Are junk food and cigarette vending machines highly accessible? Are alternatives offered? Is the use of stairways promoted? Are they accessible? Well lit? Is car pooling encouraged? Is flex time used to allow employees time to engage in wellness activities before work or during lunch? Are high quality child care services available for residents? Are buildings well ventilated and do they have adequate natural light and sufficient work/learning space?)

3. What are the cultural mix and stability of the population? (Are there one or more cultural groups living in harmony or in conflict, and how much acculturation and stress occur due to people who move in or out of the area?)

Table 9.2 (*continued*)

4.   What are the age, sex, and family groupings? (Elderly population, single-occupancy commuter group, young marrieds with children, singles, a mix?)

5.   What income levels are represented and to what extent? (Wealthy? Middle class? Poor people receiving governmental or charitable assistance for health care? Or a mix?)

6.   What are the occupational levels? (Hard driving executives who leave the family's health concerns to their wives? Action-oriented population that learns by doing? A mix? What does the occupational level tell you about the population's education, health problems, problem solving patterns, and methods of learning?)

7.   What community resources are available and where are they? (Where are the schools, hospitals, shopping areas, and clinics located in relation to available transportation? What self-help or supportive groups and services exist in the community? What facilities are there for wellness programs? What space could be developed to provide further wellness services? What skills or resources do the residents have that could be shared through a wellness program exchange? Is there any way to trade unused sick leave for a well day? Could unused sick leave be converted to cash? Do faculty, bosses, or town legislators support personal health promotion objectives? Can additional rewards or incentives be built into the current health/illness insurance programs without taking away existing benefits? If there are company or school-subsidized cafeterias, could wellness-promoting foods be subsidized more than junk foods?

How Are Needs Met?

1.   Are needs met or prevented from being met by space, culture, age, sex, family, income, occupational level, or community resource factors?

2.   What do the community's clergy, health care practitioners, welfare agencies, and clients know about what needs are not being met?

3.   What do records of health services, worker's compensation claims, and accident and safety records tell you about how needs are met and what wellness needs are not being met?

4.   What do questionnaire or survey methods tell you about what community residents say are the types of wellness activities they would participate in if offered?

5.   What specific risk factors exist in this population and how are they being addressed or not?

6.   How can family members of community residents be considered in planning wellness programs and used to provide needed support systems?

How Are Deviance and Disturbance Handled?

1.   Are those with psychiatric/mental health difficulties rejected by the community? In what way?

2.   How are delinquents or those who abuse alcohol, drugs, or food treated by community members?

3.   What political, educational, or social views lead to rejection or those who deviate from the norm?

4.   Are there humane or highly institutionalized agencies available in the community to help deal with deviate members? What are they?

5.   Does the community reject the idea of placing treatment facilities for its deviants within the community? How?

6.   Is there a prevailing view that people who deviate from accepted behavioral patterns should be punished? How is this belief put into practice?

Table 9.2 (*continued*)

How Are Identities Developed?

1. How do families, faculty, administrators, etc. teach their members to act?

2. What kinds of religious/spiritual organizations or groups exist in the community and what is their prevailing view of human motivation?

3. What youth agencies/helpers are there and how do young people relate to them?

4. What kind of formal and special education programs are available and how are they used by the community?

5. How could already existing agencies or groups be used more effectively?

How are Community Functions Accomplished?

1. Are community decisions made before adequate information has been obtained? What possible effect(s) might this have?

2. Are decisions made by default, based on the personal concerns of a few, or made by consensus? What are the consequences of this type of decision making?

3. Is communication fragmented and inefficient? How does such communication seem to affect the community?

4. Are communication messages based on a sense of community ("We're all in this together") or on stereotypes and the establishment of distance between groups ("It's us against them")? What are the effects of both types of communication messages?

5. How accurately do the local media convey information to the community?

6. Are there informal (rumor) communication channels?

7. Are problems solved informally with board and committee meetings used only to record earlier decisions? How might this affect the community or the decision-making process?

8. How are ad hoc, neighborhood, or block associations used in decision making?

9. How readily are newcomers accepted by the community?

10. Is leadership concentrated among a few groups or is it widely distributed in the community?

11. Are there wide vacillations in power or frequent changes in the power base that could affect health planning or treatment?

12. Where is power located, how is it perceived, and how is it used?

13. What overlapping areas and missing links are there in wellness services?

14. What segments in the community are receptive and hostile to outside influence?

15. Is there a sense of trust between community members and leaders?

16. Is there community disintegration? (Has a recent disaster, widespread ill health, extensive poverty, confusion of cultural values, weakening of religious affiliations, extensive migration of new groups, or rapid social change radically affected the community?)

What Are the Resistances to Change in This Community?

1. What factors in the system will be affected as a result of a change toward wellness?

2. What forces are operating to inhibit change toward wellness?

Table 9.2 (*continued*)

3.   What information or experiences must precede the change toward wellness?

4.   What new procedures or experiences will need to be developed as a result of a movement toward wellness?

5.   Who is likely to suffer from the change?

6.   How aware of the need for change are community residents ?

7.   Are community residents sufficiently involved in planning for the change?

8.   What is the relationship between the change agent and community residents?

9.   What past relationship between the change agent and the client might be influencing resistance to change now?

10.   How open have community residents been to the introduction of change in the past?

11.   How can free and open communications, administrative support of and reward for problem solving efforts, shared decision making, sufficient time to problem solve, written statements of what the change goals will be, professionalism, concern for long-term planning, cohesiveness among change agents, feelings of security among residents, timing, and resident confidence in ability to change be enhanced to lower resistance to change?

PLANNING AND IMPLEMENTING WELLNESS PROGRAMS

Worksite Wellness Programs

Parkinson (1982, p. 9) suggests that a worksite wellness program focus on all of the following: high blood pressure control, smoking control, drug/alcohol abuse control, weight control and nutrition education, exercise/physical fitness, early cancer detection, accident prevention/self-protective measures against environmental and other hazards in the workplace, and stress management.

Goldbeck (1984) contends that wellness programs at the worksite are not only focused on the individual but also the factors in the institution that decrease wellness, including emotional wellness. He states worksite wellness leaders face the following challenges:

- devising programs available to and adapted for dependents and retirees
- integrating wellness with the medical model of delivery without becoming subordinate to it
- keeping open to new research and innovation, including visualization to assist in cancer remission, etc.
- maintaining integrity when wellness clashes with the traditional rules of corporate behavior
- restricting the use of health risk appraisals, executive physicals, and other assessment tools to programs that assure education and follow-up

Factors Affecting the Success or Failure of a Worksite Wellness Program

A major factor in a successful program (or in implementing any kind of change) is the participation of those involved in planning and implementation. Although a complete program is recommended, what is developed is based on expressed employee needs. Employees can be contacted initially through questionnaires, surveys, or small group meetings to provide input. When the participants "own" the program, they will be motivated to participate in it. Many programs are beautifully planned by administrators but fail to gain acceptance because participants had no input and were not concerned with the same issues as the planners.

Canton and Monroe (1984) suggest that wellness planners must be cognizant of and learn to track and understand new work attitudes which include:

- dissatisfaction with the nature of work
- dissatisfaction with authority
- increased pursuit of leisure
- development and reinforcement of personal identity outside the workplace
- a shift from expecting work to provide security, power, and status to providing self-esteem, support, creativity, affiliation, autonomy, challenge, growth, learning, and well-being
- feelings of uncertainty, insecurity, and anxiety due to rapid societal changes
- an increasing role for women in leadership

Canton and Monroe (1984) add to the list of problems that cause failure in wellness programs and suggest ways for wellness practitioners to anticipate and work through issues before they arise. Sources of failures are *organizational* (insufficient job design, improper work tasks, lack of supervision, insufficient administration, inadequate training, lack of career development, improper work roles, lack of power, or lack of authority); *program problems* (insufficient expertise of the persons in charge, inadequate quality of the program, improper program-environment-person fit, inadequate program goals and plan comprehensiveness, insufficient availability of resources, inadequate time available to implement the program, lack of practicality of the program design and strategies or inappropriate incentive systems); *people problems* (relate to the nature of program support by top-level management or participants, the values and norms of the organizational climate, degree of interpersonal conflict in the organization and competency of program facilitators); *systemic problems* (employees feel over/underworked, burdened/unchallenged, sexually or racially harassed or powerless or are continually exposed to hazardous working conditions or toxic substances; labor-management conflicts; profit motive receives more support than human resource development).

Self-Care Produces Savings in Health Care Costs

By using a self-care guide, 30 employees at a small manufacturing company in Pennsylvania stayed away from doctors' offices and emergency rooms and lowered their company's health care costs in just one year. Participants made their own determinations about whether and how to seek medical care. By making smart decisions, they saved $21.67 per employee and dependent and achieved a nearly18% reduction in costs.

In a follow-up study conducted by Capital Blue Cross in Harrisburg, 59% said they used the self-care guide before contacting a physician, 61% said the guide prepared them for a visit with their health care provider, and 97% said the guide was a good source of wellness advice and was easy to understand.

The self-care guide was the Healthy Life Self-Care Guide developed by the American Institute for Preventive Medicine. The return on investment was projected at 19 to 1 because the guide was available for less than $2 a copy (Self-care produces savings, 1995).

Hospital Saves $1 Million by Offering Wellness Programs

Providence General Medical Center in Everett, Washington, initiated the Wellness Challenge, an outcomes-based employee health benefits program showing over $1.5 million in cost reductions in health benefits claims, sick time use, and health habit improvement over a three-year period.

Under the Wellness Challenge, employees are offered a financial incentive if they demonstrate measured responsibility for their health and fitness based on set criteria. This financial "carrot" has generated an estimated 40% greater participation level over other incentives tried. ("Hospital Saves over $1 Million in Employee Health Benefit Costs," 1995.)

The Life Gain Program: An Example of a Systems Approach to Wellness

The design and implementation of a worksite wellness program should be conceptualized as part of an overall systems approach that enhances the quality of work life as well as increases productivity and reduces absenteeism and health care costs. When viewing the work system as a whole, work and anti-wellness factors are identified, existing problems are pinpointed, total organizational participation and support is encouraged, and long-term benefit and follow-up are planned for.

When planning programs from an open systems view, interventions are based on:

- involving relevant people in a meaningful way in the planning process
- choosing powerful incentives and stating them clearly so employees will be motivated to participate

- involving employee families in programs
- encouraging employees to be responsible for wellness behaviors
- using innovative and creative approaches to relevant problems
- ensuring confidentiality
- ensuring a positive effect on teamwork, trust, communication, productivity, cooperation, and power
- affecting long-term attitudinal and behavioral changes
- choosing attainable and realistic program goals
- planning follow-up for each phase of the program
- choosing a convenient location and program length
- designing an evaluation plan prior to initiating the program
- ensuring program goals reflect a consensus of participants
- completing a needs assessment of the population at risk
- training facilitators adequately
- emphasizing free choice, participation, open communication, trust, and experiential learning
- blending individual and organizational tasks, goals, and needs
- developing a realistic timetable
- addressing the personal, occupational, familial, social, and environmental aspects of well-being
- deciding whether a prepackaged or individualized program best meets the system's needs
- identifying and intervening in resistances to introduction of a wellness program
- addressing ethical issues
- addressing labor and management issues
- identifying ways to connect wellness programs to other employee assistance programs
- ensuring an adequate budget

When two or more people share goals over time, a culture develops. Many negative norms pervade work cultures. Common sense implies that everyone wants to be well and if the appropriate information and tools are provided, people will change toward wellness. In many work cultures (including hospitals) there are pervasive feelings of helplessness and powerlessness. The culture (or "system") is conceptualized as an amorphous mass that influences the worker while it eludes change. "This pervasive feeling that we cannot do anything about it is one of the most important initial obstacles that challenges any change program" (Allen & Kraft, 1984, p. 77).

The Normative Systems approach called Life Gain (Allen & Kraft, pp. 77–78) assists employees to work on both individual and cultural variables to effect change. Small groups work together to design and modify their cultural norms until commonly shared goals are found. Through the work group members become aware of the cultural norms of the groups to which they belong and see their impact on them. They also learn they have a choice and that norms can be chosen that sustain and support them and lifestyle changes.

The method has been used effectively to change delinquent subcultures into responsible groups, supermarkets from objects of crime and pilferage to places for honesty and openness, communities that litter to clean communities, businesses from mediocrity and low productivity to places where the norm is excellence and high productivity, and police-neighborhood relations from violence to friendship and respect.

The Life Gain System for organizational and community change includes the following four phases:

• *Start-up:* obtain leadership commitment; analyze/set goals; develop task forces to tailor a program around the specific needs of the organization/community; collect baseline data to measure progress

• *Involvement:* workshops exposing participants to alternatives and participation in wellness self-assessment procedures and goal-setting procedures; workshops not begun until a supportive environment has been well established among the change agent team members; participants identify the particular norms influencing their wellness and work together to systematically change the norms that get in the way of achieving their goals; a buddy system is used for verifying progress after the workshop; modeling of wellness behaviors by leaders is an effective motivating factor; in corporate environments, the modeling effect is most effective when workshops are started with the highest level of management first

• *Initiating change*: general support groups, specialized support groups, self-help programs, task-force programs; participants freely choose groups to which to belong; information and resources are presented, but the group members select which are right for them; printed and audiovisual self-help information is available to participants; as a reinforcement mechanism, graduates of the workshop are invited to join organizational task forces created in the start-up phase; skill training in behaviors relevant to each dimension of wellness is available; incentives including awards, citations, public praise, and money are given as reinforcements; intrinsic rewards from participating are fun and the pleasure of well-being

• *Sustaining change:* family members become involved in the program; reinforcement of one's own change process occurs when participants reach out to help family members; evaluation data are gathered to discern how well the program is accomplishing its objectives; individuals receive feedback on their progress in small short report meetings, newsletters, and bulletins; the Organizational Support Indicator measure is readministered regularly to note organizational progress toward providing more supportive environments for change; an active alumni organization brings in new information in programs; regular renewal meetings are held; a range of communication devices are available to help participants keep abreast of new wellness information and maintain improvements.

Prior to implementing any major program, a pilot or small sample run-through is recommended (Brennan, 1983). Such an approach can head off any major problems, fine-tune the program, and reveal if learning methods are appropriate and if proper data are being collected.

Reducing Smoking at the Worksite

Employers are beginning to realize the impact of smoking on the health and productivity of smokers and nonsmokers. Absentee, accident, and hospitalization rates are all at least 50% higher for smoking employees than for nonsmokers. Employers have been held legally responsible for at least part of the disability costs for smoking employees who contracted smoking-related illnesses and for claims of adverse effects from nonsmoking employees (Behrens, 1985, p. 5). Other costs borne by employers due to smoking include: excess office maintenance, increased depreciation of office equipment and furniture, increased insurance costs, increased ventilation needs, lower employee morale, decreased productivity, and increased risk of fire (Behrens, 1985, p. 7).

Two studies illustrate that smokers and nonsmokers are concerned about smoking at the worksite. In one survey 75% of smokers and 87% of nonsmokers favored either designated smoking areas or a total prohibition of smoking. These numbers are impressive when compared to a Roper report revealing that 53% of the total population and 58% of smokers were unaware that smoking is the probable cause of many heart attacks, and 59% of the population and 63% of smokers did not know that there is irrefutable evidence that smoking causes most cases of emphysema (Behrens, 1985, p. 6).

A growing body of court cases and legal opinions support employee rights to a smoke-free environment and employer rights to hire only nonsmokers and ban smoking at the workplace. In Fuentes vs. Workmen's Compensation Appeals Board, 1976–1977, a smoker successfully sued his employer for one-third of the disability due to emphysema because the employer permitted him "to inflict harm on himself" by smoking during working hours. Moral and economic incentives abound for banning smoking at the worksite, and legal precedents provide further encouragement to support smoking restrictions and bans.

Nonsmokers have begun to sue for their right to a smoke-free working environment and win. In one case the court found that "The right of an individual to risk his or her health does not include the right to jeopardize the health of those who must remain around him or her in order to properly perform the duties of their job" (Shimp vs. New Jersy Bell, 1976).

It is the consensus of legal opinion that employers are fully within their constitutional and legal right in banning smoking at the workplace unless the right to smoke is specified in a union contract. According to Behrens (1985, p. 8), "There appear to be no legal grounds for the claim that smoking at work is a 'right.'"

Initially companies, agencies, or hospitals may ban smoking in specific areas. This intervention can only be considered a first step because such a policy makes smoking the norm; that is, smoking is acceptable everywhere except in areas designated as NO SMOKING. The next step in banning smoking is to identify the organization as NO SMOKING with the exception of those areas designated as SMOKING areas. This places the onus on the smoker to seek out the smoking area rather than forcing the nonsmoker to seek out a nonsmoking area for clean air.

A number of companies have successfully implemented total bans, including Provident Indemnity Insurance, Austad's Company, and Radar Electric. To be effective, the chief executive officer must be behind the policy 100%. Pro-Tec, Raven Press Ltd., and Independent Press, among others, have instituted policies of not hiring smokers.

Worksite smoking programs use cover topics, such as: the psychology of quitting, breaking addictive behaviors, using support systems, coping with smoker's nerves, smoking and nutrition (including weight gain), maintaining the nonsmoking behavior, and exercise as a substitute for smoking. Some of the successful cessation techniques that have been used are: cold turkey, gradual weaning, rapid smoking, hypnosis, and biofeedback. Group classes, small groups, self-help materials, computer-assisted instruction, and one-to-one counseling have been employed. Popular options for session lengths range from a 5-day intensive format to weekly sessions over 1 or more months. Some organizations have found including spouses and other family members useful due to the social support provided. Most programs utilize a combination of print material, audiovisuals, demonstrations, skills training, lectures, and/or group discussions. Smoking cessation programs are most successful when linked with strong smoking policy, incentives to quit, environmental changes, and a broad-based health promotion or wellness program (Behrens, 1985, pp. 13–14).

Some incentives that have been used successfully to help smokers quit include:

- Offer nonsmokers a differential rate or discount on health and life insurance.
- Offer free or reduced-rate cessation programs at the worksite.
- Pay for a portion of the cost of cessation programs taken in the community.
- Provide cessation programs on company time or on shared time with employees.
- Offer cessation programs for family members.
- Offer cash payments to quitters after 6 to 12 smoke-free months.
- Incorporate disincentives for quitters who revert to their smoking habit.
- Hold drawings for prizes for quitters.
- Provide equal incentives to long-term employees and new hires who do not smoke.
- Reward nonsmokers who "adopt a smoker" and encourage the smoker to quit.
- Participate in the "Great American Smoke Out."
- Select your own 24-hour period and encourage smokers to quit for the day.
- Distribute carrot sticks and sugarless gum to help quitters make it through the day smoke free.
- Hold a stop smoking fair with local vendors from all types of community stop smoking programs.

- Conduct stop smoking competitions among volunteer teams of employees or with neighboring companies with prizes.

The wellness practitioner may coordinate or provide the program or can use community resources including church programs, Red Cross, YMCA-YWCA, Cancer Society, Heart Association, or Lung Association. Whether in-house staff or community resources provide the program, involvement of employees in developing a smoking policy and program will facilitate its development and increase its chances for success.

Some suggestions for including employees in a smoking cessation program are:

- Survey employees to determine their smoking in general, in worksite restricted areas, and opinions about offering cessation programs at work.
- Appoint an employee committee representative of smokers and nonsmokers to make recommendations about the content of the policy and /or the implementation plan and timetable.
- Have a representative of top management hold all-staff meetings to explain the proposed policy and program, to hear input, but to remain committed to limit smoking.
- Consider offering cessation programs on neutral turf if the atmosphere is highly charged in response to company policy.
- Hold meetings with all levels of management and listen to their comments, offer support, and make suggestions concerning negotiating disputes with employees.
- Meet informally with employees to ask advice from informal leaders and request assistance from a respected employee in dealing with an especially hostile fellow worker.

One approach to smoking cessation is the use of nicotine chewing gum. In a study of its use in the general population among people who had not taken the initiative to stop smoking, there was a decline in success rates to 6% for all three groups (acupuncture, nicotine gum, and no treatment). The study makers concluded that nicotine gum would be more effective when used in special smokers' clinics than in general practice (Clave & Benhamou, 1984).

Another study showed that nicotine gum when combined with long-term follow-up appointments resulted in a 1-year abstinence rate for 27% of clients (Fagerstrom, 1984). Although nicotine gum may be useful for some smokers, especially heavy smokers, it may not be of great benefit to light smokers who may require other interventions (Glantz, 1984).

Employers are beginning to hire with a bias toward nonsmokers. Thus, the ability to stop smoking is becoming an economic as well as a wellness issue. A survey of managers in the Seattle area showed that 53% were already giving preference to nonsmoking applicants. Since the U.S. Supreme Court has verified smoking as a legal criterion for hiring, discrimination against smokers does not violate equal opportunity statutes and will probably be used as a reason for not hiring in the future (Weis, 1984).

Wellness on the Campus

Opatz (1985) points out that the philosophy of student development which has emerged in colleges and universities includes the notion that human development is continuous; occurs when change is anticipated and planned for; is most effective when an integrated approach is taken; and is enhanced when students, faculty, and staff work collaboratively to promote it. More recently the idea of intentionality (helping students determine their own needs and direct their own development) has been put forth. These ideas parallel and support the concept of wellness.

The first formally established wellness program on a university campus was developed at the University of Wisconsin at Stevens Point in 1972. Other schools have since adopted the model. The program was developed and is directed by the University's Student Life Division. Wellness has been defined as the overall mission of the division. The following areas have adopted the model: health service, counseling center, residence life, student life activities and programs, university centers and business operations; and wellness curricula have been adopted in physical education, health education, nutrition, and psychology.

Fred Leafgren, Assistant Chancellor for Student Life, suggests 11 strategies for coordinating and enhancing wellness:

- *Establish* administrative leadership (including personal involvement in the process) and support. Key staff are selected and trained to implement and coordinate wellness programs.
- *Inventory* existing programs to identify those programs presently providing wellness services and minimize overlap and duplication.
- *Identify* staff who are interested in modeling a wellness lifestyle and encourage their participation in a wellness committee.
- *Identify* students already interested in and committed to a wellness lifestyle and encourage their participation in the planning process.
- *Bring* all existing personnel resources (faculty and nonstudent affairs administrators) together for brainstorming and goal setting early in the planning process.
- *Involve* all student affairs units in a partnership for wellness program implementation.
- *Ask* each academic department to inventory its programs and services and identify those that may be related to wellness, if only tangentially.
- *Inform* students and faculty about the program and available opportunities. Use a regular publication, assessment tools, etc.
- *Establish* priorities for wellness goals and activities.
- *Provide* adequate training for professional staff and students involved in implementing the program.
- *Evaluate* wellness programs for comprehensiveness and effectiveness in assisting students in their development as persons.

Many facets of the program at the University of Wisconsin are unique and creative. Entering freshmen are given the option of a traditional physical examination or a Lifestyle Assessment Questionnaire (LAQ). Over 90% choose the LAQ. This approach introduces the student to wellness before stepping in the door. Students receive the results during group interpretation sessions in the residence halls conducted by trained residence staff. The results are filed in the student's file and used as a basis for wellness programs early in the school year.

The Student Health Center shows self-care videotypes in the waiting room, and numerous printed self-care materials are available. When students complain of symptoms, e.g., a cold, rather than being referred to a professional, they go to The Cold Clinic where they find a self-assessment program directing them to examine their throat, take their temperature, and fill out a prescription form to take to the pharmacist. Moving even further toward wellness, such a clinic might provide instruction for nutritional, stress management procedures (imagery, etc.), and fitness/movement procedures to reduce or remove symptoms and treat the original conflict/issue.

The wellness coordinator is responsible for the publication of a wellness newsletter, the food service nutrition programs, the development of wellness information materials, and the training and supervision of student Lifestyle Assistants. Approximately 10-15 students are hired each year to initiate programs for fellow students, including aerobic dancing, weight reduction, stress management, and fitness assessments.

The wellness program has had a positive effect on the campus environment. Alcohol consumption is closely regulated and smoking policies protect the rights of the nonsmokers; smoking is allowed only in designated areas, and in many of the Student Life Offices there is no smoking at all. The Food Service contract is negotiated to include provision for high quality fresh fruits, vegetables, and who grain foods. All entrees are labeled for fat, carbohydrate, and protein content. Cooks and food preparers are taught the basic principles of nutrition and new methods of cooking.

EVALUATION OF WELLNESS PROGRAMS

Evaluation issues sould be considered when programs are planned. The assessment/intervention/evaluation process is continuous and interactive. In order to design a program that will ultimately be effective, client needs must be assessed. The Windsor et al. (1984, pp. 59–60, 70) list of planning problems has been adapted below.

Evaluation Planning Begins When Program Planning Begins

1. What are the dimensions of the problem of interest —clients with diagnosed disease or relatively well people with unwell life styles—and what is the

prevalence of the problem? What is expected to be different as a result of the program?

2. What specific behaviors must clients learn or acquire or strengthen to enhance wellness?
3. What resources are needed for wellness to be enhanced?
4. What kind of support services are needed to enhance wellness?
5. Which behavior changes can and should be measured, how, and when?
6. What wider changes in conditions and situations are expected; which ones can and should be measured, how, and when?
7. What approaches will best achieve the desired effect and how can they be monitored for quality and efficacy?
8. What organizational and logistical arrangements are needed to support the program, including orientation and training of personnel?
9. What kind of budget is needed and how can it be obtained?

Most, if not all, of the questions need to be asked of "experts" *and* clients.

Types of Evaluation

Program evaluation is used to improve program planning, development, or administration. It describes accomplishments, problems, and processes, reducing uncertainty in day-to-day decision making.

Evaluation research determines the effectiveness of a program model or tests a theory; it focuses primarily on the potential effects of a new program. When designing an evaluation program, it is useful to ask, "Do I want information as the program proceeds to feed back and improve it?" (If so, use formative evaluation procedures), or "Do I want to withhold feedback and evaluate only after the program is finished?" (if so, use summative evaluation procedures). Moberg (1984, p.3) suggests that formative approaches are most relevant to prevention programs.

There are three levels of evaluation to consider: process, outcome, and impact. At the process level, activities of the program are considered (number and types of clients and staff, resources expended, services provided). Program monitoring systems measure effort, the program's capacity for success, and document level of activity. All prevention programs should establish a program monitoring system (Mober, 1984, p. 3).

A monitoring system enables an accurate count of how many people were served during the year, what services were provided, and what the characteristics of the clientele are. This kind of information indicates whether the intended population is being served and whether program content needs to be altered to meet the population being served. Consumer satisfaction surveys, participant observation, and open-ended interviewing can provide additional monitoring information.

Outcome evaluation examines the attainment of program objectives (change in participant behavior, attitude, knowledge or level of problems). Smoking prevention programs would have successful outcomes if a meaningful percentage of participants did not smoke in the future; smoking cessation programs would have successful outcomes if a meaningful percentage of participants continued not smoking for a prescribed period of time—the longer, the more successful. Cost benefit analysis (minimize costs while maximizing benefits) is another outcome measure.

Impact evaluation examines the total effect of a program, including its "spin-off" effects. Impact evaluation of an alcohol abuse prevention program might examine whether the program has reduced the incidence of alcohol abuse among youth in a community, whether there are fewer drunk driving incidents, or whether more alternatives are being used.

Attempting to examine all three levels in one evaluation effort is unrealistic and inappropriate. A level is chosen depending on resources, information needs, and accountability requirements.

Steps in Planning Program Evaluation

The following steps are useful in planning program evaluation (Moberg, 1984, pp. 7–9):

1. Identify and organize a key users group composed of an evaluator, key staff, and, if possible, clients.

2. Identify and refine relevant evaluation questions by asking diagnostic questions: What is the assessed need of the participants? What is the conceptual model the program is based on? What benefits, goals, and objectives are anticipated? What kinds of interventions are planned? What is the target population? What resources are available? Who needs information about the program and why? What data are essential for internal and external reporting? What data are currently available? What are the major issues being faced by the program? What is the political, value, and cultural context? What standards or regulations must the program comply with? Has the program model been tested elsewhere?

3. Specify program goals and objectives. Write down general goals, then list possible indicators of goal achievement. Select the best indicators and translate the indicators into measurable objectives, e.g., by the end of the program, clients will role play a 10% increase in the number of socially acceptable ways to refuse a cigarette; by 8/5/97, 90% of students will identify the wellness resource center as a viable alternative to physician visits.

4. Select evaluation methods and data collection instruments appropriate to evaluation questions. Questions to ask include:

- Should evaluation be prestructured (fixed) or vary according to the data (dynamic)?
- Are we most concerned with past participants (retrospective) or future ones (prospective)?

- Should we focus on the total program (holistic) or on specific parts of it (component)?
- Should specific hypotheses be tested (inductive) or will we develop generalizations based on the data (deductive)?
- Should groups receiving the program be compared to similar groups that do not get the program (experimental or quasi-experimental design) or look only at program participants?
- Should data be quantitative (56 participants. . .) or qualitative (the process of participating in wellness activities was. . .)?
- Should data come from existing records, observations, interviews, or questionnaires?
- Should a sample of participants be chosen (volunteers, representatives, randomly) or the entire population be examined?
- Should we ask open-ended or structured questions to obtain data?
- Should we use single-item indicators or multiple-item scales?

5. Develop an evaluation plan, including:

- a statement of the evaluation question(s);
- a description of what data will be collected from whom using what instru ments;
- a listing of who will be responsible for each evaulation task;
- a statement of conditions under which data collection will take a place and methods for standardizing data collection;
- plans for regulating the flow of evaluation data, summarizing it, and analyzing it;
- plans for protection of subjects (obtaining informed consent and limiting access to identifying information);
- time frame for data collection, analysis, reporting, and checkpoint with key user's group;
- plans for use of the findings, including a statement of level of certainty which can be placed in the findings given the research design.

6. Pilot test the evaluation system to ensure respondents understand the questions, are willing to respond, that data are coded and interpreted consistently, that data collection time allowances are accurate, and that data collectors understand the format.

7. Implement the evaluation plan ensuring that data forms are turned in and briefly examined shortly after completion; build in sanctions to enforce this.

8. Summarize and interpret the data. If the sample is small enough and of a quantitative (numbers) nature, hand tally and pocket calculator can produce frequency distributions (e.g., number of males who participated), cross tabulations (number of males vs. females who stopped smoking), or means (e.g., mean age is achieved by adding the ages and dividing the total by the number of participants). More sophisticated and/or statistical analyses may require consultation. Qualitative analyses could include reproducing the data without comment, developing

organizational categories, developing case studies, or developing typologies (e.g., isolating and categorizing the essential characteristics of successful types of participants). Throughout this process, the key user's group should be involved and provide feedback that is implemented.

9. Disseminate and use the findings. Sharing findings with other wellness programs will assist in legitimizing specific models, refining hypotheses, and improving practice.

Selecting Evaluation Tools

When selecting an existing instrument, ensure *items reflect relevant concepts,* the instrument *is the appropriate length* (too long will create resistance in participants; too short will not be reliable), *is reliable* (consistent between persons, over time, and/or internally) *and valid* (measures what it claims to measure). One consideration is determining whether the instrument has face validity (by looking at it, on the face of it, it looks as if it measures what it purports to measure) with a population similar to yours; look for a discussion of these issues accompanying the instrument.

Two (or more) methods of measurement are usually better than one. For example, if a quantitative measure and statistical methods are employed, a hypothesis may be refuted (resulting in a return to square one), but an interview with participants may still reveal useful information. Contrarily, if a post-test measure of student wellness peer facilitators reported their peers demonstrated more assertiveness after their work together and interviews with the peers independently found movement in the direction of more assertion, confidence is added to the conclusion that peer facilitation affects assertive behavior in the population under study.

When choosing a method, determine its feasibility by asking, "Are there sufficient resources available to conduct the proposed evaluation?" including budget, time (to conduct the evaluation, reasonable to expect from a client, and to carry it out in the proposed time frame), expertise, computer or data entry services, clerical time, duplicating equipment/time, and relevance to the developmental phase of the program (an impact study is not appropriate for a beginning program that is only 2 years old). At this point, statistical and computer specialist consultation can be sought if necessary.

Validity Considerations in Selecting an Evaluation Design

In addition to considering the reliability of an instrument, the *internal validity* (extent to which an observed effect can be attributed to an intervention) is of importance. Eight factors can affect internal validity:

1. *History* (unplanned internal or external events that affect the population under study, e.g., a new law banning smoking in schools interferes with a study of the effects of a smoking cessation program on smoking in school);

2. *Maturation* (normal growth and development changes, e.g., children grow out of heart murmurs);
3. *Testing or observation* (participants change their behavior because of being watched while being interviewed or taking a test);
4. *Instrumentation* (changes in the characteristics of the measures introduce bias; e.g., some observers are well-trained and others are not);
5. *Regression* (selection of a treatment or comparison group based on a very high or low level of a characteristic, e.g., those who score very high on a pretest are recruited for a weight management course);
6. *Selection* (as groups or individuals are selected or volunteer, the group(s) is not representative of all smokers, or all overweight clients, etc.);
7. *Attrition* (10% or more dropouts introduces bias into the outcome of a study);
8. *Interactive effects* (any combination of the above).

Instrumentation, selection, and attrition are the most frequent compromisers of evaluation results (Windsor et al., 1984, p. 131). Therefore, it is important to protect the results from these eight factors. A major protection is choice of evaluation design.

Program Evaluation Designs

Windsor et al. (1984, pp. 132–138) discuss five major evaluation designs:

1. *One Group Pretest and Post-test*: although it is tempting to infer that significant increases or decreases in scores on the post-test are due to an intervention, they could as likely be due to other factors, especially if there is a great deal of time between the pretest and post-test, or if maturation, historical factors, or regression interfere.

2. *Nonequivalent Control Group:* by adding a comparison group, the effects of history, maturation, testing, and instrumentation will be lessened. It is essential to make groups as comparable as possible. One way is the peer-generation method: participants are asked to identify a nonparticipant friend of the same age and sex.

3. *Time Series:* this design is usually used when a trend is being studied; up to 50 data points are used to assess an effect; the principal threat to internal validity is history; this design does not provide definitive evidence about the impact of an intervention unless it is replicated.

4. *Multiple Time Series:* outcomes are studied at differing points for a group receiving the intervention (treatment group) and for a group not receiving it (control group).

5. *Randomized Pretest and Post-test with Control Group:* this experimental design produces strong control over threats to internal and external validity (increased confidence in generalizing findings to other settings and populations with similar characteristics *if* there is confirmation that the two groups are equivalent; this can be obtained by examining each of the effects of the threats to internal validity for both groups). In many settings, it may not be ethical or feasible to withhold treatment from a control group; in some cases the intensity, duration,

methods, materials, or frequency can be varied for the control group; when a new program is being established, the old method of treatment can be administered to the control group and the new program to the experimental group.

Determining Sample Size

When quantitative designs are used, the sample size is crucial to ensure sufficient statistical power in data analysis. The appropriate size for groups is determined prior to an intervention. *Statistical power* is the probability of rejecting a null hypothesis if it is false (Type I error). The null hypothesis asserts the two groups (treatment and control) are not significantly different.

To determine the efficient sample size, parameters must be defined. Statistical significance (α) is usually set between .01 and .05. Next, the ß level, or probability of accepting a null hypothesis when it is false (Type II error), is computed. ß should be equal to $1-4\alpha$; if $\alpha = .05$, $\beta = 1-4\,(.05)$ or .80 (Windsor, 1984, p. 139). Finally, the current median level of expected effectiveness is calculated. A search of the literature or an examination of ongoing program data should reveal the expected effectiveness of a particular program. For example, the literature indicates that the self-initiated cessation rate for smokers is approximately 10% ($p = .10$). A reasonable expectation of impact for a smoking-cessation program at a 6- to 12-month follow-up is about 30% cessation, or 0.30. Standard size statistical tables can then be consulted to find how many participants are needed for each group to test the significance of a difference (Windsor, 1984, p. 139).

Problems in Program Evaluation

In addition to the obvious problems of evaluation such as lack of sophistication of the researcher, there are other problems that may be encountered. Frequently it is difficult, if not impossible, to meet the criteria for experimental control that would lend greater confidence to findings. School-based programs are the exception; it is relatively easy to randomly select classrooms for treatment.

Issues of interest to employers, such as productivity and morale, are difficult to measure with any degree of confidence. Yet management may demand that researchers relate results to "the bottom line" (profits) in order to continue funding wellness programs. The costs associated with researching the benefits of wellness may be considerable. The evaluation process itself is not considered profitable and therefore the wellness practitioner may have difficulty convincing management that they should invest in data analysis.

Some of the best worksite wellness evaluation studies include Browne et al. (1984), Cady et al. (1985), Spilman et al. (1986), Bly et al. (1986), Blair et al. (1986), Gibbs et al. (1985), Wood et al. (1989), Shepard (1992), and Henritze et al. (1992). Study their designs for further information.

INTEGRATIVE LEARNING EXPERIENCES

Beginning Level

1. Use the case study of the Block family below to make recommendations for wellness interventions regarding nutrition, fitness/exercise, stress management, positive relationships, environmental wellness, and self-care.

The Block family lives in a small house with little privacy from their neighbors or one another. The windows have heavy curtains that allow little light or air in. *Jim Block,* the father, age 42, is a management consultant for a large corporation. He is overweight, "out of shape," travels a lot, and seems emotionally and physically removed from the rest of the family. He once mentioned that he doesn't want to be like his father and die of a heart attack. *Wanda Block,* the mother, is 40 years old. She is just beginning to pursue her own life and has enrolled as a freshman at the local college; she feels guilty about being away from the twins so much and having to leave the house before breakfast. She smokes cigarettes continually and drinks coffee whenever you visit. *Mrs. Suzanna Block,* Jim's mother, age 60, has diabetes. She came to live with her son's family when her husband died last year. She alternates between being depressed and telling her daughter-in-law how to run the household. There are angry scenes at dinner between Wanda and Mrs. Block. *Gregory Block,* one of the twins, is 10 years old. He is doing poorly in school. His mother calls him "the bad one." He subsists on chocolate bars and cokes. You noticed him standing on the corner near school talking to the local drug dealer. *Glenda Block,* Gregory's twin, does the food shopping for the family and cooks some meals; these consist of hamburgers, cokes, french fries, and store bought cakes and cookies. *Ramona Block,* age 17, is unmarried and lives at home with her 6-month-old infant, Randy. You saw Ramona in a hot embrace with her date in a car near the house. *Randy Block,* age 6 months, was born with multiple physical defects. Ramona pays little attention to Randy; he is being raised by his grandmother.

2. Complete a community assessment using Table 9.2, (see p. 296)

Advanced Level

1. Develop and implement a smoking cessation program with three clients or a group of clients. Summarize your results.
2. Develop a blueprint for the assessment, implementation, and evaluation of a wellness program in a hospital, school, or corporation, including your justification for such a program. Expand your practitioner role by approaching administrators in three hospitals, schools, or corporations and discussing the feasibility of adopting your plan.

REFERENCES

Allen, R., and Kraft, C. (1984). The importance of cultural variables in program design. *Health Promotion in the Workplace,* M. O'Donnell and T. Ainsworth, Eds. New York: John Wiley & Sons.

Anderson, D., Brink, S., & Courtney, T. (1995). *Health Risks and Their Impact on Medical Costs.* Brookfield, WI: Milliman & Robertson, Inc.

Angotti, C., and Levine, M. (1994). Review of 5 years of combined dietary and physical fitness intervention for control of serum cholesterol. *J Amer Diet Assoc* 94: 634–638.

Arbeit, M.L., Johnson, C.C., Mott, D.S., et al. (1992). The Heart Smart Cardiovascular School Health Promotion. *Prev Med* 21 (1): 18–32.

Behrens, R. (1985). A Decision Maker's Guide to Reducing Smoking at the Worksite. Washington, D.C.: U.S. Department of Health and Human Services.

Blair, S. et al. (1986). Health promotion for educators: Impact on absenteeism. *Prev Med 15*: 166–175.

Bly, J., et al. (1986). Impact of worksite health promotion on health care costs and utilization: Evaluation of Johnson & Johnson's life for life program. *J Am Med Assoc* 256(23): 3235–3240.

Brennan, A. (1983). How to set up a corporate wellness program. *Management Rev* May:41–47.

Browne, D., et al. (1984). Reduced disability and health care costs in an industrial fitness program. *J Occu Med* 26(11): 806–816.

Cady, L., et al. (1985). Program for increasing health and physical fitness of fire fighters. *J Occup Practitioner Med* 27(2): 110–114.

Cancer risks found for hospital workers. (1982). *WOHRC NEWS* 4(4):1,6.

Canton, J., and Monroe, T. (1984). The importance of worker involvement in program design. In *Health Promotion in the Workplace,* M. O'Donnell and T. Ainsworth, Eds. New York: John Wiley & Sons, p. 58.

Clavel, F., and Benhamon, S. (1984). Nicotine chewing gum in general practice. *Brit Med J* 289(6454):1308.

Gibbs, J., et al. (1985). Worksite health promotion: Five-year trend employee health care costs. *J of Occup Med* 27(11): 826–830.

Glantz, L. (1984). Nicotine chewing gum not for all smokers. *Clin Pharm* 3(3):236.

Glanz, K. (1994). Reducing breast cancer through changes in diet and alcohol intake: From clinic to community. *Ann Behav Med* 16(4): 334–346.

Goldbeck, W. (1984). Forward. *In Health Promotion in the Workplace,* M. O'Donnell and T. Ainsworth, Eds. New York: John Wiley & Sons, p. viii.

Health risks and their impact on medical costs. n.a. (1995). Brookfield, WI: Milliman & Robertson, Inc.

Healthy People 2000, National Health Promotion and Disease Prevention Objectives (1990). Washington, DC: U.S. Department of Health and Human Services, Public Health Service.

Heirich, M.A., Foote, A., & Erfurt, J.C. (1993). Worksite physical fitness programs: Comparing the impact of different program designs on cardiovascular risks. *Journal of Occup Med 35:* 510–517.

Henritze, J., et al. (1992). LIFECHECK: A successful low-touch, low-tech in-plant cardiovascular disease risk identification and modification program. *Am J Hlth Promotion* 7(2): 129–136.

Hospital saves over $1 million in employee health benefit costs (1995). *Worksite Wellness Works* November: 5

Kagan, N.I., Klein, H.K., and Watson, M.G. (1995). Stress reduction in the workplace: The effectiveness of psychoeducational programs. *J Counseling Psychol* 42(1); 71–78.

Moberg, D. (1984). *Evaluation of Prevention Programs: A Basic Guide for Practitioners.* Madison, WI: WI Clearinghouse.

National Cancer Institute. (1980). *Everything Doesn't Cause Cancer.* Washington, D.C.: NIH. NIH publication 80–2039.

Olds, D.L., Henderson, C.R., Phelps, C., et al. (1993). Effects of prenatal and infancy nurse home visitation on government spending. *Med Care* 31(2): 155–174.

Opatz, J. (1985). Wellness in colleges and universities. In *Proceedings of the Ninth Annual Community Health Nursing Conference: Maximizing Wellness in a High Tech Age: Focus for Community Health Nursing,* M. Assay, Ed. Chapel Hill NC: Department of Community Health Nursing.

Parkinson, R. (1982). *Managing Health Promotion in the Workplace.* Palo Alto, CA: Mayfield Publishing Co.

Ruffing-Rahal, M.A., (1994). Evaluation of a group health promotion with community dwelling older women. *Pub H Nurs* 11(1): 38–48.

Self-care produces savings (1995). *Worksite Wellness Works* November: 4.

Shepard, R. (1992). Twelve years experience of a fitness program for salaried employees of a Toronto life insurance company. *Am J Hlth Promotion* 6(4): 292–301.

Spilman, M.A., et al. (1986). Effects of a corporate health promotion program. *J of Occup Med* 28(4): 285–289.

Vickery, D., et al. (1983). Effect of a self-care education program on medical visits. *JAMA* 250(21):2952–2956.

Weiss, W. (1984). Giving smokers notice, going public with policies against hiring smokers. *Management World* July:44, 41.

Windsor, R., et al. (1984). *Evaluation of Health Promotion and Education Programs.* Palo Alto, CA: Mayfield Publishing Co.

Wood, E.A. et al. (1989). An evaluation of lifestyle risk factors and absenteeism after two years in a worksite health promotion program. *Am J Hlth Promotion* 4(2):128–133.

10

RESEARCH AND WELLNESS THEORY

This chapter discusses the following topics:

- Turning illness-oriented research questions into wellness-oriented ones
- Research methods especially suited to wellness theory
- Research providing support for wellness theory
- Developing relationship statements and testing theoretical relationships

Planning and carrying out wellness-focused research implies the reader already has a working knowledge of conventional research methods. Research from a wellness focus also implies a wellness framework from which to practice. Without it the research that will be produced may be more illness-oriented than wellness-oriented. This chapter attempts to provide the reader with information necessary to begin generating wellness questions, suggests some methods that may be most useful in studying wellness-oriented questions, supplies a report of some evolving research to support wellness theory, and suggests some wellness relationship statements that can be used to test the theory.

TURNING ILLNESS-ORIENTED RESEARCH QUESTIONS INTO WELLNESS-ORIENTED ONES

There are a number of ways to turn illness-oriented research questions into wellness-oriented one. One way is to focus on a well population. Although it is possible to use a problem orientation with a well population, it is easier to see how to structure questions to focus on wellness concerns. An example of research focusing on a well population appears in the section "Research Providing Support for Wellness Theory" later in this chapter.

Another way to turn illness-oriented questions into wellness ones is to begin to relate problems or human responses to the dimensions of wellness. For example, instead of focusing on the pain or illness experience of otitis media, the focus would be on the prevention and minimization of pain using self-care strategies. Some questions that might be asked are:

- What is the relationship between level of exercise and otitis media?
- What is the relationship between positive expectations about the outcome of otitis media and healing?
- What is the effect of eating additional amounts of high vitamins C, A, and zinc-containing foods on the otitis media process?
- What is the effect of progressive relation and healing imagery measures on the otitis media process?
- What is the effect of color, full spectrum light, or noise on the otitis media process?
- What is the effect of peer or family supportive communication on the otitis media process?

A variant of this procedure is to take some of the indicants of whole person wellness (Figure 1.2, Chapter 1, p. 5) and begin to formulate them into research questions, especially those related to manageability, comprehensibility, and meaningfulness. Antonovsky (1984) has been developing a model based on the sense of coherence as a determinant of health. His work has relevance for wellness research because he has begun to examine health as a process, not merely as the absence of disease. Additionally, he conceives of the process as one of moving toward greater order and meaningfulness; this idea, too, is relevant for wellness.

His model is most relevant for wellness dimension of stress but can be expanded to encompass other dimensions. Antonovsky's "sense of coherence" is formed from a cluster of attitudes that he calls:

- comprehensibility (perceiving stimuli as making cognitive sense as information, as opposed to finding them unpredictable, random, noisy, and chaotic);
- manageability (having resources at one's disposal either directly under one's control, or having access to resources controlled by dependable others);
- meaningfulness (feeling life makes sense in emotional terms so that some life problems are viewed as worth investing energy in).

Using Antonovsky's (1984) concept of coherence, the following wellness-oriented questions could be formulated:

- What is the relationship between the belief in the ability to influence the level of fitnesss either directly or with the help of others and fitness activities?
- What is the relationship between believing the solution to life problems is worth investing energy in and preventive nutrition?
- What is the relationship between believing one is able to make sense out of

new and risk-requiring situations and attempts to form positive relationships with others?

The Intersystems Wellness Practitioner Model (Figure 1.1, Chapter 1, p. 3) could also be used to generate wellness-oriented research questions. For example:

- The more the practitioner serves as a wellness role model, the more likely the client will be to move toward a wellness orientation.
- The greater the movement toward a wellness belief system, the more wellness-oriented behaviors will be exhibited.
- The more the client participates in wellness self-assessment, the greater the movement toward wellness.

Another idea is to use the conceptual framework developed by Mehl (1981), a proponent of a holistic approach to research. He pointed out the fallacy of thought that underlies the medical model in which an adverse factor or factors is believed to "cause" an illness or disease. Such a model ignores why one particular, unique human being becomes ill; until recently this kind of question has been defined as irrelevant because it is outside the paradigm. Psychoneuroimmunology, a new field spawned from the interrelationship of three disciplines, promises to address some of the most important questions in the area of understanding the mind/body link (O'Regan, 1983). However, until these links are established and accepted by traditional medicine, many scientific studies will continue to address parts of bodies or organs and to infer effect on the whole person.

Because of the uniqueness of individuals, Mehl questions whether randomization procedures used in quantitative research are valid. If each person has a unique position in time and space, how can randomization of space/time units be appropriate? A holistic model, such as wellness, is based upon the significance of the individual. Theory construction is systematic, is based on the assessment of factors effecting individuals, and does not require that the same factor affect every individual in exactly the same way to be considered significant (Mehl, 1981).

Using this method, a researcher might begin with a detailed description of the life of individuals with a life problem, such as diabetes: childhood events, stresses pre-illness, spiritual beliefs, life events, emotional changes, paralleling changes in their illness and their general world view. Only after one individual's pathway to diabetes is understood would the practitioner researcher begin to look for similarities and differences among different individual pathways. Theory might be formulated for each individual regarding how diabetes functioned in his or her personal system. Continuing with the research, it would be important to observe if diabetes changed for each person as factors changed.

Using Mehl's model, an example of a wellness-oriented question might be: What are the interactions of exercise on the development of client Jones related to diabetes, spirtual beliefs, life events, emotional changes, paralleling changes in her view of diabetes and her general world view, stresses and ability to use stress management procedures, positive relationships with others, preventive nutrition, and amount of full-spectrum light exposed to?

According to Mehl (1981), a holistic approach to research begins with a description of all possible factors in the life of an individual with a particular disease or problem. Only then would other individuals be studied and similarities and differences be noted. Theory would then accumulate regarding the many possible individual pathways of development of the problem.

This kind of approach emphasizes the interactive nature of variables rather than the isolation and proof of one effect. It is also congruent with a systems approach that focuses on interactive factors and in which there are many paths to one outcome; in systems terms, this is referred to in systems theory as *equifinality* (Putt, 1978).

Mehl (1981) is also supportive of the emphasis on the meaning and quality of life so essential to a wellness model. He discusses the importance of value clarification by the individual and support of that person's right to decide on his or her own values. Additionally, Mehl gives precedence to observation and description of client behavior over statistical procedures.

Another method of turning illness-oriented research questions is to search current research reports for ideas. For example, in looking through abstracts of research on mind and immunity, the following studies were found: Achterberg and Lawlis (1977) found that blood chemistries tended to reflect ongoing or concurrent disease states in those with cancer; that there was a statistical relationship between psychological variables and blood chemistries; and that psychological factors were predictive of subsequent disease status. The researchers concluded that blood chemistries offered information about the current status of disease, whereas the psychological variables offered future, and perhaps preventive, insights. Some questions this research might raise about wellness research are:

- What is the practitioner's role in assisting clients to identify the feelings that are interfering with their wellness or supporting their disease?
- What feelings are interfering with this client's healing processes?
- How can client feelings about disease be used to prevent further development of the disease?

A study by McClelland et al. (1980) focused on the need for power and its relationship to illness. The researchers noted that previous research reported that individuals high in the need for power, high in inhibition, and high in power stress were more likely than other individuals to report more severe illness. The McClelland study found that the high power group had above average urine excretion of epinephrine and below average concentrations of immunoglobulin A in saliva. They interpreted the findings as consistent with the hypothesis that when a strong need for power is inhibited, there is an immunosuppressive effect making individuals more susceptible to illness. From a wellness perspective, the following questions might be asked:

- Which clients most need to maintain a sense of power and control over themselves and/or their disease process?
- How can the nurse identify these clients readily?
- What interventions would be useful in increasing immune responses in these clients and in clients in general?

A number of researchers have noted the correlation between inability to express anger and poor prognosis in cancer (Bageley, 1979; Bieliauskas et al., 1979; Morris et al., 1981; Borysenko, 1982). Such studies may raise the following issues from a wellness perspective:

- What clients are suppressing angry feelings?
- What effect is suppressed anger having on their lifestyle and/or disease process?
- What interventions can be used to enhance anger expression?
- What is the effect of anger expression on well-being and/or ability to heal?

RESEARCH PROCEDURES FOR HOLISTIC, COMPLEX PROCESSES

Studying wellness requires research procedures that allow the researcher to examine holistic, interactive processes. Two kinds of research approaches are especially suited: qualitative research and action research.

Qualitative Research

Qualitative research taps the context and meaning of observed behaviors. Qualitative research is most apropos for the discovery of theory and understanding. Its scope is holistic; its methods emphasize interactions of variables (Mullen & Iverson, 1982).

Recently, more and more researchers in fields with a traditional quantitative (numbers) emphasis, such as psychology, sociology, educational research, and others have shifted to a more qualitative paradigm. This shift is in line with a trend toward holism. Qualitative data are well-grounded in real world observations and contain rich descriptions and explanations of processes. Quantitative data tend to isolate findings and make analysis difficult if one does not find what one is hoping to find.

For example, a pair of students were searching for correlations between anxiety, loneliness, and grade point average in their classmates. They did a multiple regression correlation (used to understand the effects of two or more independent variables on a dependent measure), but there was so much variance unaccounted for that all they were able to conclude was that there was no significant relationship between the three. What if they had gathered some qualitative data such as interviewing a focused sample of students with low or high grade point averages to find out other variables that the students thought might be involved? Their discussion of findings would have been much richer and they would have untangled more of the puzzle of the relationship of the variables.

Quantitative research often does not have meaning for the practice world because researchers isolate variables to a single dimension to look at direct relationships between them. Such an approach overlooks the highly complex and diverse nature of practice and frequently falls short of providing direction for interventions (Swanson & Chenitz, 1982).

Additionally, it provides little understanding of the context that gives meaning to actions. Noting that the family planning literature on male contraception has large theoretical gaps, Swanson and Chenitz (1982) set out to find out what prevented men from using contraceptives, rather than to simply count men and their contraceptive use. They found that the "hassle" of using contraception was mentioned frequently by the men being interviewed. One of the major advantages of a qualitative method is that it allows the researcher to analyze data while collecting it. This quality permitted Swanson to further explore the concept of "hassle" and found that if contraception did not fit into their lifestyles, they did not use it.

As she continued her study, Swanson began to interview couples and found that lifestyle factors influenced contraceptive use.

> Although contraceptive use appears to be a simple matter, it embodies a complex activity which is influenced by many social, sexual, and physical variables. How one feels about one's self, one's partner, what is acceptable sexually, is convenient, valued, approved by others and tolerated by institutions are but a few factors represented by "contraceptive" use. (1982, p. 244)

The grounded theory method of qualitative research has been written about by a number of researchers, but never with such lucidity as by Stern (1980). She studied stepfather families and their integration into an existing family. She began by conducting intensive interviews with 30 stepfather families from a variety of social classes and ethnic groups. She also observed the families interacting and coded all data according to their main substance, eventually clustering them into categories. Two of the categories noted were family rules and enforcement techniques.

As Stern moved to the second phase of concept formation, she began to develop a conceptual framework that represented integration from the family member's point of view. The framework chosen was discipline because the topic elicited strong emotional responses when discussed with families.

During the next step, concept development, categories were linked together to define key variables, e.g., categories of teaching, accepting, and copying were included in the larger category of affiliating actions or those actions that seemed to bring the stepfather and child closer together. As relationships became clearer, Stern returned to the literature and formulated the question, "Under what conditions do the variables discipline and integration co-exist?" (p. 22). She returned for another look at the data to clarify this relationship. She found that integration and discipline occurred together only when affiliating actions were also present. This is the point at which statement synthesis (Walker & Avant, 1983, p. 83) occurred; a statement about the relationship between phenomena under observation was made by Stern. Her thinking became consolidated and she proposed the term "integrative discipline" as the core variable that explained integration of stepfathers into families around the issue of child discipline.

Stern continued refining the concept by coding data in terms of theoretical ideas. She wrote memos to herself as she coded data. Memo writing is a useful technique in qualitative studies. The researcher writes a sentence, paragraph, or a few pages about a momentary idea that occurs while looking at data.

> Memos are always *conceptual* in intent. They do not just report data, but they tie
> different pieces of data together in a cluster, or they show that a particular piece of
> data is an instance of a general concept. (Miles & Huberman, 1984, p. 69)

Finally, memos were reorganized and used to produce a research report. The final report presented theoretical outcomes substantiated by examples from data.

Action Research

Action research is the use of research methodology to solve problems. Social change can be brought about at the same time that there is a valuable contribution made to science. An underlying assumption of action research is that members of our organization are better able than anyone else to define their problems and propose solutions for them because they are best acquainted with their own situations. This assumption implies that it is desirable, and even necessary, for clients to possess decision making skills (Cunningham, 1976).

Clients are assisted to define the problem as they see it and then to generate hypotheses. They learn to specify and define terms, decide on a way to measure change, decide how change will be implemented, decide how to interpret data to see if they support or refute their hunches or hypotheses, and infer generalizations (Corey, 1953, p. 29).

In action research, hypotheses are ways of stating objectives; they predict the consequences of carrying out actions and move participants toward those actions (Corety, 1953, p. 133). An overriding theme is that people are more likely to change "if they participate in exploring the reasons for, and means of, change. . .The action training and research process releases the interpersonal energies that are stifled in most authority-bound systems" (Gardner, 1974).

Action research tends to enhance the position of the individual and to diffuse sources of power. Clients are given freedom, meaningful activity, opportunity to participate, recognition of their worth, needed decision making and problem solving skills, and growth and security opportunities (Gardner, 1974). Each of these seems likely to enhance wellness also.

There may be language barriers between researchers and clients and interviews or mailed questionnaires may be inappropriate, because each group has its own perspective and understanding of the major parameters of the problem areas. The nominal group may be the best way to help all involved understand the problem (Van de Ven & Delbecq, 1972).

For example, participants studying the problem of obtaining wellness services in a community would be asked to list the subjective (personal feelings and emotions that were barriers to attaining wellness services) and objective (organizational or environmental difficulties which interfered with movement toward wellness) barriers. The next steps are as follows:

1. 15 minutes for the participants to silently generate ideas.
2. In round robin, each person shares one problem and each is written on a large pad of paper by number alternating between subjective and objective columns. No ideas are discussed or critiqued, but participants are encouraged to write new ideas as they are stimulated by others' ideas.
3. 30 minutes to discuss, clarify, elaborate, dispute, or add new items; no items are eliminated.
4. 15-minute break.
5. The group ranks the priority of items, choosing the 10 most critical elements, writing on each on a 3 × 5 card and ranking them in order of importance.
6. A spontaneous discussion follows in which participants can reclarify, elaborate, defend, or dispute the preliminary vote. Some problems are now redefined at this point.
7. The priority of times is changed by individuals as they rerank them on their own sheets, assigning a value of 100 to his or her most important item and values between 0 and 100 to the other items.
8. The researcher collects the final ratings and reports the votes to the group. A 20-minute discussion period follows.

The *nominal group process* technique allows for multiple individual inputs simultaneously while keeping participation balanced. The method also controls variance; a major source of error or variance can arise when there is incongruence between the researcher and/or practitioner system and the client or user system. The nominal group reduces incongruence.

Cunningham (1976) suggested that participants in action research begin to generate action hypotheses that describe the possible actions that could be taken to solve a problem and the necessary resources that implement them. In developing an action research plan, the action researcher helps the participants to allot time into segments and to outline the activities to be done in each time segment, noting how responsibilities will be assigned. The action researcher facilitates the transfer of information and decisions to the participants, and serves only as a watchdog or conscience for the group (Cunningham, 1976).

Traditional research is judged for value in terms of the amount of dependable knowledge it adds to that which has already been recorded and is available to anyone who wants to be familiar with it. The value of action research is "determined primarily by the extent to which findings lead to improvement of the practices of the people engaged in the research" (Corey, 1953, p. 13).

The issue of random selection (so difficult to attain in the real world) is not a problem because action researchers only want to discover generalizations that will help them work effectively together on the same situation as that in which the studies were conducted (Corey, 1953, p. 14).

Traditional research can dehumanize those being studied because the data that have been collected may never yield any benefit for them. Nalekoff (1994) described an action research project for preventing substance abuse and promoting social competency. The central theme of investigation was local youths' perceptions of drug and alcohol abuse in their lives. A group of youths, in partnership with professionals, surveyed their contemporaries with a questionnaire of their own creation. The community meeting that followed was designed to stimulate the youths through reflection, dialogue, and planning for action.

A wellness perspective implies the consumer of services is responsible and deeply involved in the wellness process. Therefore, an action research approach that involves clients in the study of their own wellness processes would be relevant.

Action research might raise some of the following questions:

- How well are we accomplishing our wellness goals?
- How might we make our work more expeditious?
- How do we feel about ourselves and what we are accomplishing?
- What should we accomplish in the next wellness group meeting?
- How can wellness programs be improved?
- What kind of assistance would help us develop our potential?
- What are the problem areas in wellness programs that should be changed?
- What is the planning process we used to develop wellness programs?
- What hypotheses about wellness can be formulated?
- What is the best way to introduce change to facilitate wellness behaviors?
- What tools should be used to identify our progress?
- What reactions to our wellness programs do our family members have?
- What reactions to our wellness behaviors do our supervisors at work have?

RESEARCH PROVIDING SUPPORT FOR WELLNESS THEORY

One of the main issues in wellness practice is how the practitioner assists the client to move toward wellness. It is relatively easy to teach wellness procedures. What is difficult is facilitating clients to regularly engage in wellness.

Fleury (1991) developed a grounded theory of empowering potential for wellness motivation. She found the process of empowering potential consisted of three stages: appraising readiness, changing, and integrating change. Two processes—imaging the self in desired and undesired states, social support systems—occurred throughout the process. One of the roads to bridging the difficulty is understanding what facilitates and prevents clients from engaging in wellness behaviors. Therefore, this study is presented as an example of how researchers may begin to develop wellness theory.

To begin moving in this direction, the author began a study of students and their reports of what facilitated and prevented them from engaging in wellness behaviors, using qualitative methods. A semistructured questionnaire was developed based on the wellness dimensions and was revised based on feedback from the students. Results were fed back to students to assist them in understanding factors that affect their participation (as a group) in wellness activities.

Fifty-five students participated in various phases of the study. As questionnaires were completed, they were analyzed by the researcher for common categories. During the first phase of the study, the issues identified as preventing students from engaging in wellness behaviors included: time, fear, guilt, low self-esteem, cravings, overeating, negative environment, lack of motivation, giving up, isolating oneself, being depressed, and inconvenience. Factors that were identified as encouraging participation in wellness activities were:

- someone with good communication skills who listens ("encourages me to discuss what's bothering me"; "is patient"); gives feedback ("tells me I'm appreciated"; "helps me confront issues"; "points out my progress toward goals"; "points out my potentials");
- is persistent ("reminds me of my goals"; doesn't nag"; "reassures me I can be honest"; "reminds me how good it will feel if I exercise, etc."; "pushes me to do more");
- encourages ("asks me to list what I do well"; "asks me how I'm doing on my goal"; "talks calmly");
- provides information ("gives me educational materials"; "reinforces benefits of wellness"); "tells me how other people have coped"; "suggests helpful activities");
- has a sense of humor (laughs and makes wellness fun);
- shares wellness activities or role models wellness;
- provides touch ("shows they care with touch"; "gives me a hug when I'm low"; "gives me a massage when I'm tense");
- activities are convenient or affordable;
- when own success is acknowledged;
- when important to others' wellness activities ("when I know he depends on me to go jogging with him, it's easier to get up").

Further isolating categories, the following skills were identified:

- time management
- assertiveness
- access to wellness information/knowledge
- change skills, especially those assisting in attitude change

An additional factor, which held across the board, was the presence of a peer who provided support and a problem-solving, accepting, assertive relationship; in some, but not all, cases, the presence of caring touch was identified.

By examining the data again, the relationship between peer facilitator and self-esteem became clearer. It appeared that what the peer facilitator provided for those with low self-esteem was an external source of self-esteem; someone who "cares enough to devote time to me and who shows me it's O.K. to care about myself and take time to do this."

Other relationships became evident. A patterning of self-esteem, a well thought out plan or wellness goal, regularity in working toward it, feedback from a peer, from oneself, or one's body fell into a set of promoting conditions for each respondent. These conditions did not seem to be phases, but rather interacting variables. There was always action toward pursuing a wellness goal, but depending on the participant it was irregular, unplanned, mechanical ("I do it because I think I should"; "Someone else thinks I should"), or positively reinforcing ("I want to do it because I know I'll feel good during or afterwards").

The issue of self-esteem and wellness is paradoxical. Earlier research has shown that people who regard themselves highly are more likely to set aside time for wellness activities than those with low self-esteem, and that self-esteem or self-concept is enhanced through participation in physical fitness activities (Hanson & Nedde, 1974; Sidney & Shephard, 1976; Sonstroem, 1978). Some unanswered questions include:

- How can those who need external motivation to participate in wellness activities be identified?
- What is the individual mix of self-esteem, plan, regularity and feedback that leads to wellness?

According to Borba and Borba (1982), indicants of low self-esteem include: fearfulness and timidity, aggressiveness (bullying, bragging, derogating others), expectations of failure, reluctance to express feelings, and difficulty making decisions. In re-examining the data, the students, who reported evidence of one or more of these indicants did have difficulty regularly pursuing a wellness goal unless they had a peer facilitator who provided structure for pursuing the goal and positive feedback and ongoing encouragement.

Using the data from 55 students, additional relationship statements were developed based on further reading and thought, including:

- Participation in regular wellness activities exists when (a) the person has learned the benefits of participation and receives self-reinforcement to participate, or (b) the person has a peer to encourage, share, initiate, remind, push, etc.
- If the person has low self-esteem (tends to label oneself as "lazy" or lacking in persistence to engage in wellness activities), then a peer who provides regularity, encouragement, and positive feedback leads to increased participation in wellness activities.
- If the person has inconsistent belief systems so that thoughts, feelings, and actions are not supportive of one another, there will be less participation in wellness activities unless peer support is provided. (Breaks in belief systems were identified when participants responded with comments such as "I should. . ." and /or "I'm lazy" and then reported irregular participation in wellness activities. Consistent belief system was indicated when a participant stated, "I want to . . ." or "It makes me feel confident and strong" and then reported regular participation in the wellness activities.)

Figure 10.1 (p. 331) shows the interaction of variables that appear to facilitate or prevent students from engaging in wellness behaviors.

Another issue in wellness practice is the elusiveness of wellness. If wellness has to do with quality of life, it is important to explore this concept further. To do so, the author asked 20 students the following questions:

1. In your opinion, what does the phrase "quality of life" mean? (Be as specific as you can; give any examples of how you measure your quality of life.)
2. What specific things do you think increase your quality of life?
3. What things can you do to enhance your quality of living?
4. What things do you think others can do to enhance your quality of life?
5. Is there anything else that might increase your quality of life?

Results provided support for the wellness dimensions presented in Chapter 1. Examples of responses providing support for each dimension are found in Table 10.1.

Table 10.1 Examples of Quality of Life Responses and Wellness Dimensions

Fitness Dimension: Regular exercise; healthy body

Nutrition Dimension: Eating appropriately

Belief Systems and Relationship with Self: Feeling confident; feeling good about myself; sense of accomplishment; maximizing potential; existing as a total being; mind/body/spirit; positive outlook; setting goals; being kind to myself; self-awareness; sense of humor; peaceful; self-acceptance

Stress Management: Stop worrying; put things in perspective; learn not to react to pressure; 7–8 hours of sleep; taking time out for myself

Relationships with Others: Sharing laughter and fun; being understood; being liked; being appreciated; firm spiritual base; being supported; being accepted; caring and being cared for;

Table 10.1 (*continued*)

being able to compromise; standing my ground; giving to others; being open to others; sharing opinions and criticisms; noncompetitiveness; being respected; sharing experiences; being reliable; encouraging others; listening without being critical; being a role model; allowing independence

Environment: Peaceful; recharges me; allows privacy and sufficient space; pleasant; allows choice; encourages learning; presents a challenge; is aesthetically pleasing; safe; allows full participation; is organzed; is clean and nonpolluted; provides the proper amount of stimulation; allows pride in possessions

DEVELOPING RELATIONSHIP STATEMENTS AND TESTING THEORETICAL RELATIONSHIPS

According to Chinn and Jacobs (1983, pp. 96–97) theories can only be tested when a translation is made from the theoretical to the concrete.

> The activity of testing of theoretical relationships involves three subcomponents: (1) formulating the specific statement of relationship, often a hypothesis, (2) determining the operational definitions necessary to validate the statements, and (3) validating the statement through systematic methods.

To accomplish the first subcomponent, empirical indicators must be substituted for abstract concepts. Some possible relationship statements for testing wellness theory might be:

1. When fitness goals are written, there is a greater likelihood that action toward fitness will follow.
2. When fitness goals are systematically evaluated, there is a greater likelihood that new fitness goals will be set as previous ones are met.
3. When fitness goals are attained, there is a greater likelihood that movement toward wellness in other dimensions will occur.
4. When preventive nutrition goals are attained, there is a greater likelihood that movement toward wellness in other dimensions will occur.
5. There is an inverse relationship between time spent specifying fitness goals and time needed to act on them.
6. There will be a positive relationship between frequency of wellness goal facilitation and progress toward goal attainment.
7. The more the practitioner serves as a wellness role model, the more the client will move toward wellness.
8. The more the practitioner resolves his or her inconsistent belief systems, the more helpful he or she will be to the clients' ability to move toward wellness.
9. The greater the movement toward a wellness belief system, the more wellness behaviors will be exhibited by the client.
10. The more the client participates in self-assessment, the greater the movement toward wellness.

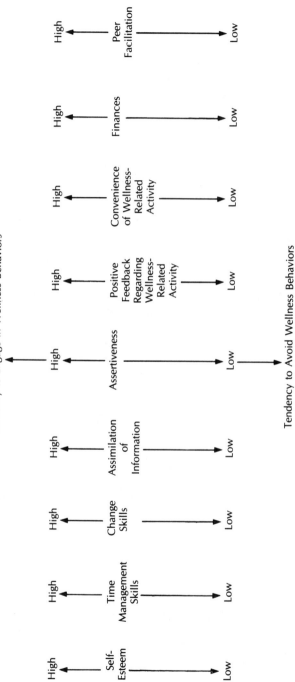

Figure 10.1 Variables facilitating and preventing students from engaging in wellness behaviors.

INTEGRATIVE LEARNING EXERCISES

Beginning Level

1. Develop research questions from a wellness perspective based on your area of clinical practice focused on:
    A. A well population
    B. The dimensions of wellness
    C. Antonovsky's concept of coherence
    D. The Intersystems Wellness Model
    E. Mehl's conceptual framework
    F. A search of current research reports or publications
2. Write in your journal regarding what motivates you to engage in wellness behaviors.
3. Write in your journal about what quality of life means to you.

Advanced Level

1. Complete 1 above.
2. Look at the list of questions you developed in number 1 and decide which could be approached from a qualitative and /or action research method. Give rationale for your choices.
3. Use a survey or questionnaire to elicit responses from 10-30 well people about what encourages and discourages them from engaging in wellness behaviors. Compare your responses to the ones found from a student population.
4. Interview 10-30 well people about what "quality of life" means to them. Compare your answers with those found in this chapter.

REFERENCES

Achterberg, J. et al. (1977). Psychological factors, blood factors and blood chemistries as disease outcome predicators for cancer patients. *Multivariate Experimental Clinical Research* 3:107-122.

American Nurses Association. *Nursing, a social policy statement* (1980). Kansas City, MO : ANA.

Antonovsky, A. (1984). The sense of coherence as determinant of health. *Advances* 1(3)(Summer):37-50.

Bageley, C. (1979). Control of the emotions, remote stress, and the emergence of breast cancer. *Indian J Clin Psychol* 6:213–220.

Bieliauskas, L., et al. (1979). Psychological depression and cancer mortality. *Psychosom Med* 41 : 77–78.

Borba, M., and Borba, C. (1982). *Self-Esteem: A Classroom Affair.* Minneapolis, MN: Winston Press, pp. 2–3.

Borysenko, J. (1982). Behavioral-physiological factors in the development and management of cancer. *Gen Hosp Psychiatry* 4:69–74.

Chinn, P. L., and Jacobs, M. (1983). *Theory and Nursing.* St. Louis: C.V. Mosby.

Clark, C. C. (1984). What encourages and prevents students from engaging in wellness activities. *The Wellness Newsletter* 5(6):3–4.

Corey, S. (1953). *Action Research to Improve School Practices*. New York: Teachers College Press.

Cunningham, B. (1976). Action research: Toward a procedural model. *Human Rels* 29(3):215–238.

Dunn, H. L. (19977). *High Level Wellness*. Thorofare, NJ: Charles B. Slack.

Fleury, T. D. (1991). Empowering potential: A theory of wellness motivation. *Nursing Research* 40(5):286–291.

Gardner, N. (1974). Action training and research: Something old and something new. *Public Admin Rev* March/April:106–115.

Hanson, J. S., and Nedde, W. H. (1974). Longterm physical training effect in sedentary females. *Journal of Applied Physiology* 37:112–116.

Malekoff, A. (1994). Action research: An approach to preventing substance abuse and promoting social competency. *Health Social Work* 191:46–53.

McClelland, D., et al. (1980). Stressed power motivation, sympathetic activation, immune function and illness. *Journal of Human Stress* 6:11–19.

Mehl, L. (1981). *Mind and matter: Foundations for holistic health*. Berkeley, CA: Mindbody Press.

Miles, M., and Hiberman, A. (1984). *Qualitative data analysis*. Beverly Hills, CA: Sage.

Morris, T., et al. (1978). Psychological response to breast cancer: Effect on outcome. *Lancet* 2:785–787.

Mullen, P., and Iverson, D. (1982). Qualitative methods for evaluative research in health education programs. *Health Education* May/June:11-18.

O'Regan, B. (1983). Psychneuroimmunology: The birth of a new field. *Investigations* 1(2):1–2.

Putt, A. (1978). *General systems theory applied to nursing*. Boston: Little, Brown.

Sidney, K.H., and Shephard, R. J. (1976). Attitudes toward health and physical activity in the elderly. Effects of a physical training program. *Medicine and Science in Sports* 8:246–252.

Sonstroem, R.J. (1978). Physical estimation and attraction scales: Rationale and research. *Medicine and Science in Sports* 10:97–102.

Stern, P. (1980). Grounded theory methodology: Its uses and processes. *Image* 12:20–23.

Swanson, J., and Chenitz, W. C. (1982). Why qualitative research in nursing? *Nursing Outlook* 30(April) : 241–245.

Van de Ven, A., and Delbecq, A. (1972). The nominal group as a research instrument for exploratory health studies. *Am J of Pub Hlth* 62(March):337–342.

Walker, L., and Avant, K. (1983). *Strategies for theory construction in nursing*. Norwalk, CT: Appleton-Century-Crofts.

APPENDIX: RESOURCES

Environmental Wellness

American Horticulture Society. 1-800-777-7931 for a free brochure on composters. (Take care of your yard waste in an environmentally friendly way.)

Concern Inc. 1794 Columbia Road, NW, Washington, DC 20009. (202) 238-8160. Publishes the *Community Action Guide* on water, pesticides, waste, farmland, and household waste.

Congress. Write to your representatives and let them know how you feel.U.S. Senate, Washington, DC 20510. U.S. House of Representatives, Washington, DC 20515.

Co-op America. 1850 M Street NW, #700, Washington, DC 20036. 202-872-5307. Harnesses economic power for positive change to educate people to use their spending and investing power to bring the values of social justice and environmental sustainability into the economy; helps socially and environmentally responsible businesses thrive, and pressures irresponsible businesses (sometimes through boycotts) to adopt socially and environmentally responsible practices. Publishes *Co-op America Quarterly, National Green Pages, Socially Responsible Financial Planning Handbook,* and *Boycott Action News.*

Environmental Action. 1525 New Hampshire Avenue, NW, Washington, DC 20036. (202) 745-4870. National membership group that researches clean air, water and solid waste, as well as lobbies for bills before Congress. Two bimonthly magazines.

Environmental Defense Fund. 257 Park Avenue South, New York, N.Y. 10010. (212) 595-2100. Encourages its members to take action to contact Congress (and others) to protect the environment. EDF lawyers fight for environmental safety. Publishes the monthly, *EDF Letter.*

Environmental Protection Agency. (EPA). (800) 424-4000

Environmental Working Group. 1718 Connecticut Avenue, NW, Suite 600, Washington, DC 20009. (202) 667-6982. Provides information on scientific studies, including women's health, breast cancer, and pesticides.

Free Brochure: *Thirty Ways to Save the Environment.* Garden Way Inc., 102nd Street, Ninth Avenue, Troy, NY 12180.

Greenpeace. 1611 Connecticut Avenue, NW, Washington, DC 20009. (202) 462-1177. Publishes newsletter and fact sheets and sponsors regional environmental libraries. Focuses on acid rain, ocean dumping, and toxic wastes.

Indoor Air Quality Information Clearinghouse. P.O. Box 37133, Washington, DC 20013-7133. (800) 438-4318. Provides information, referrals, publications, and database searches on indoor air quality.

Inform. 381 Park Avenue South, New York, NY 10016. (212) 689-4040. Research and educational group that specializes in solid-waste management, alternative vehicle fuels, and irrigation in the West. On the cutting edge.

Jemarco. Judith Miley, President. Conducts seminars on designing and adapting homes to prevent accidents, trauma, and premature death.

Natural Resources Defense Council. (**NRDC**) 40 West 20th Street, New York, NY 10011 (212) 727-2700. Provides publications, journal, and newsletter on many environmental concerns. A public-interest advocacy group whose lawyers go to court to protect the environment.

Office on Smoking and Health (OSH). Technical Information Center, Park Building, Room 116, 5600 Fishers Lane, Rockville MD 20857. (301) 443-1690. Serves as a clearinghouse for information about the health risks of smoking and how to quit. Provides computerized literature searches and copies of up to 10 specific articles.

Seventh Generation. Department 60M89, 10 Farrell Street, South Burlington, VT 05403. A mail-order business that offers environmentally safe household products, such as nontoxic cleaners and solar-powered accessories, and environmental books.

Sierra Club Legal Defense Fund. 2044 Fillmore Street, San Francisco, CA 94115 (415) 567-6100. Quarterly newsletter on environmental law focusing on member activities.

Toxnet. Specialized Information Services Division, National Library of Medicine, 8600 Rockville Pike, Bethesda, MD 20894. (301) 496-6351. A 24-hour database leading callers step-by-step through the process of cleaning up toxic spills, small or large. CompuServe telecommunications networks.

Union of Concerned Scientists. National headquarters: 2 Brattle Square, Cambridge, MA 02238. Washington Office: 1616 P Street NW, Washington, DC 20036. West Coast Office: 2397 Shattuck Avenue, Berkeley, CA 94704. A nonprofit organization that advances responsible public policies in areas where technology plays a role. Publishes *Nucleus*, a quarterly journal.

U.S. Consumer Product Safety Commission Hotline. Washington, DC 20207. (800)638-2772 and (800) 638-8270. Conducts investigations of unsafe/defective products and establishes product safety standards. Publications. Spanish-speaking operator available.

Fitness

President's Council on Physical Fitness and Sports. 701 Pennsylvania Avenue, NW, Suite 250, Washington, DC 20004 . (202) 272-3430. FAX: (202) 504-2064.

Better Backs. P.O. Box 13, Washington, DC 20044. Consumer information series from the Better Sleep Council. For specific back exercises write to: *Back Exercises*, American Academy of Orthopaedic Surgeons, P.O. Box 1998, Des Plaines, IL 60017; or the American Physical Therapy Association, Attn: Back, P.O. Box 37257, Washington, DC 20013; or the Arthritis Foundation, Attn: Back Information, P.O. Box 19000, Atlanta, GA 30326 (and enclose a written request).

Nutritional Wellness

American Dietetic Association. 216 W. Jackson Boulevard, Chicago, IL 60606. Offers cookbooks and other materials to educate about food and nutrition.

American Institute for Cancer Research. (800) 843-8114. Toll Free Nutrition Hotline M-Th, 9–10 p.m. EST and F 9–6 EST. Educational pamphlets on diet, nutrition, and cancer prevention. Funds research.

Food Market Institute. Free Copies of *Nutrition and Your Health: Dietary Guidelines for Americans*. Write to Consumer Information Center, Department 514-X, Pueblo, CO 81009.

Organic Farms. l0726B Tucker Street, Beltsville, MD 20705. (800) 222-6244. One of the nation's largest distributors of organically grown foods. Also provides nationwide listing of restaurants serving organically grown food.

Physicians Committee for Responsible Medicine. P.O. Box 6322, Washington, DC 20015. (202) 686-2210. Nutrition, preventive medicine.

Self-Care

Lift It Safe, Prevent Broken Hips. Available FREE call (800) 824-BONES American Academy of Orthopaedic Surgeons, 6300 North River Road, Rosemont, IL 60018.

National Headache Foundation. (800) 843-2256; (800) 523-8858 in IL. Offers membership information and sends written materials on headaches and their treatment.

PMS Access. (800) 222-4767. (800) 833-4767 in WI. Provides information, literature, and counseling on all aspects of premenstrual syndrome. Gives referrals to physicians and clinics in the caller's locale.

Wellness Programs/Practitioners

Community Service, Inc. P.O. Box 243, Yellow Springs, OH 45387. Publishes the *Community Service Newsletter* six times a year to promote the small community as a basic social institution involving organic units of economic, social, and spiritual development. Offers conferences and publications on sustainable development.

Life Balancing Center. Peter Reuter, LNC. Works with clients on nutritional aspects, especially cancer and AIDS. l950 Sandra Drive, Clearwater, FL 34624-4772. (813) 447-6305.

National Health Information Center. P.O. Box 1133, Washington, DC 20013-1133. (800) 336-4797. FAX: (301) 984-4256. Helps the public and health professionals locate health information through identification of health information sources, an information and referral system, and publications.

National Wellness Institute. l045 Clark Street, Suite 210/PO Box 827, Stevens Point, WI 54481-0827. Phone: (715) 342-2969. Fax: (715) 342-2979. Toll free access to Resource Referral Center, Subscription to *Wellness Management, National Wellness Institute Wellness Resource Directory*, National Wellness Conference, Membership Directory, Monthly Job Opportunities Bulletin.

Pathways to Wellness. Janet Hand, MA, RN. Relaxation, seminars, psychotherapy, meditation, body work, guided imagery, therapeutic touch, wellness counseling. 96B Glenwood Rd., Glenwood Landing, NY ll547. (516) 671-7584.

Public Citizen. Ralph Nader's nonprofit organization based in Washington, DC at 2000 P Street, NW, Suite 605, 20077-6488. (202) 293-9142. Monitors legislation on Capitol Hill, documents campaign financing abuses, tracks House and Senate voting records, and lobbies for the public interest; fights for protection against unsafe foods, drugs, and workplaces, and for greater consumer control over health decisions; brings precedent-setting lawsuits on behalf of citizens against the government and large corporations to enforce rights and ensure justice; works for safe, efficient, and affordable energy and enables consumers to exercise their economic leverage in the marketplace.

Summex Corporation. Larry S. Chapman, MPH, P.O. Box 55056, Seattle, WA 98155. (206) 364-3448.

Wellness Resources. Carolyn Chambers Clark, EdD, ARNP. Provides seminars, consultation, self-study programs, and wellness services (nutrition, fitness, relationship, environmental, self-care, stress management). 3451 Central Avenue, St. Petersburg, FL 33713. (813) 821-8567 (M–Th, 9–6:30 p.m EST.) Fax: (813) 321-0841.

Wellness Works. Carol Roberts, MD. 1209 Lakeside Drive, Suite B. Brandon, FL 33510. (813) 661-3662 Fax: 661-0515. Offers free community presentations. Clinical services include wellness evaluation, mental health counseling, weight management, acupuncture, smoking cessation, hypnotherapy, massage, electrotherapy, yoga, Tai Chi, low-impact aerobics, and personal weight training.

INDEX

Research (*cont.*)
  designing wellness research questions
    and, 318-322
  integrative learning exercises, 332
  procedures for, 322-326
  progressive relaxation, 74-75
  qualitative, 322-324
  quality of life and, 329-330
  relationship statements and, 330
  theoretical relationships and, 330
  wellness behavior variables and, 331
  wellness theory and, 318-332
Right brain, 36
Rights, standing up for, 52-65
Rotter, J., 31
Ruffling the field, 193, 215
Running
  shoes for, 174
  walk-job program and, 174-178

Salt, blood pressure and, 101
Schedule of Recent Experience stress
    assessment (Holmes), 69
School for Body/Mind Centering, 155-156
Screening
  as a preventive measure, 199
  questionable procedures of, 206
Selenium, cancer and, 104, 115, 121
Self-assessments
  of assertiveness, 55
  of empathy, 49-51
  of fitness, 164-165
  of sexual experiences, 200-201
  of stress, 69-72
  of wellness, 27-31, 91-93
Self-care
  detection tests and preventive measures
    and, 202-205
  health care costs and, 302
  movement of, 4
  questionable screening procedures and,
    206
  resources on, 337
  theoretical frameworks for, 190-198
  wellness promoted through, 27-30;
    See also Self-assessments; Self-care
    interventions; Wellness interven-
    tions
Self-care interventions
  aromatherapy and, 237-240

  herbal remedies, 234-237;
    See also Wellness interventions
Self-differentiation. *See* Differentiation of
    self
Self-esteem, 11, 64
Self-examination
  of abdomen, 200
  of breast, 198, 261-262
  of fitness, 164-165
  of lymph nodes, 199
  of vagina, 201, 261-262
Self-hypnosis
  for allergies, asthma, colds, 78
  behavior and, 41
  children and, 78
  coaching clients in, 76
  definition of, 75
  emotional disturbance and, 77
  instructions for, 76
  for itching, 77-78
  for pain, 78-80
  positive/negative suggestions and, 75,
    77
  vs. psychotherapy, 77
  for stress, 75
  symptoms treatable through, 77
Self-talk, 82-84
Senate Select Committee on Nutrition and
    Human Needs, 96, 98
Setpoint theory, of weight loss, 142-143
Sexual experiences
  assessments of, 261-262
  communicating about, 200-201
Shingles, self-care measures for, 257
Shoulder stand, in yoga, 217
SIDS. *See* Sudden Infant Death Syndrome
    (SIDS)
Sinusitis, self-care measures for, 257
Smoking
  cancer and, 266-267
  cessation of, 77, 293, 305-306
  community wellness and, 291-292
  environmental wellness and, 265, 266-
    268, 283
  self-care intervention and, 211-212
  worksite wellness programs and, 304-
    307
Solid waste, 265, 266, 280
Soybeans, amino acids and, 127
Spinal movement, 155

Wellness Interventions *(cont.)*
hypoglycemia, 230
immune deficiencies, 4, 68-69, 133,
135, 191-192, 195-198, 213-214,
236, 239, 240
impaired physical mobility, 74
incontinence, 237
indigestion, 71, 80, 208, 210, 215-216,
226, 230, 233, 235, 246, 248-249
ineffective breathing, 74
ineffectual coping, 74
infection, 108, 111, 112, 209, 226, 236,
239, 240
infertility, 226, 236
insect bites, 235, 239
insomnia, 71, 73, 215-216, 226, 230
irritability, 72
itching, 77-78, 106, 107, 226
jet lag, 226, 230
kidney disorders, 130, 133, 205, 226,
230, 236, 250
labor, 230
lead poisoning, 236
legs, cramping, swelling, 105, 106, 230,
236
leukemia, 230
lip disorders, 107
liver disorders, 112, 226, 236, 239,
250-251
lock jaw, 226
mastectomy, 230
memory loss, 105, 106, 183-184, 251
Ménière's syndrome, 252
menopause, 106, 230, 236, 239, 240,
252
menstrual disorders, 106, 193, 209,
226, 230, 235, 236, 239, 240
mental retardation, 205
migraines, 73, 239, 253
mitral valve prolapse, 253
morning sickness, 209, 236, 254
motion sickness, 226, 227, 230, 236,
254
mouth sores, 107, 236, 239
multiple sclerosis, 192, 254
muscle pain, 72, 73, 107, 209, 219-220,
226, 230, 239, 240
muscle spasm, 71, 73, 105, 106, 209,
219-220, 226, 230, 239, 240
nausea and vomiting, 107, 114, 192,

208, 210, 226, 230, 233, 236
neck and shoulder tension, 71, 216,
225, 226, 231, 258
neural tube defect, 134
neurasthenia, 215-216
nightmares, 230
obesity, 71, 82, 100, 121, 137-145, 169,
216
osteoarthritis, 209
osteoporosis, 109, 121, 130-131, 255
overeating, 77, 99
pain, 73, 74, 77, 78-80, 89, 109, 119,
135, 192-193, 194, 225, 231, 236
paralysis, 231
parasites, 236
Parkinson's disease, 231, 255
peptic ulcer, 192
peristalsis, 182
phobias, 71, 73, 82, 84, 192
poison ivy, 236
powerlessness, 73, 74
premenstrual tension, 132, 192, 231,
236, 239, 240, 256
progressive relaxation as a, 74
prolapsed viscera, 226
prostate problems, 216, 231, 236, 239,
256
psoriasis, 238
relationship improvement, 48, 52-64
respiratory disorders, 80, 105, 107,
209, 226, 230, 236, 240
sciatic relief, 209, 226, 231
seizures, 226
self-esteem, low, 11, 64, 71
self-hypnosis as a, 75
senility, 236
sexual dysfunction, 200-201, 240
sexual passion, 237, 239, 240
shingles, 231, 257
shock, 226, 231
sinuses, 210, 226, 231, 233, 237, 239,
257
skin disorders, 105, 135, 237, 238, 239,
240
sleep disorders, 74, 80, 85, 106, 240
smoking cessation, 77, 211-212, 265,
266-268, 283, 291-292, 293, 304-
307
snoring, 231
sore throat, 237

S *Springer Publishing Company*

THE NURSE AS GROUP
LEADER, *3rd Edition*

Carolyn Chambers Clark, EdD, RN, ARNP, FAAN

This book is useful in a wide range of settings—from teaching groups to supportive or therapeutic groups to committee work with other health care providers. Simulated exercises in the book provide opportunity for practice. New to this edition are chapters on working with the elderly in groups, and on working with groups with specific problems, such as eating disorders, rape, or depression.

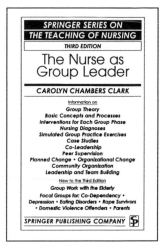

SPRINGER SERIES ON
THE TEACHING OF NURSING
THIRD EDITION
The Nurse as
Group Leader
CAROLYN CHAMBERS CLARK
Information on
Group Theory
Basic Concepts and Processes
Interventions for Each Group Phase
Nursing Diagnoses
Simulated Group Practice Exercises
Case Studies
Co-Leadership
Peer Supervision
Planned Change • Organizational Change
Community Organization
Leadership and Team Building
New to the Third Edition
Group Work with the Elderly
Focal Groups for: Co-Dependency •
Depression • Eating Disorders • Rape Survivors
• Domestic Violence Offenders • Parents
SPRINGER PUBLISHING COMPANY **S**

Contents:

- Introduction to Group Work
- Basic Group Concepts and Process
- Working to Achieve Group Goals
- Special Group Problems
- Beginning, Guiding, and Terminating the Group
- Supervision of Group Leaders and Co-leadership
- Behavioral Approaches for Group Leaders
- Recording
- Groups for the Older Adult
- Working With Focal Groups
- When the Organization is the Group
- When the Community is the Group

Springer Series: Teaching of Nursing
1994   304pp   0-8261-2333-3   softcover

536 Broadway, New York, NY 10012-3955 • (212) 431-4370 • Fax (212) 941-7842